Medical Implications of Basic Research in Aging
Volume 2

Andrew R. Mendelsohn, PhD
James W. Larrick, MD, PhD

with a Foreword by Aubrey de Grey, PhD

Eosynth Press

Cover and Illustration provided by Jasmine W. Larrick.
Editorial support provided by Ashley Kay Hoffman.

Publisher: Eosynth Press

Editors: Andrew R. Mendelsohn and James W. Larrick

ISBN-13: 978-0-9912162-2-2

1. Aging 2. Longevity 3. Health 4. Immortality

DEDICATION

J.W.L: Dedicated to my wife and life companion, Jun CHEN, and our beautiful daughter, Jasmine.

A.R.M: Dedicated to my lovely wife, Katalin, and to our daughter, Anna.

TABLE OF CONTENTS

FOREWORD

In the eleven years since my publication of *Ending Aging* (New York: St. Martin's Press), numerous advances have been made in basic biomedical science that impact the possibility of controlling biological aging. Unfortunately, as I predicted, increasing understanding of the mechanisms of aging has so far had limited impact on extending longevity. *Medical Implications of Basic Research in Aging* provides a sampling of the most important discoveries of the past several years relevant to aging research in the context of extending human healths pan and thereby lifespan.

Andrew and Jim have assembled in this volume a number of the commentaries they previously authored for "Rejuvenation Research." The presentations are clearly written, jargon-free and thus accessible to those with minimal background in biology and medical science. Thorough referencing provides an opportunity for further in-depth reading, and a variety of suggestions for increasing health span are provided. As the appreciation spreads that aging may be brought under genuine medical control quite soon, these commentaries are precisely what the educated layman, as well as the professional biologist, needs in order to understand how those at the cutting edge of the held believe that this will come about. As "Rejuvenation Research"'s editor-in-chief, I feel privileged to have had the opportunity to publish these articles, and I am especially grateful to Mary Ann Liebert, Inc. for participating in this means of bringing them to a new audience. I am sure that you will share my enthusiasm.

Aubrey de Grey PhD
SENS Research Foundation
Mountain View, California

ACKNOWLEDGEMENTS

We appreciate the support and encourage of our colleagues. Among those most important are: Greg Adams, Mark Alfenito, Mark Allen, Ramesh Baliga, Bob Balint, Annelise Barron, Gale Bergado, Andrew Bradbury, John Cambier, Luis Carbonell, Casey Chan, Chris Chen, Ben Chen, John Chen, George Church, David Collier, Josefina Coloma, Jim Crowe, Mark de Boer, Dennis Burton, Jorge Gavilondo, Aubrey de Grey, Jeff Fang, Rafal Farjo, Elliott Fineman, John Furber, Eva Harris, Lance Harter, Jeng Her, Eric Hoang, Ashley K. Hoffman, Daotian Fu, Sean Hu, Manley Huang, Tom Huang, Jim Huston, Nael Kassar, Miria Kaname, Matt Kerby, Brad Keller, Jin Kim, Nety Krishna, Eric Kunkel, John Lambert, John Latera, Donald Larrick, Andrew Larrick, Randy Lee, Isabelle Lehoux, Stuart Lipton, Joyce Liu, Leslie Loven, Larry Lum, Jennifer Lei, Jian-xiang Ma, Julian Ma, Jim Marks, Donnie McCarthy, Mike Melnick, Tom Niedringhaus, Paul Parren, Andrew Perlman, Andreas Pluckthun, Jeff Price, Cary Queen, Janice Reichert, Anie Roche, Ed Schnipper, Howard Schulman, Jamie Scott, Peter Schulz, Peter Senter, Vikram Sharma, Ronnie Shaw, Dean Sheppard, Mark Tepper, Ian Tomlinson, Frank Torti, Lotay Tshering, Carl Vogel, John Wages, Hong Wang, Jianming Wang, Shan Wang, Yuqiang Wang, H. Shaw Warren, Cheng-I Wang, Qishen Wei, Louis Weiner, Greg Went, Robert Whalen, Dane Wittrup, Cees Wortel, Keith Wycoff, Geoff Yarranton, Heng Yu, Bo Yu, Gaia Zhao, and Xiaoming Zhang.

The front and back cover was kindly designed by Ms. Jasmine Larrick. Other illustrations were the work product of Wolfgang Arlo Scatman.

We especially wish to thank Susan Jensen and Mary Ann Liebert Inc. for permission to reprint our papers from *Rejuvenation Research*.

OVERVIEW AND INTRODUCTION

Aging Research and Healthspan Engineering

"Death comes to all."

A notable line from a very old famous book remains as true today as the day it was first written more than 2000 years ago. What is different today is the fact that many people will live long enough to experience old age before death. Everyone reading these words, if they don't succumb to some unfortunate accident or illness will grow old before they die. Yet, no one looks forward to the loss of physical vigor that accompanies aging. And rightly so, who wants to see their body and mind slowly disintegrate.

But what can be done after all? Most of us deal with this conundrum in two ways: denial before it happens and then finally during our dotage, acceptance, – because nothing can be done. Or can it?

The revolution in biomedical research and biotechnology over the past 40 years makes possible what was previously unthinkable: changing the very substance our biological nature. However, a recent U.S. Pew poll suggests that a large majority of people are <u>not</u> in favor of ending death or "curing" aging. Even so, Google sponsored the creation of a biotech company, Calico, whose long-term goal is apparently to do just that, although there is likely as much hype as reality to their goals. However, the idea of reducing or even eliminating the dysfunction and illness that accompanies aging is a more popular idea and one that likely will be accomplished gradually. In other words, healthspan is more directly addressable than lifespan. Increasing healthspan has been the great success of modern medicine, as many of the diseases that have plagued human beings through the centuries can now be prevented by modern public health practices, cured with drugs or surgery or even eliminated like smallpox and polio via a worldwide vaccination campaign.

The problem of declining health in old age remains the key hurdle for further increases in healthspan. Such improvements are closely linked to our understanding of aging and its associated diseases. We have entered an era where advances in biotechnology, synthetic biology and basic biomedical research will fuel engineering of healthspan. Although enhanced healthspan will probably lead to increased lifespan. As a consequence, it is important to realize that although the processes are connected, significant lifespan enhancement is a far more difficult problem. For example, it has been estimated that eliminating cancer will only add three years on average to a person's lifespan.

To make significant progress on both healthspan and lifespan enhancement requires understanding aging, which in turn requires understanding the underlying biological processes that regulate our development from a fertilized egg to an adult, and the homeostatic processes that keep us alive. <u>However, there is one key simplifying idea: use new parts to replace old or broken ones.</u> The same idea which we use to maintain our cars and other mechanical and electrical devices directly applies to biological systems as well. Damaged or old tissues can be replaced by new ones. At some point in the near future we will develop the tools to enhance, reprogram and even create regenerative biological mechanisms to allow replacement of old or diseased tissue.

So the future sounds great. We can dream of curing cancer and growing new tissues and organs to replace old ones. But what can we do NOW? We have been reviewing the basic medical literature to find hints of what might one do to increase healthspan by preventing age-associated diseases or possibly even slowing fundamental aging processes. This second volume of **Medical Implications of Basic Research in Aging** based on our papers published in *Rejuvenation Research* helps elucidate the state of the art of our knowledge of how to rationally treat aging as a "disease." Our suggestions follow in subsequent pages, but they are couched in cautionary words and for good reason: many potentially beneficial drugs and nutraceuticals may turn out not to be, and many will have unexpected effects that may even be counterproductive. But for those of you just dying to know what they can do now, here is a sneak peak.

One can likely increase healthspan by a program of moderate exercise, a smart balanced diet that avoids regular consumption of sugar, red meat, etc., and attempting countermeasures for age-associated diseases that one is likely to suffer. The last point is the most difficult as it requires calculating personal medical risk. It is advisable that one obtain a physician's advice in making any final determination, but risk can be crudely estimated by combining personal and family medical history with inexpensive personal genomics data (from such services as 23andme) to determine which age-associated diseases one is most likely to suffer. Armed with foreknowledge of possible future diseases, it might be possible to use an understanding of the underlying biological processes to select drugs and compounds found in supplements to delay or even prevent their occurrence. One extreme example of this approach are women carrying dominant mutations in the BRCA1 or BRCA2 tumor suppressor genes, who elect prophylactic surgery to remove their breasts and/or ovaries in order to ward off likely breast or ovarian cancer. Prospective dear reader, are you disappointed? Were you expecting Dr. Heidegger to give you a magical rejuvenation elixir? Well, one may yet be found, but we urge caution based on the very science that promises so much.

There is a natural human tendency to breathlessly read the latest news of potential scientific or medical breakthroughs in uncritical ways. That is especially true when such news appears to promise fulfillment of a wish to live longer or healthier. But before one ends up as disappointed as Ponce de Leon was in his quest to find the Fountain of Youth, it is very useful to have a framework into which to place such potentially significant discoveries. Such a framework requires understanding a) how well discoveries in cells and animals translate to humans, b) that potential therapeutics may often involve tradeoffs, and c) the mechanism(s) by which aging works.

It is very important to understand that it is difficult to predict how well any discovery made in cell culture or in animal models will translate to benefit human beings. That's because isolated cells often behave differently than in their normal milieu and because worms, flies, mice and rats are not humans. Biologists like to focus on the impressive unity and conservation of biochemical pathways between organisms. For example, mice and men are about 90% similar genetically, however there are obvious important differences. Human beings are simply "built better" than mice and that is why they will live on average 40 times longer. The road to fame and riches has been littered by the carcasses of biotech and pharma companies that thought they had an important therapeutic based on preclinical animal data, only to find translation had limited activity in humans or even worse was harmful. If medically trained experts with years of experience can be so wrong, don't doubt for a minute that a non-expert is even on more treacherous ground.

Here are some principles that we apply throughout this book:

• Experiments in cell culture or invertebrates need to be confirmed by experiments in animal models.

• Results from studies of invertebrates or microorganisms are less reliable than mammals in predicting human responses. Although mice and rats are the most frequently used animal models they often poorly predict human responses, especially for inflammatory diseases, neurodegenerative diseases and cancer.

• Many published studies are more anomalous than they appear and must be independently confirmed.

• Human studies are better than animal studies, but even preliminary human trials, especially Phase I and II clinical trials, which tend to be small, often do not have the statistical power to predict how well a therapeutic will really work or whether an observed effect is real. Even large Phase III clinical trial data can overlook serious problems, that are sometimes discovered later, after a drug is approved by the FDA.

Taken together these limitations mean that one should be very careful in applying results from basic medical research to one's own life: *caveat emptor!*. Determination of one's comfortable level with personal risk is critical.

It's been said that life is a series of tradeoffs. Not so remarkably, there are inherent tradeoffs in using almost every drug, in choice of diet and even in the amount and kind of exercise one pursues. Although this may sound almost trivial, the effects are profound and are based on the fundamental way biological systems work. For example, there are numerous studies that suggest that a daily low dose of aspirin somewhat lowers the risk of heart attack and colon cancer. However, the same mechanism that aspirin mediates to protect against heart attacks, by blocking platelet aggregation, i.e., blood clotting, also increases the risk for internal bleeding and ulcers. Furthermore aspirin may also cause hearing loss in some people by destroying the sensory cells of the inner ear, and has been associated with Reye's syndrome in children. One recent paper has linked aspirin to increased risk of skin cancer. Current medical practice suggests that the decision to take aspirin be made by one's physician.

Why are there tradeoffs? Some tradeoffs may be due to the inherent biological processes designed by evolution to create organisms to maximize successful reproduction. Some tradeoffs result from the specificity of action of a drug or treatment. For example, aspirin has multiple molecular mechanisms of action. Aspirin inhibits prostaglandin and thromboxane synthesis through inhibition of cyclooxygenase, which in turn inhibits platelet aggregation.

By reversibly inhibiting COX-2, aspirin can uncouple oxidative phosphorylation (energy production) inside the mitochondria, with activation of AMP-activated protein kinase (AMP kinase). Tradeoffs can result from the complex linkage of biological and biochemical pathways, where affecting one component of one pathway can cause a multitude of downstream effects, not all of which are beneficial. Although not the case for aspirin, *per se*, some of the downstream effects of one compound may even block the beneficial effects of another as has been shown for the ability of vitamin C and other antioxidants to block the beneficial effects of exercise on blood sugar and muscle metabolism. Another critical type of tradeoff is that many biochemical pathways are subject to homeostatic feedback control mechanisms, which alter the ability of a drug or treatment to affect the body. Homeostasis may modulate potentially beneficial drug-based physiological alterations. Sometimes this can make the drug ineffective over time, other times this activity may augment the danger of withdrawal of the drug. Aspirin provides an example of the latter: ending long term use of aspirin is associated with an increased short-term risk of heart attack due to increased cyclooxygenase expression and clotting resulting from the body's attempt to compensate.

Understanding the biological bases of aging helps to place the potential benefits of any treatment designed to impede or reverse aging in perspective. Because aging results from the decay in homeostasis and functional reserve of normal physiological and biochemical processes in an organism the transmission of pain information to the brain, modulation of the body's internal thermostat in the hypothalamus, and inflammation.

Over time, it is likely that a complete description of the mechanisms by which humans age will require a complete understanding of how humans function at the molecular, cellular, organ, and systemic levels. Luckily, we do understand enough today to potentially intercede and to choose productive directions for future research.

So first the big question: <u>Why do we age?</u> The answer is that we (and all other life on earth) have been selected by evolution to accomplish one great task: reproduction. Our body is just a supporting player. It's a well-built supporting player with the capacity to live as long as 120 years in some cases, but it still remains a supporting player for the cells that really count: the germ cells (sperm and egg cells). These cells have a degree of immortality in that they can potentially produce a new man or woman, who in turn can produce offspring and so on. However, the rest of the body, including our brains which encode our precious consciousness is made of cells that have not been selected to endure. Evolutionary selection to maintain a sexually mature individual diminishes with time as the probability of prior successful reproduction increases.

There are also controversial theories that promote the idea that aging may be a programmed process selected by evolutionary processes on a group of organisms to maximize reproductive success of the group. Regardless of the merits of this argument, even if such a programmed "aging" mechanism evolved, for example, a sudden death mechanism such as that that exists for some semelparous species (which only mate once within their lifetimes) such as anadromous salmonids, which die shortly after mating, there would be no selective pressure to maintain homeostasis after that point, and even had the animals been previously "immortal," (for which there is no evidence by the way) they would soon be lacking homeostatic mechanisms necessary for continued life.

The second big question is: <u>How do we age?</u> This is the subject of a great amount of work and speculation. It is our opinion that the most useful way to look at aging is that adult human beings (and all but a few animals) lack rejuvenative homeostatic maintenance mechanisms. In a typical animal's life, a developmental program is executed, when it is finished the organism is dependent on pre-existing homeostatic mechanisms. In multicellular animals these mechanisms require maintaining cell differentiation state, specialized cell function, and eliminating any damage from biochemical processes and the environment. That damage to cellular biomolecules, organelles, and the cells themselves occurs over time is well understood, and precise characterization of that damage is ongoing. Because we know that germ cells are capable of a kind of indirect immortality, the question arises, what is absent from somatic cells that permits such damage to accumulate limiting cellular lifespan. As a crude example consider the moth born without a mouth, in this case we know exactly what is missing to cause the "damage," although here the very idea of "damage" clearly misses the mark. <u>We hypothesize that absence of critical homeostatic mechanisms is the key to aging, and among those mechanisms that are absent, cell and tissue replacement (regeneration) is the one most often critically absent.</u> Furthermore, besides direct biomolecular damage, the intrinsic strength of the underlying biochemical networks to stochastic noise probably plays an important role in the loss of cellular and tissue function observed with aging, especially that relating to changes in the epigenetic state and cell differentiation. In other words, cells undergo a process of gradual amnesia of who they are and what should they do.

So why does this matter? Because this logic points to ways in which diseases of aging might occur and to why simplistic interventions that target just one type of damage, regulatory molecule, cell type, such as so-called senescent cells whose targeted destruction by senolysis is considered one of the most promising anti-aging strategies, or just one epigenetic change such as enhancing telomere length are unlikely to be as significant as they may first appear. Correctly understanding how aging occurs is quite important to interpreting the implications of basic research results.

We have organized reviews of basic research into three sections that correspond to the basic processes that can be altered to affect aging:

    1)   Repairing intracellular substructures (mitochondria/telomeres)
    2) Modulating metabolism and growth regulation
    3) Altering epigenetics and cell differentiation and engineering rejuvenation.

Please note the conspicuous absence of enhanced regeneration, which we earlier indicated to be perhaps the most promising means to achieve a breakthrough in health and lifespan. Unfortunately, safely engineering new regenerative processes has not yet been reported, although Belmonte's group has demonstrated significant benefit to transiently inducing IPS reprogramming factors to increase regenerative capacity and lifespan in a mouse model of premature aging. This approach will require significantly more sophisticated biotechnology than is now attempted clinically.

Models of aging are of more than academic interest, because they have profound impact not only on the research community, but also on the public. A cottage industry of models of aging exists in the scientific literature. Like the blind men of legend describing an elephant each model tends to focus on one aspect of aging, often coming to radically different conclusions. Eventually a consensus will be reached in which the correct aspects of each model will be unified and an "elephant" of a theory may emerge.

The best example of a highly influential damage theory of aging is Harmon's free-radical theory of aging. Metabolic activity leads to generation of harmful reactive oxygen species (ROS) that then damage biomolecules, cells and beyond leading to aging and death. This theory was extended to the mitochondrial free radical theory of aging, which localizes the primary source of damaging free radical production to the mitochondria. Data has accumulated to show that reduction of oxidative stress is associated with prolongation of life expectancy in animals, especially invertebrates. These theories logically led to the idea that antioxidants might be able to prolong lifespan and healthspan. This idea has become very widespread and popular both in and outside of scientific circles. However, many studies have found a lack of correlation between antioxidants and human health benefits. Some reports even suggest that human consumption of antioxidants may promote cancer or increase incidence of diseases associated with aging. One very interesting effect of antioxidants is that they appear to block the beneficial effects of exercise in humans, in some cases contrary to their effects in mice.

Current Perspective

Presently there are only a few clear-cut strategies to promote healthspan: moderate exercise, 7 to 8 hours of quality sleep, a smart balanced diet that avoids regular consumption of red meat (carnitine) and excessive sugar, and possibly caloric restriction. Extended periods of sitting or inactivity should be avoided, since lack of activity has been correlated with as much as a 50% increase in all-cause mortality, even in individuals who engage in leisure time physical activity [1]. The advent of fitness watches that remind the wearer to move more often should be a useful tool to reduce inactivity for desk workers. Beyond a complex patchwork of poorly studied supplements that are claimed to promote longevity, several studies have suggested that intermittent fasting cam slow aging in model organisms and has rejuvenative potential on stem cell function. For example, work from Prof. Longo's laboratory suggests that reducing caloric intake for five days to near fasting levels results in a prolonged fasting-like effect which in mice promotes neurogenesis, hematopoietic stem cell function, delays cancer onset, slowed bone mineral loss, and even modestly increased mean lifespan. In humans, this approach improved diabetes and inflammation associated biomarker levels. However, intermittent fasting may not be universally beneficial, as maximum lifespan increase was not observed by Longo and colleagues. Furthermore, fasting is known to increase cortisol levels, a key stress hormone, whose over-expression is actually used by several semelparous animals such as salmon to kill themselves rapidly. Thus, it is possible that fasting is a two-edged sword-- generally benefit but with a hidden downside.

Attempting countermeasures for age-associated diseases that one is likely to experience is a reasonable idea. How to go about it? Reconciling known family medical history with personal genomics data (from such services as 23andme or Veritas Genomics) to establish some quantitative risk for critical age-associated diseases like for example type II diabetes, hypertension and Alzheimer's disease. Armed with foreknowledge of possible future diseases, it might be possible to use understanding of the underlying biological processes to select drugs and compounds found in supplements to delay or even forestall occurrence of pathological conditions. For example, some female carriers of BRCA mutations elect prophylactic surgery, but there are many possible examples. For illustration, a person with a family history of type II diabetes, at high risk according to a personal genomics analysis or already exhibiting borderline elevated blood sugar levels (so-called prediabetes), might reasonably consult a physician to obtain a prescription for a low dose of metformin to be taken prophylactically. Metformin may have other benefits as well, as the recent clinical trial to delay aging associated diseases with metformin attests (NCT03309007). There is evidence that treatment with rapamycin, transfusions of plasma or microvesicles from the young or newborns have anti-aging effects in mice. Human trials of the possible benefits of young plasma in Alzheimer's disease are ongoing. Positive assessment of anti-aging activity in humans would be enlightening.

Removal of senescent cells by blocking anti-apoptotic regulators such as Bcl-2/Bcl-XL, AKT/PI3K, p53/p21, and chaperonin HSP90, appears to have anti-aging and pro-regenerative effects in a variety of mouse models of osteoarthritis, liver fibrosis, pulmonary fibrosis and atherosclerosis for example {4}. In one normal mouse model, but not another, a senolytic therapy extended maximum lifespan significantly. A related strategy has identified senomorphics, drugs that suppress the senescent phenotype without killing senescent cells. Senomorphic targets include IkB kinase, NF-kappaB, ROS and Janus kinase JAK inhibitors. Interestingly rapamycin acts partially as a senomorphic by reducing the senescence-associated secretory phenotype (SASP) as does caloric restriction. While decreasing cell senescence is beneficial to healthspan, it's limited ability to extend lifespan suggests it plays a secondary role in homeostatic processes related to aging-- which might be expected given the likelihood that senescent cells may have evolved partially to serve as beacons for repair after tissue damage.

One of the great advances since our first edition has been the development of biomarkers that correlate well with chronological and perhaps biological age. The best of these biomarkers for humans appears to be DNA methylation clocks of varying types. Several chapters address the advances in this technology. Although the DNA methylation clocks that best correlate with chronological age are useful, those that have been designed to better predict biological age, like DNAm PhenoAge [5] are likely to be most useful in the development of anti-aging therapeutics.

The Future

Some might apply the old adage about the last refuge of scoundrels to the art of predicting the future. But it is so easy and entertaining that more and more scientists can't help but succumb to temptation. And we are no better than our starry-eyed colleagues.

The biological sciences are in the midst of a revolution as biotechnology has advanced to the point, where unparalleled power to understand and alter biological material is within reach. These advances have brought into existence numerous new fields, the most important of which with regards to aging are systems biology, synthetic biology and regenerative biology.

Systems biology involves elucidating how the various parts of biological systems are connected and interact to make a living organism. In the appendix of Volume One, we discussed the hierarchical nature of biological systems, which is just one of the many subjects of systems biology. Large scale initiatives to map and model the genome, proteome, transcriptome, etc. fall under this rubric. Especially important is the increasing ability to computationally model dynamic living systems on computers. _Employing the boatloads of new bioinformation to create increasingly realistic dynamic simulations of biological systems by leveraging large networks of powerful computers will be the key to progress. Artificial intelligence technologies such as deep learning may be able to accelerate the creation of such powerful models and/or identify key targets for intervention._ Precise knowledge is essential to be able to determine what changes might extend health and lifespan.

Synthetic biology is really a mishmash of biological fields that could just as well be called "Biotechnology 2.0." Essentially this encompasses every biotechnological advance beyond expressing or engineering a protein or drug.

This involves using the knowledge obtained from systems biology to alter, program and create new organisms or biologically related entities. Hard core synthetic biology is based on using good engineering practices such as "standardized parts" to build interoperable systems, although the field is currently far broader in scope. Already it has been possible to program bacteria to act as photographic emulsion, or to identify and destroy some cancer cells (at least in a research lab). The scourge of cancer will likely fall, when synthetic biologists program a subset of one's own cells to seek out tumors by interacting with and querying cells for altered gene expression patterns, and then destroying the abnormal cancer cells Synthetic biology will also provide the tools to program cells to perform tasks necessary to replace aging tissue most efficiently by encouraging regenerative processes. Since the publication of our first edition, the discovery of the CRISPR genome editing tools has created new tools which can not only insert or delete specific DNA sequences, but induce specific base changes or alter specific epigenetic states such as CpG methylation at defined genomic locations.

Scientists studying regenerative biology and medicine seek to understand and then use knowledge of natural regenerative processes to replace damaged, missing or aged tissues. Regenerative biology is the most likely path leading to engineering greater lifespan and healthspan. Why? Because evolution itself has used regenerative processes to endow some organisms with a form of "negligible senescence," better known as immortality. Specifically, some organisms use their incredible regenerative powers to rebuild their body at will. Asexual planaria and hydra are the best understood examples. Hydra are capable not only of regenerating their bodies continuously, as old cells are simply sloughed off and replaced by new ones, but can actually reassembly themselves into an intact organism from their component cells after dissociation into single cells. Asexual planaria can rebuild their entire body from as small a fraction as 1/297th of the parent. These organisms carry pluripotent stem cells called neoblasts within their body, that can be activated to make any needed tissue or body structure at will. Research is ongoing to understand how this works, perhaps so that our own cells can be similarly engineered using systems and synthetic biology. It's not difficult to see that a confluence of genetics, regenerative biology, systems biology and synthetic biology will revolutionize medicine in the coming years. But like most revolutions, it will take time.

What is the current state of the art in regenerative biology?

We know the exact molecular recipes to transform somatic cells into pluripotent stem cells, which can become any cell type. We are learning the recipes to change these pluripotent cells back into specific cell types, tissues and organs. Advances in the study of regeneration have already begun to identify key regulators of stem cell maintenance and regeneration itself. For example, mice lacking cell cycle inhibitor and tumor suppressor gene p21 have regenerative capacities not normally seen in mammals, such as healing a puncture wound to the earlobe using a structure called a blastema, where epithelial cells surround mesenchymal cells. The blastema is the hallmark of limb regeneration in newts and axolotls, and of planarian regeneration as well. A more substantial model of the cell and molecular networks involved in regeneration and in normal development will be of great utility to creating conventional therapeutics and then advanced therapies based on synthetic biology. Researchers around the globe are pursuing work to make regenerative medicine therapies a reality. One of us (ARM) founded Regenerative Sciences Institute, for the express purpose of catalyzing research combining systems, synthetic and regenerative biology and we encourage our readers to visit our website to learn more: www.regensci.org.

So why can't we have these wondrous advances NOW (which will be transformative outside of the narrow focus of aging)?

The answer is we are getting closer all the time. Of the objections we raised in our first edition only the first problem of gathering critical information and learning how to create dynamic models to integrate the information to predict biological function and dysfunction remains as the most important. The continuous improvements to AI-based technology will likely revolutionize our ability to achieve this goal.

For therapies based on synthetic biology, we need gene therapy. Although molecular machines may be built such that they don't use the transcription/translation machinery of the host (DNA automatons have been developed to deliver a drug payload to cells carrying a specific receptor), and other informational biomolecules such as RNA may be used, DNA is the most natural choice as "wetware" for synthetic biology "programs." DNA-based programs invariably require some form of gene therapy, in which foreign DNA enters and interacts with human cells to accomplish a therapeutic purpose. Gene therapy, although technically possible [2] since the early 1980s, was moving forward at a snail's pace, especially since the unexpected death of Jesse Gelsinger in a clinical trial in 1999, but that has changed with the advent of successful clinical trials for gene therapies for cancer using engineered "chimeric antigen T cells". Regulatory infrastructure to permit development of synthetic biology-based, and stem cell-based therapies had not been established five years ago, but that has been changing. The FDA recently announced new guidelines for stem cell therapies. Importantly, inertia from both regulators and from organizations (Big Pharma) that have the huge financial resources to conduct clinical trials necessary to prove safety and efficacy is being overcome by increased enthusiasm for anti-aging therapeutics.

So what will happen in the near term, that is, the "adjacent possible?' Better targeted small molecules, antibodies, proteins, formulated siRNA and perhaps more complex hybrid "smart" molecules will be developed to treat numerous specific diseases, including those associated with aging. Reprogrammed young adult stem cells and smart cells will begin to appear subsequently. In fact, allogenic "young" mesenchymal stem cells derived from IPS cells are already in development by one biotechnology company. Some of these will be capable of enhancing regeneration as well as slowing some aspects of aging. The future of anti-aging therapeutics looks bright indeed.

References

1. Numerous studies support this conclusion. Reviewed by Dunstan DW, Howard B, Healy GN, Owen N. Too much sitting--a health hazard. Diabetes Res Clin Pract. 2012 97:368-76.
2. This should be qualified by noting that technically possible does not imply practicality or safety.
3. Brandhorst S, Choi IY, Wei M, Cheng CW, Sedrakyan S, Navarrete G, Dubeau L, Yap LP, Park R, Vinciguerra M, Di Biase S, Mirzaei H, Mirisola MG, Childress P, Ji L, Groshen S, Penna F, Odetti P, Perin L, Conti PS, Ikeno Y, Kennedy BK, Cohen P, Morgan TE, Dorff TB, Longo VD. A Periodic Diet that Mimics Fasting Promotes Multi-System Regeneration, Enhanced Cognitive Performance, and Healthspan. Cell Metab. 2015 Jul 7;22(1):86-99.

4. Childs BG, Gluscevic M, Baker DJ, Laberge RM, Marquess D, Dananberg J, van Deursen JM. 2017. Senescent cells: an emerging target for diseases of ageing. Nat RevDrug Discov. 16:718-735.

5. Levine ME, Lu AT, Quach A, Chen B, Assimes TL, Bandinelli S, Hou L, Baccarelli AA, Stewart JD, Li Y, Whitsel EA, Wilson JG, Reiner AP, Aviv A, Lohman K, Liu Y, Ferrucci L, Horvath S. 2018. An epigenetic biomarker of aging for lifespan and healthspan. bioRxiv 276162; doi: https:// doi.org/10.1101/276162.

Section I

Repairing intracellular substructures (mitochondria, telomeres)

Chapter 1

Uncoupling Mitochondrial Respiration for Diabesity

Until recently the mechanism of adaptive thermogenesis was ascribed to the expression of uncoupling protein 1 (UCP1) in brown and beige adipocytes. UCP1 is known to catalyze a proton leak of the inner mitochondrial membrane resulting in uncoupled oxidative metabolism with no production of ATP and increased energy expenditure. Thus increasing brown and beige adipose tissue with augmented UCP1 expression is a viable target for obesity-related disorders. Recent work demonstrates an UCP1-independent pathway to uncouple mitochondrial respiration. A secreted enzyme, PM20D1, enriched in UCP1+ adipocytes exhibits catalytic and hydrolytic activity to reversibly form N-acyl amino acids. N-acyl amino acids act as endogenous uncouplers of mitochondrial respiration at physiological concentrations. Administration of PM20D1 or its products, N-acyl amino acids, to diet induced obese mice improves glucose tolerance by increasing energy expenditure. In short term studies treated animals exhibit no toxicity while experiencing 10% weight loss primarily of adipose tissue. Further study of this metabolic pathway may identify novel therapies for diabesity, the disease state associated with diabetes and obesity.

Introduction

Adipose tissue has been characterized by color: abundant white fat, which stores calories, and mitochondria-packed brown or beige fat cells that burn energy and produce heat. In humans, until as recently as 2009, it was thought that only babies had deposits of brown fat. At that time small amounts of brown fat were identified in adults, while individuals with lower body mass indexes (BMIs) tended to have more brown fat. Brown fat helps babies — who don't yet have the ability to shiver — to stay warm. In adults exposed to cold temperatures, brown fat may serve as an "internal heating jacket" to keep blood warm as it flows back to the heart and brain from cold extremities. PET-CT scans have since shown that most individuals have small amounts of brown fat in the neck and the shoulders with other deposits in the chest and along the axial skeleton.

Brown and beige fat express uncoupling protein 1 (UCP1) which dissipates stored chemical energy in the form of heat [1-4]. Knockout of the Ucp1 gene [5] or genetic ablation of brown or beige cells increases susceptibility of the rodents to diabetes and/or obesity, while augmentation of the activity or numbers of these cells can be protective against metabolic disease and obesity [6-8].

In a process called oxidative phosphorylation, the electron transport chain (ETC) pumps protons across the inner mitochondrial membrane into the matrix to generate a proton gradient. This gradient drives a molecular machine, the ATP synthase to form ATP. The UCP1 protein catalyzes a "proton leak" that "uncouples" oxidative respiration resulting in a futile cycle, producing heat but no ATP [1,4]. Augmentation of UCP1 levels was thought until recently to be the primary mediator of so-called adaptive thermogenesis [9].

However, Kazak *et al.* described a creatine-driven substrate cycle that enhanced energy expenditure and thermogenesis in beige fat [10] and now Long *et al.* describe a unique enzyme (PM20D1) secreted by beige and brown fat cells that catalyzes the formation of N-acyl amino acids [11]. Increasing expression of PM20D1 or administration of N-acyl amino acids directly activate mitochondrial energy expenditure in diet-induced obese mice resulting in significant weight loss. Novel enzyme from UCP1+ adipocytes promotes energy expenditure.

Adipose tissue, once thought to be a simple depot for fat storage, is now known to play a key role in energy balance by producing numerous bioactive proteins and "adipokines" such as adiponectin, adipsin, leptin, etc. [12]. Long *et al.* sought to identify signature proteins secreted by UCP1+ brown and beige adipocytes [11]. Out of an initial panel of 32 candidates, one, called PM20D1, contained a signal peptide without any transmembrane domains [13]. To evaluate the potential activity of PM20D1, mice fed a high fat diet (so-called diet-induced obesity, DIO) were injected with adeno-associated viral (AAV) vectors expressing PM20D1 and compared to individuals receiving negative control AAV-green fluorescent protein (GFP) [15]. After 40 days the PM20D1-treated mice gained 9-10% less body weight. Body composition analysis revealed that the weight difference was due exclusively to a 30% reduction in fat mass with no effect on lean body mass. The PM20D1-treated animals had significantly elevated VO2 and VCO2 indicative of increased energy expenditure with no change in food intake or activity (a potential effect of adrenergic stimulation) [11].

PM20D1 generates N-lipidated amino acid *in vivo*. Surprisingly, the increased metabolic rate was not accompanied by an induction of UCP1 nor the recently described futile creatine phosphorylation cycle [10]. PM20D1 is one of five members of the mammalian M20 peptidase family. LC-MS profiling of plasma from the mice injected with AAV-GFP or AAV-PM20D1 revealed a novel metabolite at m/z = 428 which corresponded to N-oleoyl phenylalanine (C18:1-Phe). Subsequently, other related N-acyl amino acids were found in plasma at concentrations ranging from 1-100 nM. Both short (6 hours or 2 days) and longer (16 day) exposure to cold increased the plasma concentration of PM20D1 as well as several N-acyl amino acid products (e.g. C18:1-Leu/Ile and C18:1-Val).

N-acyl amino acids are endogenous uncouplers of respiration acting directly on the mitochondria.

In vitro studies of brown adipose tissue (BAT) adipocytes revealed that a product of PM20D1, C18:1-Phe stimulated maximum oxygen consumption rates (OCR) by almost 200%. This effect was seen with wild type cells as well as UCP1-KO cells suggesting that UCP1 was not required for this biochemical effect. Structure-activity relationship (SAR) studies revealed a need for a free amino acid carboxylate. Many, but not all, amino acids were active as conjugates and N-acyl amino acids were much more active that free fatty acids alone. Tetramethylrhodamine methyl ester (TMRM) fluorescence was used to directly measure the mitochondrial membrane potential in live cells. The N-acyl amino acids directly decreased TMRM fluorescence by ~45%. Because the uncoupling effects were observed on isolated mitochondria efforts were made to identify the mitochondrial target. A UV light-activated conjugate of an N-acyl amino acid was used to identify potential targets in mitochondria. The mitochondrial SLC25A4 and SLC25A5 proteins, also known as ANT1 and 2, may be the targets [16]. Although the consensus function of these proteins is to transport ADP/ATP, they have previously been demonstrated to translocate protons across the inner membrane of the mitochondrion. The N-acyl amino acids generated from the cold-induced PM20D1 enzyme may increase uncoupled respiration by modulating the activity of SCL25-mediated proton flux into the mitochondrial matrix [11].

N-acyl amino acids improve glucose homeostasis and energy expenditure in mice.

DIO mice weighing ~40 g were treated daily for 8 days with vehicle, oleate, or C18:1-Leu (25 mg/kg, i.p.). The N-acyl amino acid-treated mice lost 4.1 g vs. 0.3 and 0.6 g for the vehicle and oleate controls. MRI studies of the mice showed that all of the weight loss was due to a difference in fat mass. The N-acyl amino acid-treated animals exhibited reduced food intake (17%), an improvement in their glucose tolerance and significantly augmented energy expenditure (measured as VO2, VCO2). The respiratory exchange ratio was significantly lower in mice receiving the C18:1-Leu indicating a switch to fats as the metabolic fuel type. Several other N-acyl amino acids (e.g. C18:1-Phe, C20:4-Gly) demonstrated the general property of this class of molecules to uncouple respiration. Finally, plasma liver enzymes, cytokines, etc. were not elevated in the treated animals demonstrating that the N-acyl amino acids are DIRECTLY augmenting whole body energy expenditure, reducing fat mass and improving glucose metabolism in the DIO mice by this novel mechanism [11].

Medical Implications

Long *et al.*'s results suggest a model in which exposure to cold activates UPC1 AND activates PM20D1 to catalyze the formation of N-acyl amino acids, which in turn cause proton to leak back across the inner mitochondrial membrane, dissipating the proton gradient thereby uncoupling oxidative phosphorylation (**Figure 1.1**).

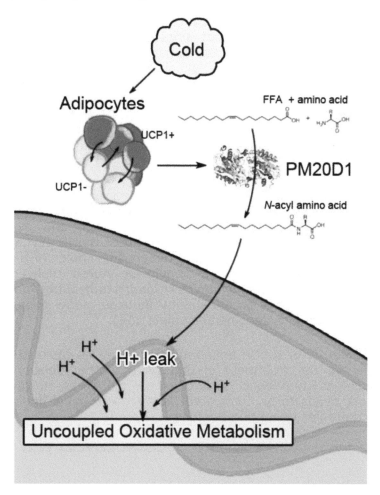

Figure 1.1 N-acyl amino acids uncouple oxidative phosphorylation. Exposure to cold activates UPC1 AND activates PM20D1 to catalyze the formation of N-acyl amino acids, which in turn cause proton to leak back across the inner mitochondrial membrane, dissipating the proton gradient thereby uncoupling oxidative phosphorylation.

Given our current lack of understanding of PM20D1 regulation and its relevance to human physiology, more detailed information about whether the components of N-acyl amino acids, i.e. fatty acids and amino acids, regulate its function will be important.

Interestingly, PM20D1 could not acylate all amino acids to the same extent: phenylalanine is the preferred substrate by far with the branched chain amino acids, leucine, isoleucine and valine having some activity. This latter observation has to be reconciled with the known association of branched chain amino acids (BCAA) with type 2 diabetes [17], although there is some evidence that it is actually the metabolites of BCAA's that may be more important. Methionine, whose restriction has been reported to confer anti-aging effects [18], is a weak substrate of PM20D1, and its absence is unlikely to affect the overall formation of other N-acyl amino acids. In any case, it is quite likely that amino acid concentration itself is not rate limiting for PM20D1, which would explain the apparent discordance. Similarly, it is unlikely that fatty acid levels per se, which play a complex role in diabetes and NASH, control the formation of N-acyl-amino acids. Of note is that some FFA's are known to act beneficially, including short chain amino acids [19] by activation of free fatty acid receptors 2 and 3 [20] and mono-unsaturated (e.g., oleic acid, C18:1), and polyunsaturated long-chain FFAs via FFA1 or other LCFAs, including α-linolenic acid (α-LA) and docosahexaenoic acid (DHA) acting via LFA4 [20].

What else do we know about N-acyl amino acids themselves? Arachidonoyl serine is known to be vasodilatory and neuroprotective. Arachidonoyl glycine inhibits the sensation of pain, and oleoyl serine reverses bone lost. These diverse activities suggest that N-acyl amino acids have other important biological roles and the specific choice of N-acyl amino acid is probably important [21]. It should be noted that Long *et al.* predominately used oleoyl phenylalanine in their studies, but that exposure of mice to cold for 16 days predominantly induced oleoyl conjugates with alanine, glycine, leucine, isoleucine and valine [11].

Either PM20D1 or N-acyl amino acids themselves could be developed therapeutically for the treatment of obesity and other obesity-associated disorders such as metabolic syndrome or diabetes. However, much preclinical work needs to be completed before these novel findings can be translated to therapies benefiting humans.

Among the questions to be answer are:

• How relevant is this enzyme and metabolic pathway to humans?
• What are the characteristics of the human enzyme?
• What about N-acyl amino acid activities on human cells?
• What governs its activity, induction, etc.?
• How is it regulated?
•What controls the balance between PM20D1's synthase and hydrolase activities?
• Does administration of exogenously administered N-acyl amino acids have any toxicity?
• What is the metabolism and pharmacokinetics of the enzyme or the N-acyl amino acid products in primates and then humans?
• Are the N-acyl amino acids orally available?
• Does dysregulation of PM20D1 or its product N-acyl amino acids play a role in the pathogenesis of diabetes, obesity, or non-alcoholic steatohepatitis (NASH) etc.?

The fact that the general findings of Long *et al.* were performed in two laboratories independently supports the veracity of the claims made about the rodents. What remains in the exciting translation of this work to the specific physiology of brown and beige fat and to the general field of human metabolic disease. It is expected to be safer than earlier attempts to uncouple oxidative phosphorylation [22].

Conclusion

Studies in mice have identified a novel enzyme pathway that generates N-acyl amino acids that uncouple mitochondrial respiration. Administration of N-acyl amino acids directly or the secreted enzyme, PM20D1, that generates them to DIO mice results in significant weight loss primarily of fat tissue in a short period of time. Discovery of this novel, completely unexpected pathway may provide novel insights into the pathogenesis of diabetes and obesity while being exploited for novel therapies that are much needed for the global pandemic of diabesity.

References

1. Nicholls DG, Bernson VS, Heaton GM. The identification of the component in the inner membrane of brown adipose tissue mitochondria responsible for regulating energy dissipation. Experientia Suppl 1978;32:89–93.

2. Cannon B, Nedergaard J. Brown Adipose Tissue: Function and Physiological Significance. Physiol Rev 2004;84:277–359. doi:10.1152/physrev.00015.2003.

3. Harms M, Seale P. Brown and beige fat: development, function and therapeutic potential. Nat Med 2013;19:1252–63. doi:10.1038/nm.3361.

4. Rousset S, Alves-Guerra M-C, Mozo J, Miroux B, Cassard-Doulcier A-M, Bouillaud F, et al. The Biology of Mitochondrial Uncoupling Proteins. Diabetes 2004;53:S130–5. doi:10.2337/diabetes.53.2007.S130.

5. Feldmann HM, Golozoubova V, Cannon B, Nedergaard J. UCP1 Ablation Induces Obesity and Abolishes Diet-Induced Thermogenesis in Mice Exempt from Thermal Stress by Living at Thermoneutrality. Cell Metab 2009;9:203–9. doi:10.1016/j.cmet.2008.12.014.

6. Seale P, Conroe HM, Estall J, Kajimura S, Frontini A, Ishibashi J, et al. Prdm16 determines the thermogenic program of subcutaneous white adipose tissue in mice. J Clin Invest 2011;121:96– 105. doi:10.1172/JCI44271.

7. Cohen P, Levy JD, Zhang Y, Frontini A, Kolodin DP, Svensson KJ, et al. Ablation of PRDM16 and Beige Adipose Causes Metabolic Dysfunction and a Subcutaneous to Visceral Fat Switch. Cell 2014;156:304–16. doi:10.1016/j.cell.2013.12.021.

8. Lowell BB, S-Susulic V, Hamann A, Lawitts JA, Himms-Hagen J, Boyer BB, et al. Development of obesity in transgenic mice after genetic ablation of brown adipose tissue. Nature 1993;366:740– 2. doi:10.1038/366740a0.

9. Ukropec J, Anunciado RP, Ravussin Y, Hulver MW, Kozak LP. UCP1-independent thermogenesis in white adipose tissue of cold-acclimated Ucp1-/- mice. J Biol Chem 2006;281:31894–908. doi:10.1074/jbc. M606114200.

10. Kazak L, Chouchani ET, Jedrychowski MP, Erickson BK, Shinoda K, Cohen P, et al. A creatine-driven substrate cycle enhances energy expenditure and thermogenesis in beige fat. Cell 2015;163:643–55. doi:10.1016/j.cell.2015.09.035.

11. Long JZ, Svensson KJ, Bateman LA, Lin H, Kamenecka T, Lokurkar IA, et al. The Secreted Enzyme PM20D1 Regulates Lipidated Amino Acid Uncouplers of Mitochondria. Cell 2016;0. doi:10.1016/j.cell.2016.05.071.

12. Kershaw EE, Flier JS. Adipose tissue as an endocrine organ. J Clin Endocrinol Metab 2004;89:2548–56. doi:10.1210/jc.2004-0395.

13. Veiga-da-Cunha M, Chevalier N, Stroobant V, Vertommen D, Van Schaftingen E. Metabolite proofreading in carnosine and homocarnosine synthesis: molecular identification of PM20D2 as β- alanyl-lysine dipeptidase. J Biol Chem 2014;289:19726–36. doi:10.1074/jbc. M114.576579.

14. Cravatt BF, Giang DK, Mayfield SP, Boger DL, Lerner RA, Gilula NB. Molecular characterization of an enzyme that degrades neuromodulatory fatty-acid amides. Nature 1996;384:83–7. doi:10.1038/384083a0.

15. Zincarelli C, Soltys S, Rengo G, Rabinowitz JE. Analysis of AAV serotypes 1-9 mediated gene expression and tropism in mice after systemic injection. Mol Ther J Am Soc Gene Ther 2008;16:1073–80. doi:10.1038/mt.2008.76.

16. Brand MD, Pakay JL, Ocloo A, Kokoszka J, Wallace DC, Brookes PS, *et al.* The basal proton conductance of mitochondria depends on adenine nucleotide translocase content. Biochem J 2005;392:353–62. doi:10.1042/BJ20050890.

17. Giesbertz P, Daniel H. Branched-chain amino acids as biomarkers in diabetes. Curr Opin Clin Nutr Metab Care 2016;19:48–54. doi:10.1097/MCO.0000000000000235.

18. Lee BC, Kaya A, Gladyshev VN. Methionine restriction and life-span control. Ann N Y Acad Sci 2016;1363:116–24. doi:10.1111/nyas.12973.

19. Canfora EE, Jocken JW, Blaak EE. Short-chain fatty acids in control of body weight and insulin sensitivity. Nat Rev Endocrinol 2015;11:577–91. doi:10.1038/nrendo.2015.128.

20. Watterson KR, Hudson BD, Ulven T, Milligan G. Treatment of Type 2 Diabetes by Free Fatty Acid Receptor Agonists. Front Endocrinol 2014;5. doi:10.3389/fendo.2014.00137.

21. Hanuš L, Shohami E, Bab I, Mechoulam R. N-Acyl amino acids and their impact on biological processes. BioFactors Oxf Engl 2014;40:381–8. doi:10.1002/biof.1166.

22. Grundlingh J, Dargan PI, El-Zanfaly M, Wood DM. 2,4-dinitrophenol (DNP): a weight loss agent with significant acute toxicity and risk of death. J Med Toxicol Off J Am Coll Med Toxicol 2011;7:205–12. doi:10.1007/s13181-011-0162-6.

Chapter 2

Telomerase Reverse Transcriptase and Peroxisome Proliferator-Activated Receptor γ Co-Activator-1α Cooperate to Protect Cells from DNA Damage and Mitochondrial Dysfunction in Vascular Senescence

Reduced telomere length in dividing cells with increasing age has been implicated in contributing to the pathologies of human aging, which include cardiovascular and metabolic disorders, through induction of cellular senescence. Telomere shortening results from the absence of telomerase, an enzyme required to maintain telomere length. TERT, the protein subunit of telomerase, is expressed only transiently in a subset of adult somatic cells, which include stem cells and smooth muscle cells. A recent report from Xiong and colleagues demonstrates a pivotal role for transcription cofactor, peroxisome proliferator-activated receptor gamma coactivator-1α (PGC-1α) in maintaining TERT expression and preventing vascular senescence and atherosclerosis in mice. Ablation of PGC-1α reduced TERT expression, increased DNA damage and ROS, resulting in shortened telomeres and vascular senescence. In the APOE-/- mouse model of atherosclerosis, forced expression of PGC-1α increased expression of TERT, extended telomeres, reversed genomic DNA damage, vascular senescence and the development of atherosclerotic plaques. Alpha lipoic acid (ALA) stimulated expression of PGC-1α and TERT, and reversed DNA damage, vascular senescence and atherosclerosis similarly to ectopic expression of PGC-1α.

ALA stimulated cyclic AMP signaling, which in turn activated CREB, a cofactor for PGC-1a expression. The possibility that ALA might induce TERT to extend telomeres in human cells suggests that ALA may be useful in treating atherosclerosis and other aging related diseases. However, further investigation is needed to identify whether ALA induces TERT in human cells, which cell types are susceptible, and whether such changes have clinical significance.

Introduction

The protein component of telomerase, TERT, is not expressed in most somatic cells in adult mammals [1]. However, TERT is inducibly-expressed in hematopoietic stem cells (HSC), mesenchymal stem cells (MSC) and satellite cells, as well as cells undergoing many cell divisions such as smooth muscle cells and endothelial cells. Down-regulation and absence of TERT is associated with induction of cellular senescence in cultured cells [2] and severe aging-like phenotypes in mice and other experimental organisms. These TERT-dependent phenotypes arise from cells undergoing a large number of divisions which shorten telomeres sufficiently for the cells to recognize the telomeric DNA as damaged. In mice lacking telomerase, up to 4 generations may be required for such effects to be observed [3]. However, even in mice, shortened telomeres arise and characterize certain pathologies, such as atherosclerosis [4]. Telomeres of humans are significantly shorter than in mice: on the one hand it is thought that short telomeres may contribute to aging-related immune dysfunction, but on the other hand protect humans from cancer [5]. However, it is likely that a small subpopulation of human cells with short telomeres themselves are precursors of cancer, since short telomeres destabilize the genome [6].

Inactivation of TERT leading to pathologically shortened telomeres in mice has been shown to reduce mitochondrial biogenesis and transcription co-activator factor PGC-1α via induction of p53. P53 antagonizes PGC-1a expression, causing mitochondrial and metabolic dysfunction which can be rescued by ectopic expression of PGC-1α or TERT [3]. Thus, PGC-1a can be viewed as a suppressor of telomere-mediated pathology.

Deleting one copy of PGC1-α in an atherosclerotic ApoE-/- mouse strain reduces expression of PGC-1α by 50%. This effect results in more severe atherosclerosis, as well as vascular senescence characterized by reduced TERT, SIRT1 and catalase, as well as increased p53 expression. Thus PGC-1α may play a key role in preventing vascular senescence and atherosclerosis [4].

TERT1 and PGC-1α cooperate to protect cells from DNA damage and mitochondrial dysfunction.

In a recent study, Xiong *et al.* [7] extend previous work to identify mechanisms by which PGC-1α and TERT cooperate to protect cells from mitochondrial dysfunction, DNA damage and vascular senescence beyond stimulating SIRT1 transcription [4]. This group [7] discovered that the APOE-/- mouse model of atherosclerosis, in which old mice develop atherosclerotic plaques similar to human atherosclerosis, can be augmented by knocking out both copies of the gene encoding PCG-1α. They constructed a new double knockout mouse model (ApoE-/-, PGC-1α/-), in which old (18 to 20-month-old) mice fed a standard diet develop more severe atherosclerosis and increased vascular senescence than the ApoE-/-mice, suggesting that PGC-1α helps protect the vasculature from development of atherosclerosis [7].

Based on previous work in which TERT deficiency reduced PGC-1α expression [3], Xiong et al hypothesized that levels of TERT, which is known to be expressed in vascular smooth muscle cells, would be reduced. Indeed, western blot analysis showed reduced TERT expression, while telomerase assays showed a consistent 50% reduction of activity in the aortas of middle aged mice. In old mice, a further 50% reduction in TERT expression and activity was observed. At the same time, vascular senescence, as measured by age- associated beta-galactosidase (AABG) expression increased inversely with decreased TERT expression. As expected, telomere length was shortened significantly to an average of 6KB using Southern blot analysis in primary mouse aortic smooth muscle cells (MASMs) [7]. The authors do not mention that "short" 6KB mouse telomeres are still twice as long as average adult human telomeres, However, forced expression of a constitutively active PGC-1alpha or TERT using an adenovirus gene therapy vector reduced expression of AABG to normal levels, while at the same time restoring telomere length to 10 to 12KB, similar to normal control cells.

Although these results suggest that telomere length may matter, they beg the question of how such "short" telomeres in mice, that are actually relatively long in humans, behave so differently across species. The answer may lie in the extent of telomere associated DNA damage would result from increased reactive oxygen species (ROS), which is associated with the atherosclerotic phenotype and PCG-1alpha deficiency. They observed moderately increased ROS in PGC-/- aortas and MASMs, as well as increased levels of 8-hydroxy-deoxyguanosine (8-HG), a characteristic of oxidatively damaged DNA. Moreover, comet assays detected single and double DNA strand breaks. Consistent with data on restored telomere length, ectopic expression of either TERT or PGC-1alpha restored 8-HG levels to normal [7]. But what about possible telomere DNA damage? Xiong et al suggest that these data support the idea that the absence of PGC-1α causes TERT down-regulation which in turn causes DNA damage and telomere shortening/dysfunction.

Increased ROS was hypothesized to cause the observed DNA damage. To test this idea, Xiong *et al.* treated cells with N-acetylcysteine, a strong antioxidant, in order to reduce ROS levels. 5 mM NAC decreased levels of ROS in PCG-1α-/- ApoE-/- MASMs in culture to that of wild-type MASM controls. As expected, there was a beneficial effect of NAC, with about 50% reduction in senescence biomarker AABG, a 2.5-fold induction of TERT/telomerase activity and a 3-fold reduction of 8-HG. However, even after NAC treatment, there was still 50% more AABG, 5-fold less TERT and 2-fold less damage as assessed by the comet assay, suggesting that the defects associated with the absence of PGC-1α were due to more than just increased ROS and oxidative DNA damage. Tellingly, telomere length increased moderately with NAC treatment, but still was not restored to wild-type levels. This raised the possibility of telomere dysfunction and associated DNA damage. To investigate possible telomere DNA damage, cells were immuno-fluorescently stained with antibodies to gamma-H2AX, a histone which accumulates at double-stranded breaks. At the same time cells were stained with fluorescently-labeled telomere-specific peptide nucleic acid probes to determine the location of the telomeres. Gamma-H2AX staining showed significant evidence of DNA damage in PCG-1α-/- ApoE-/- MASMs (7-fold more) compared with wild-type cells, split almost evenly between telomeric and non-telomeric foci. Treatment with NAC reduced non-telomeric damage to within 2-fold of normal levels, but only reduced DNA damage at telomeric foci by about 10%, so that telomere DNA damage remained at least 4-fold greater than controls. They conclude that oxidative stress associated with loss of PGC-1α strongly contributes to genomic DNA damage and moderately contributes to telomere shortening and telomeric DNA damage. But clearly there is some other factor causing telomeric DNA damage, most likely reduced TERT. They hypothesize that reduced TERT expression is not only due to ROS, but to loss of PGC-1α directly [7]. This makes sense, and may explain the species difference between mice and humans alluded to earlier: TERT is not only lengthening telomeres, but stabilizing them to confer protection from DNA damage. Also, it has been reported that telomerase can protect mitochondrial DNA from damage [8], which may also play a role in how PGC-1α and TERT reverse senescence, although mitochondrial DNA damage was not assayed by Xiong and colleagues. So the absolute length of telomeres is only one factor. This idea could be tested by making cells conditional for TERT expression.

To test the hypothesis that PCG-1α directly regulates TERT transcription, Xiong *et al.* analyzed the TERT promoter and found evolutionarily-conserved DNA-binding elements of transcription factors (TFs) PPAR-gamma as well as FoxO1, Nrf-2, p53, CREB, ER-a/ERR-a and YY-1. PGC-1α controls the expression of all these TFs [9]. In support of this idea, over- expression of constitutively active PGC-1α in rat aortic smooth muscle (RASMs) cells increased TERT in a dose dependent manner [7]. Surprisingly, similar evidence from MASMs or human aortic smooth muscle cells was not provided.

Moreover, multiple pathways with anti-inflammatory and pro-mitochondrial activity were stimulated: Nrf-1, Nrf-2, mitochondrial transcription factor A (TFAM), SIRT1, heme oxygenase-1 (HO-1), and MnSOD. Of special interest were Nrf-2 and HO-1, which are important for antioxidant/electrophile-responsive element (ARE/ERE) adaptive electrophilic responses [10].

Xiong *et al* postulated that alpha lipoic acid (ALA), a compound that previously was observed to reduced atherosclerosis and increase PGC-1α expression in mice [11], would increase TERT and ARE/ERE signaling to decrease DNA damage and improve telomere function. In normal RASMs, ALA induces PGC-1α about 3-fold and TERT about 2-fold, confirming their hypothesis.

Moreover, treatment of young ApoE-/- mice with 3-10 mg/kg ALA increases telomerase activity 2.5 fold, increases TERT and ARE/ERE signaling significantly over background and reduces p53, which is known to reduce TERT expression levels by 2-fold in a dose and time dependent manner. To confirm that PGC-1α is required, Xiong *et al* repeated this experiment on PGC1-α -/- MASMs and found no stimulation of TERT, or ARE/ERE signaling [7].

Xiong next tested the hypothesis that CREB, the cAMP response element binding protein, mediates the effects of ALA on PGC-1α. CREB is known to enable PGC-1α transcription [12] and its down-regulation is associated with atherosclerosis [13]. ALA strongly stimulates cAMP is mice aortas and smooth muscle cells for 2 days after treatment, and activating phosphorylation at Ser133 of CREB, although CREB expression levels were unchanged, suggesting that ALA may stimulate PGC-1α through increased cAMP via CREB [7].

A high fat diet (HFD) is known to be pro-atherosclerotic in ApoE-/- mice [14]. Xiong et all observed that ApoE-/- mice fed a HFD for 2-4 weeks exhibited reduced PGC1-α, SIRT1 and TERT/telomerase activity, but increased p53. Treatment of youthful HFD ApoE-/- mice with injected ALA for 7 days, completely blocked the reduction of PGC1-α, SIRT1 and TERT/telomerase activity, and the increase in p53, while reducing DNA damage to background levels. Vascular aging, as assessed by AABG and atherosclerotic plaques, was reduced to below background levels after ALA treatment [7].

It should be noted that these studies were performed not only in rodents, but mostly in genetically manipulated mouse models, which are not physiological, and that careful biochemical studies in normal animals and humans are needed to extend the applicability of this work. Xiong et al suggest that these data are consistent with a model wherein TERT and PGC-1α form an inhibitory positive feedback loop, whereby loss of either one promotes the loss of the other (**Figure 2.1**).

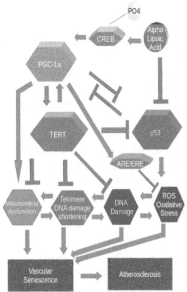

Figure 2.1. PGC-1a stimulates TERT to mitigate telomeric and genomic DNA damage, ROS, mitochondrial dysfunction and senescence in vascular smooth muscle cells. PGG-1α stimulates transcription of TERT which in turn reduces genomic and telomeric DNA damage, and mitochondrial dysfunction reversing vascular senescence and atherosclerosis. PGC-1α stimulates multiple anti-inflammatory pathways (not shown) including ARE/ERE, which promote mitochondrial function. Mitigation of DNA damage and ROS, lower p53 levels to allow increases in TERT and PGC1-α expression. ALA stimulates PGC-1α transcription via phosphorylation of transcription factor CREB, to stimulate TERT expression and relieve vascular senescence and atherosclerosis.

It is intriguing that the DNA regulatory elements that control PGC-1α are conserved into humans, and suggest that these results or at least this control loop may translate to humans, although confirmatory experiments on human cells and subsequently in humans are required.

Medical Implications

There is great interest to stimulate telomerase expression to alleviate shortened telomeres that are associated with aging, especially in lymphocytes [15]. Because ALA augments telomerase in rat MASMs and mouse aortas, its ability to stimulate TERT and telomerase activity in corresponding human cells and especially lymphocytes should be investigated. Should ALA increase telomere length in humans, it may prove to be a relatively safe way to control telomere length. ALA is available over-the-counter as an oral supplement and has been used in clinical trials for diabetes and other ailments. In Germany injected ALA is a prescription medicine to treat type II diabetes [16, 17]. On the other hand, clinical trials with ALA have failed to produce data that are consistent with the results reported by Xiong et al, although specific endpoints consistent with this report have not explored [18-21].

Preventing replicative senescence and/or telomere DNA damage during aging could be of benefit, since elimination of some senescent cells has been reported to rejuvenate some tissues, which presumably are affected by the secreted associated senescent phenotype (SASP) [20, 21].

If ALA can actually stimulate TERT in a wide variety of human cells, then it may have serious benefit to maintain quality of life during aging. However, supplementation with ALA in adult mice did not lead to increases in health span or lifespan [23], casting some indirect doubt on its capability to affect TERT in a large variety of cells, since ectopic TERT expression in normal mice promotes health span [24].

It will be interesting to elucidate how permissive most adult somatic cells that do not normally express TERT are to TERT induction. Furthermore it will be useful to understand the mechanism that underlies how ALA stimulates PGC-1α. If ALA stimulation of cAMP, activates CREB, which in turn promotes the expression of PGC-1a (**Figure 2.1**), then how does ALA stimulate cAMP?

At least one report suggests that ALA stimulates cAMP through G-coupled membrane receptors [25]. If true, how universal are cAMP stimulation, CREB activation, and induction of PGC-1α and TERT?

It is informative that increased DNA damage and senescence are associated with reduced expression of master transcription factor like PGC-1α, through its interaction with TERT. That PGC-1α can suppress senescence and DNA damage, and is some cases reverse these phenotypes suggests that therapies based on stimulating PGC1-a could have benefit in aging.

However, it is quite premature to believe that enhanced expression of PGC1-alpha will increase human longevity. To date, studies in people have found no correlation of longevity with PGC-1α levels or with mitochondrial biogenesis [26]. In fact, data suggest that mitochondrial biogenesis in "successful" old age is reduced and that transcription factor Ying-Yang 1 (YY1) has a negative correlation with longevity [26]. Moreover, no SNPs have been reported in the PGC-1α gene that associate with longevity, although several polymorphisms associated with Parkinson's disease in one study [27], but were not confirmed in another [28].

Conclusion

PGC1-α expression prevents vascular senescence in a mouse model of atherosclerosis by maintaining TERT levels through an inhibitory positive feedback loop. ALA is able to induce PGC1-α, TERT and other pro-mitochondrial signaling pathways possibly by activation of CREB via phosphorylation. ALA may be a general purpose treatment to increase telomere length, although this idea requires further investigation.

References

1. Choudhary B, Karande AA, Raghavan SC. Telomere and telomerase in stem cells: relevance in ageing and disease. Front Biosci Sch Ed 2012;4:16–30.
2. Jeyapalan JC, Sedivy JM. Cellular senescence and organismal aging. Mech Ageing Dev 2008;129:467–74. doi:10.1016/j.mad.2008.04.001.
3. Sahin E, Colla S, Liesa M, Moslehi J, Muller FL, Guo M, et al. Telomere dysfunction induces metabolic and mitochondrial compromise. Nature 2011;470:359–65. doi:10.1038/nature09787.
4. Xiong S, Salazar G, Patrushev N, Ma M, Forouzandeh F, Hilenski L, et al. Peroxisome Proliferator- Activated Receptor γ Coactivator-1α Is a Central Negative Regulator of Vascular Senescence. Arterioscler Thromb Vasc Biol 2013;33:988–98. doi:10.1161/ATVBAHA.112.301019.
5. Donate LE, Blasco MA. Telomeres in cancer and ageing. Philos Trans R Soc Lond B Biol Sci 2011;366:76–84. doi:10.1098/rstb.2010.0291.
6. Shay JW, Wright WE. Role of telomeres and telomerase in cancer. Semin Cancer Biol 2011;21:349–53. doi:10.1016/j.semcancer.2011.10.001.
7. Xiong S, Patrushev N, Forouzandeh F, Hilenski, L, Alexander RW. PGC-1α Modulates Telomere Function and DNA Damage in Protecting against Aging-Related Chronic Diseases. Cell Rep 2015;12:1391–9. doi:10.1016/j.celrep.2015.07.047.
8. Haendeler J, Dröse S, Büchner N, Jakob S, Altschmied J, Goy C, et al. Mitochondrial Telomerase Reverse Transcriptase Binds to and Protects Mitochondrial DNA and Function From Damage. Arterioscler Thromb Vasc Biol 2009;29:929–35. doi:10.1161/ATVBAHA.109.185546.
9. Patten IS, Arany Z. PGC-1 coactivators in the cardiovascular system. Trends Endocrinol Metab 2012;23:90–7. doi:10.1016/j.tem.2011.09.007.
10. Vriend J, Reiter RJ. The Keap1-Nrf2-antioxidant response element pathway: a review of its regulation by melatonin and the proteasome. Mol Cell Endocrinol 2015;401:213–20. doi:10.1016/j.mce.2014.12.013.
11. Zhang W-J, Bird KE, McMillen TS, LeBoeuf RC, Hagen TM, Frei B. Dietary α-Lipoic Acid Supplementation Inhibits Atherosclerotic Lesion Development in Apolipoprotein E–Deficient and Deficient Mice. Circulation 2008;117:421–8. doi:10.1161/CIRCULATIONAHA.107.725275.

12. St-Pierre J, Drori S, Uldry M, Silvaggi JM, Rhee J, Jäger S, et al. Suppression of Reactive Oxygen Species and Neurodegeneration by the PGC-1 Transcriptional Coactivators. Cell 2006;127:397–408. doi:10.1016/j.cell.2006.09.024.

13. Reusch JEB, Klemm DJ. Cyclic AMP Response Element-Binding Protein in the Vessel Wall Good or Bad? Circulation 2003;108:1164–6. doi:10.1161/01.CIR.0000084296.45158.50.

14. Wang JC, Bennett M. Aging and Atherosclerosis Mechanisms, Functional Consequences, and Potential Therapeutics for Cellular Senescence. Circ Res 2012;111:245–59. doi:10.1161/CIRCRESAHA.111.261388.

15. Larrick JW, Mendelsohn AR. Telomerase redux: ready for prime time? Rejuvenation Res 2015;18:185–7. doi:10.1089/rej.2015.1695.

16. Nebbioso M, Pranno F, Pescosolido N. Lipoic acid in animal models and clinical use in diabetic retinopathy. Expert Opin Pharmacother 2013;14:1829–38. doi:10.1517/14656566.2013.813483.

17. Han T, Bai J, Liu W, Hu Y. A systematic review and meta-analysis of α-lipoic acid in the treatment of diabetic peripheral neuropathy. Eur J Endocrinol Eur Fed Endocr Soc 2012;167:465– 71. doi:10.1530/EJE-12-0555.

18. Pagano G, Aiello Talamanca A, Castello G, Cordero MD, d'Ischia M, Gadaleta MN, et al. Current experience in testing mitochondrial nutrients in disorders featuring oxidative stress and mitochondrial dysfunction: rational design of chemoprevention trials. Int J Mol Sci 2014;15:20169–208. doi:10.3390/ijms151120169.

19. Ajith TA, Jayakumar TG. Mitochondria-targeted agents: Future perspectives of mitochondrial pharmaceutics in cardiovascular diseases. World J Cardiol 2014;6:1091–9. doi:10.4330/wjc.v6.i10.1091.

20. Koufaki M. Therapeutic applications of lipoic acid: a patent review (2011-2014). Expert Opin Ther Pat 2014;24:993–1005. doi:10.1517/13543776.2014.937425.

21. Park S, Karunakaran U, Jeoung NH, Jeon J-H, Lee I-K. Physiological effect and therapeutic application of alpha lipoic acid. Curr Med Chem 2014;21:3636–45.

22. Zhu Y, Tchkonia T, Pirtskhalava T, Gower AC, Ding H, Giorgadze N, et al. The Achilles' heel of senescent cells: from transcriptome to senolytic drugs. Aging Cell 2015:n/a – n/a. doi:10.1111/acel.12344.

23. Lee C-K, Pugh TD, Klopp RG, Edwards J, Allison DB, Weindruch R, et al. The impact of alpha-lipoic acid, coenzyme Q10 and caloric restriction on life span and gene expression patterns in mice. Free Radic Biol Med 2004;36:1043–57. doi:10.1016/j.freeradbiomed.2004.01.015.

24. Bernardes de Jesus B, Vera E, Schneeberger K, Tejera AM, Ayuso E, Bosch F, et al. Telomerase gene therapy in adult and old mice delays aging and increases longevity without increasing cancer. EMBO Mol Med 2012:n/a – n/a. doi:10.1002/emmm.201200245.

25. Salinthone S, Schillace RV, Tsang C, Regan JW, Bourdette DN, Carr DW. Lipoic acid stimulates cAMP production via G protein coupled receptor dependent and independent mechanisms. J Nutr Biochem 2011;22:681–90. doi:10.1016/j.jnutbio.2010.05.008.

26. van Leeuwen N, Beekman M, Deelen J, van den Akker EB, de Craen AJM, Slagboom PE, et al. Low mitochondrial DNA content associates with familial longevity: the Leiden Longevity Study. Age 2014;36. doi:10.1007/s11357-014-9629-0.

27. Clark J, Reddy S, Zheng K, Betensky RA, Simon DK. Association of PGC-1alpha polymorphisms with age of onset and risk of Parkinson's disease. BMC Med Genet 2011;12:69. doi:10.1186/1471-2350-12-69.

28. Shibata N, Motoi Y, Tomiyama H, Ohnuma T, Kuerban B, Tomson K, et al. Lack of Genetic Associations of PPAR-γ and PGC-1α with Alzheimer's Disease and Parkinson's Disease with Dementia. Dement Geriatr Cogn Disord EXTRA 2013;3:161–7. doi:10.1159/000351419.

Chapter 3

Telomerase Redux: Ready for Prime Time?

By maintaining genome integrity, controlling cell proliferation, and regulating tissue homeostasis, telomerase plays a critical role in the pathology of aging and cancer. Telomerase is composed of telomerase RNA, or telomerase RNA component (TERC), which serves as a template for telomeric DNA synthesis, and a catalytic subunit, telomerase reverse transcriptase (TERT). The canonical function of TERT is the synthesis of telomeric DNA repeats and the maintenance of telomere length. Recent studies suggest that adeno-associated virus (AAV)-expressed TERT in adult mice can increase life span and health span. Because TERT physically interacts with proteins that regulate gene expression, and because TERT's expression at high levels is associated with oncogenic transformation, its synthesis needs to be carefully regulated. Due to safety concerns, transient expression of TERT mRNA may be preferred for tissue engineering and adoptive stem cell therapy.

Introduction

Increasing telomere length to slow or prevent aging is a popular idea, especially in some segments of the lay community, but the science is controversial. The absence of telomerase from most somatic cells of mammals has significant consequences for aging. First, by limiting the number of potential cell divisions, active telomerase sets limits on both life span and cancer cell proliferation. Second, shortened telomeres are known to result in physiological dysfunction and play a role in human diseases such as Werner syndrome [1] and ataxia telangiectasia [2]. Ectopic expression of the catalytic subunit of telomerase, telomerase reverse transcriptase (TERT), has been reported to extend life span by as much as 40% in cancer-resistant mice [3]. On the other hand, ectopic expression of TERT promotes cancer in normal mice.

Ectopic expression of TERT using adeno-associated virus serotype 9 (AAV9)-based gene therapy in adult mice increases both health span and life span without increasing cancer incidence, [4,5] although increased cancer incidence is clearly an issue in transgenic animals ectopically expressing TERT [3,6]. In addition, transient induction of TERT by an astragalus-derived compound increases health span without an apparent increase in cancer incidence in mice [7]. Available evidence suggests that increases in life span may require both elongated telomeres and the continuous presence of telomerase to stimulate various signaling pathways [6]. The canonical function of TERT is the synthesis of telomeric DNA repeats and the maintenance of telomere length. However, accumulating evidence indicates that TERT may also have some fundamental non-canonical functions that are independent of its enzymatic activity. TERT has been reported to physically interact with many proteins including nuclear factor-$^{\kappa}$ β (NF-$^{\kappa}$β), [8] DNA methytransferase I, [9] RNA helicase BRG1/SMARC4A,[10] nucleostemin/GNL, [10] and β-catenin. [11] TERT's interaction with BRG1 and nucleostemin has been reported to alter microRNAs (miRNAs) that can affect expression of multiple downstream genes [10]. TERT may even play roles in non-dividing cells, where, for example, its expression has been reported to protect neurons from Alzheimer's disease by preventing accumulation of pathological phosphorylated tau protein [12]. Moreover, ectopic expression of TERT via an AAV gene therapy vector increases survival after myocardial infarction in mice, partly through its effects on cardiomyocytes [13].

However, the interaction of β-catenin with TERT has recently been shown to be artifactual, [14] suggesting that some care must be taken in predicting the implications of TERT expression. For example, the recent observation that WNT/β-catenin signaling can stimulate TERT expression raised the possibility of a positive feedback loop between TERT and WNT/β-catenin [15]. Such a positive feedback loop suggested that safety must be carefully considered in the development of drugs that stimulate telomerase activity. However, if the reciprocal interaction of TERT with β-catenin does not occur, the regulation may actually be uni-directional, with β-catenin driving TERT expression.

Will Extending Telomeres Lead to Longer, Healthier Lives?

In the short term, we predict that extension of telomeres will facilitate tissue engineering, paving the way for future *in vivo* applications. Whereas some success has been re- ported using AAV, telomere extension by non-viral, non- integrating methods remains inefficient. A recent report from Helen Blau's lab at Stanford University shows that delivery of modified mRNA encoding TERT to human fibroblasts and myoblasts increases telomerase activity transiently (24–48 hr) and can rapidly extend telomeres, which was associated with increased cell proliferation [16].

Modified mRNA encoding TERT was administered to four groups of cells. The modified mRNA used pseudo-uridine and 5-methylcytidine. To increase mRNA stability, the full-length human TERT open reading frame was flanked by the 59- and 39- untranslated regions (UTR) of the human β-globin gene, a 5' cap, and a 151-nucleotide 3' poly(A) tail [17]. The mRNA was transfected via a cationic lipid carrier into primary human fibroblasts and myoblasts, cells known to have limited proliferative capacity [18,19]. Transfection efficiency was determined using flow cytometric single-cell quantitation of fluorescence following delivery of green fluorescent protein (GFP) mRNA, which showed that most cells (~90%) were transfected even at relatively low concentrations of modified mRNA (0.1 ug/mL).

Group 1 received modified mRNA encoding TERT, and the other three control groups received either: (1) mRNA encoding an inactive form of TERT, (2) TERT buffer solution, or (3) no treatment. Telomeres of the first group (telomere-extending treatment group) rapidly lengthened over a period of a few days, whereas the telomeres of the three control groups were not extended. Group 1 exhibited more cell divisions, compared to the controls. Regarding the safety of this approach, the telomeres of group 1 cells resumed shortening after they were extended. Ultimately, all of the cell populations stopped dividing, indicating that they were not immortalized. This approach has been tested on fibroblasts and myoblasts and is now being tested on stem cells. Importantly, the research showed that cells could be treated several times with enhanced effects on the capacity for cell division. Because the increase in numbers is compounded with each treatment, a small sample of cells, for example from a small biopsy, might be amplified to very large numbers. The authors claim up to 1012-fold amplification is possible! [16]

However, the estimated 1012-fold increase was only ob- served for primary fibroblasts, a cell type known to be subject to immortalization by ectopic expression of TERT [20]. With myoblasts, Ramunas *et al.* only observed an increase of a few population doublings, in line with the inability of human myoblasts to be immortalized by TERT [21, 22]. Unfortunately, many cell types are refractory to TERT immortalization, reducing the possible benefit of delivery of modified TERT- encoding mRNA to preventing senescence-associated changes in gene expression. On the other hand, many adult stem cells do express TERT, albeit at levels sufficient to slow, but not prevent, telomere loss, suggesting that extension of telomere levels by transient expression of TERT could be of benefit.

Medical Implications

Transient delivery of TERT mRNA provides an advantageous alternative to previous approaches because the "therapy" is brief, rapidly extends telomeres, can be repeated in an iterative manner, and apparently does not risk insertional mutagenesis. Of great interest may be application to expansion of adult stem cells of diverse tissues to model diseases, screen for drugs, or use for cell therapy. In this case, loss of stem cell phenotype over time in culture remains a problem that is partially addressable by this brief and repeated exposure. How differentiated or stem cell phenotype beyond proliferation is affected by shortened telomere length is an open question. The telomere position effect [23] and p53 activation [24] are two known mechanisms. The transient non-integrating nature of modified mRNA with finite increase in proliferation may render this method safer than viral or DNA vectors. In the short term, the method has enormous potential in tissue engineering and could be applied for ex vivo treatment of cell types currently transplanted, such as skin, hair, hematopoietic stem cells, or bone marrow progenitors. Numerous patients receive these therapies for immunosenescence and/or bone marrow failure, during plastic surgical procedures, and for cosmeceutical reasons. Unfortunately, despite some success with delivery of modified mRNA to certain tissues *in vivo*, [25] safe delivery remains a significant technical challenge. Issues related to targeting and toxicity must be overcome for the method to be applied therapeutically.

Overcoming problems associated with telomere shortening, such as the loss of proliferative capacity and potential induction of the senescent phenotype, is but a first step in maintaining stem cell function. Remaining unsolved problems include loss and alteration of cell differentiation potential with increasing cell division.

The safe enabling of tissue engineering with stem cells shares a problem with the use of inducible gene therapy constructs to express telomerase for the same purpose (although it avoids generic problems with gene therapy). This problem is related to the observation that telomerase does not immortalize many cell types, including many adult stem cell types. Where immortalization does not occur, telomerase barely extends the Hayflick limit—i.e., TERT has very limited benefit [21]. Perhaps other aging/cell proliferation clocks are running in parallel. Alterations in DNA methylation associated with cell proliferation have been proposed and a DNA methylation signature observed [26]. It remains a formal possibility, although unlikely, that telomerase itself might induce another senescence clock.

The limited immortalization capability of TERT is apparently why combinations of factors such as ectopic c-myc and anti-p16ink4a RNA interference (RNAi) are needed to immortalize many progenitor and stem cells [27]. Combining these factors with modified RNA lipofection is expected to overcome this obstacle to support the tissue engineering. However, transient expression of a proto-oncogene and knockdown of a tumor suppressor might result in even a greater risk of oncogenic transformation than with TERT alone. Work to address this challenge is ongoing in many laboratories.

References

1. Crabbe L, Verdun RE, Haggblom CI, Karlseder J. Defective telomere lagging strand synthesis in cells lacking WRN helicase activity. Science 2004;306:1951–1953.
2. Metcalfe JA, Parkhill J, Campbell L, Stacey M, Biggs P, Byrd PJ, Taylor AM. Accelerated telomere shortening in ataxia telangiectasia. Nat Genet 1996;13:350–353.
3. Tomas-Loba A, Flores I, Fernandez-Marcos PJ, Cayuela ML, Maraver A, Tejera A, Borras C, Matheu A, Klatt P, Flores JM, Vin~a J, Serrano M, Blasco MA. Telomerase reverse transcriptase delays aging in cancer-resistant mice. Cell 2008;135:609–622.
4. Bernardes de Jesus B, Vera E, Schneeberger K, Tejera AM, Ayuso E, Bosch F, Blasco MA. Telomerase gene therapy in adult and old mice delays aging and increases longevity without increasing cancer. EMBO Mol Med 2012;4: 691–704.
5. Mendelsohn AR, Larrick JW. Ectopic expression of telomerase safely increases health span and life span. Rejuvenation Res 2012;15:435–438.
6. Vera E, Bernardes de Jesus B, Foronda M, Flores JM, Blasco MA. Telomerase reverse transcriptase synergizes with calorie restriction to increase health span and extend mouse longevity. PLoS One 2013;8:e53760.
7. De Jesus BB, Schneeberger K, Vera E, Tejera A, Harley CB, Blasco MA. The telomerase activator TA-65 elongates short telomeres and increases health span of adult/old mice without increasing cancer incidence. Aging Cell 2011;10: 604–621.
8. Ghosh A, Saginc G, Leow SC, Khattar E, Shin EM, Yan TD, Wong M, Zhang Z, Li G, Sung WK, Zhou J, Chang WJ, Li S, Liu E, Tergaonkar V. Telomerase directly regulates NF-jB-dependent transcription. Nat Cell Biol 2012;14: 1270–1281.

9. Young JI, Sedivy JM, Smith JR. Telomerase expression in normal human fibroblasts stabilizes DNA 5-methylcytosine transferase I. J Biol Chem 2003;278:19904–19908.

10. Lassmann T, Maida Y, Tomaru Y, Yasukawa M, Ando Y, Kojima M, Kasim V, Simon C, Daub CO, Carninci P, Hayashizaki Y, Masutomi K. Telomerase reverse transcriptase regulates microRNAs. Int J Mol Sci 2015;16: 1192–1208.

11. Park J-I, Venteicher AS, Hong JY, Choi J, Jun S, Shkreli M, Chang W, Meng Z, Cheung P, Ji H, McLaughlin M, Veenstra TD, Nusse R, McCrea PD, Artandi SE. Telomerase modulates Wnt signaling by association with target gene chromatin. Nature 2009;460:66–72.

12. Spilsbury A, Miwa S, Attems J, Saretzki G. The role of telomerase protein TERT in Alzheimer's disease and in Tau- related pathology *in vitro*. J Neurosci 2015;35:1659–1674.

13. Bar C, Bernardes de Jesus B, Serrano R, Tejera A, Ayuso E, Jimenez V, Formentini I, Bobadilla M, Mizrahi J, de Martino A, Gomez G, Pisano D, Mulero F, Wollert KC, Bosch F, Blasco MA. Telomerase expression confers cardioprotection in the adult mouse heart after acute myocardial infarction. Nat Commun 2014;5:5863.

14. Listerman I, Gazzaniga FS, Blackburn EH. An investigation of the effects of the core protein telomerase reverse transcriptase on Wnt signaling in breast cancer cells. Mol Cell Biol 2014;34:280–289.

15. Zhou J, Ding D, Wang M, Cong Y-S. Telomerase reverse transcriptase in the regulation of gene expression. BMB Rep 2014;47:8.

16. Ramunas J, Yakubov E, Brady JJ, Corbel SY, Holbrook C, Brandt M, Stein J, Santiago JG, Cooke JP, Blau HM. Transient delivery of modified mRNA encoding TERT rapidly extends telomeres in human cells. FASEB J 2015; doi:10.1096/fj.14-259531.

17. Tavernier G, Andries O, Demeester J, Sanders NN, De Smedt SC, Rejman J. mRNA as gene therapeutic: How to control protein expression. J Control Release Off J Control Release Soc 2011;150:238–247.

18. Webster C, Blau HM. Accelerated age-related decline in replicative life-span of Duchenne muscular dystrophy myoblasts: Implications for cell and gene therapy. Somat Cell Mol Genet 1990;16:557–565.

19. Hayflick L, Moorhead PS. The serial cultivation of human diploid cell strains. Exp Cell Res 1961;25:585–621.

20. Bodnar AG, Ouellette M, Frolkis M, Holt SE, Chiu C-P, Morin GB, Harley CB, Shay JW, Lichtsteiner S, Wright WE. Extension of life-span by introduction of telomerase into normal human cells. Science 1998;279:349–352.

21. Di Donna S, Mamchaoui K, Cooper RN, Seigneurin-Venin S, Tremblay J, Butler-Browne GS, Mouly V. Telomerase can extend the proliferative capacity of human myoblasts, but does not lead to their immortalization. Mol Cancer Res MCR 2003;1:643–653.

22. Zhu C-H, Mouly V, Cooper RN, Mamchaoui K, Bigot A, Shay JW, Di Santo JP, Butler-Browne GS, Wright WE. Cellular senescence in human myoblasts is overcome by human telomerase reverse transcriptase and cyclin- dependent kinase4: Consequences in aging muscle and therapeutic strategies for muscular dystrophies. Aging Cell 2007;6:515–523.

23. Robin JD, Ludlow AT, Batten K, Magdinier F, Stadler G, Wagner KR, Shay JW, Wright WE. Telomere position effect: Regulation of gene expression with progressive telomere shortening over long distances. Genes Dev 2014;28: 2464–2476.

24. Wang H, Chen Q, Lee S-H, Choi Y, Johnson FB, Pignolo RJ. Impairment of osteoblast differentiation due to proliferation-independent telomere dysfunction in mouse models of accelerated aging. Aging Cell 2012;11:704–713.

25. Kormann MSD, Hasenpusch G, Aneja MK, Nica G, Flemmer AW, Herber-Jonat S, Huppmann M, Mays LE, Illenyi M, Schams A, Griese M, Bittmann I, Handgretinger R, Hartl D, Rosenecker J, Rudolph C. Expression of therapeutic proteins after delivery of chemically modified mRNA in mice. Nat Biotechnol 2011;29:154–157.

26. Koch CM, Reck K, Shao K, Lin Q, Joussen S, Ziegler P, Walenda G, Drescher W, Opalka B, May T, Brummendorf T, Zenke M, Saric T, Wagner W. Pluripotent stem cells escape from senescence-associated DNA methylation changes. Genome Res 2013;23:248–259.
27. Garbe JC, Vrba L, Sputova K, Fuchs L, Novak P, Brothman AR, Jackson M, Chin K, LaBarge MA, Watts G, Futscher BW, Stampfer MR. Immortalization of normal human mammary epithelial cells in two steps by direct targeting of senescence barriers does not require gross genomic alterations. Cell Cycle 2014;13:3423–3435.

Section II

Modulating Metabolism and Growth Regulation

Chapter 4

ATP Synthase: A Target for Dementia and Aging

Advancing age is the biggest risk factor for development for the major life-threatening diseases in industrialized nations accounting for >90% of deaths. Alzheimer's dementia (AD) is among the most devastating. Currently approved therapies fail to slow progression of the disease, providing only modest improvements in memory. Recently reported work describes mechanistic studies of J147, a promising therapeutic molecule previously shown to rescue the severe cognitive deficits exhibited by aged, transgenic AD mice. Apparently, J147 targets the mitochondrial alpha-F1-ATP synthase (ATP5A). Modest inhibition of the ATP synthase modulates intracellular calcium to activate AMP-activated protein kinase to inhibit mammalian target of rapamycin, a known mechanism of lifespan extension from worms to mammals.

Our story begins with turmeric (*Curcuma longa*) an herbaceous perennial plant of the ginger family native to the Indian subcontinent and Southeast Asia and widely used in traditional Chinese and Ayurvedic medicine to treat various diseases.*

Although limited high-quality clinical evidence supports the use of turmeric or its main constituent, curcumin (**Figure 4.1)**, in medical therapy, [1, 2] medicinal chemists warn that curcumin is a textbook example of both a "PAINS" (panassay interference compound), which means that it tends to be false positive in drug screens, and IMPS (invalid metabolic panaceas) compound, a compound that has bioactivity in every bioassay studied [3, 6].

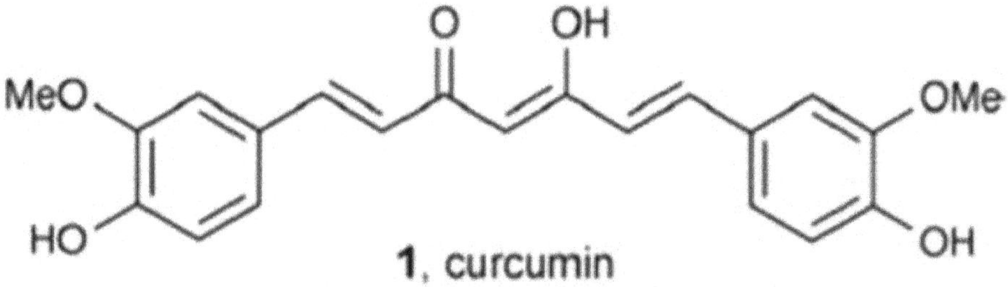

1, curcumin
(60-70% of turmeric extract)

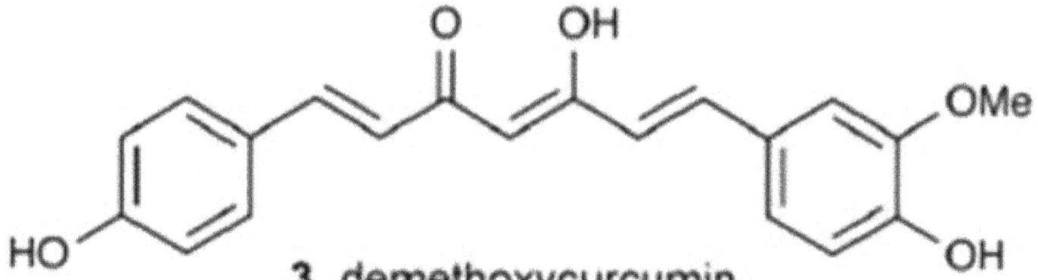

3, demethoxycurcumin
(20-27% of turmeric extract)

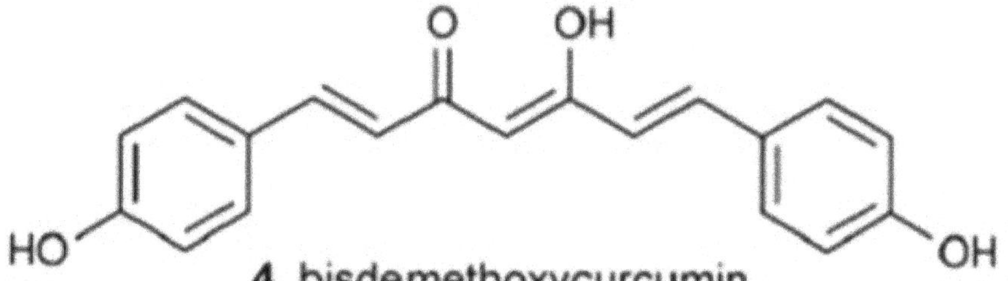

4, bisdemethoxycurcumin
(10-15% of turmeric extract)

**Figure 4.1. Curcumin-related constituents from extracts of
Curcuma longa.**

The Salk Institute laboratory of David Schubert citing earlier work on the purported efficacy of curcumin in murine models of Alzheimer's disease [7,8] utilized this pharmacophore to synthesize and evaluate a series of neurotrophic and neuroprotective molecules [9]. To improve the potency and pharmacokinetic properties of curcumin, hybrid molecules between curcumin and cyclohexyl-bisphenol A, a molecule, itself exhibiting neurotrophic activity, were prepared [10]. One derivative, CNB-001, exhibited improved stability over curcumin and was neuroprotective in multiple neurotoxicity assays in which curcumin was inactive [9].

Additional medicinal chemistry produced J147 (**Figure 4.2**), [11] a potent, orally active, neurotrophic molecule that facilitates memory in normal rodents, and prevents the loss of synaptic proteins and cognitive decline when administered preventatively to 3-month-old APP/PSEN1ΔE9

Alzheimer disease model mice for 7 months [12] or given therapeutically to 3–20-month-old aged mice [13]. Administration of J147 augmented CNS levels of brain-derived neurotrophic factor and nerve growth factor, enhanced long-term potentiation, preserved synaptic proteins, reduced markers of oxidative stress and inflammation, and reduced amyloid plaques with lower levels of soluble Abeta1-42 and Abeta1-40. However, the molecular target of J147 was elusive until now [14].

J147 Targets Mitochondrial ATP Synthase

Goldberg *et al.* [14] determined the protein target of J147 using drug affinity responsive target stability (DARTS), a method that relies on the protection against proteolysis conferred on the target protein by interaction with a small molecule [15]. Separately, Goldberg *et al.* performed a pull-down experiment in which a biotinylatedderivative of J147, BJ147,is bound to cell extracts, interacting peptides are captured with streptavidin, and these are analyzed by LC/MS/MS to identify coprecipitating proteins. The most highly enriched protein in both the DARTS and affinity precipitation experiments was ATP5A, the alpha subunit of the mitochondrial ATP synthase (**Figure 4.3**). J147 incubated with mitochondria isolated from bovine heart exhibited potent (EC50 @ 20 nM) although only partial modest inhibition (~24%) of ATP synthase activity [14].

Figure 4.3. Schematic of ATP synthase, Complex V. The ATP synthase comprises two "rotary nanomotors," each powered by a different fuel. The membrane-embedded motor, termed F0, is powered by the flow of hydrogen ions across the membrane. As the protons flow through the motor, (a) they turn a circular rotor (c) (shown in green). This rotor is connected to the second motor, termed F1. The F1 motor is a chemical motor, powered by ATP. The two motors are connected together by a stator (b) (left). The F0 motor uses the power from the proton gradient generated by other complexes of the respiratory chain to force the F1 motor to generate ATP. The vacuolar ATPase working in reverse, uses an ATP-driven motor to pump protons across a membrane. Work of Goldberg et al. demonstrated that J147 is bound to the alpha subunit of the ATP synthase. Earlier work of Chin et al. demonstrated that alpha-ketoglutarate mediated ATP synthase inhibition through the beta subunit.

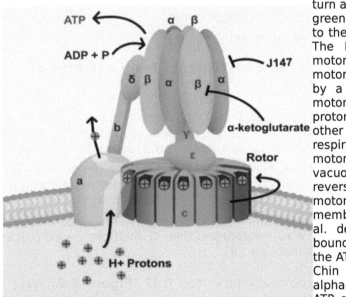

It should be noted that several other mitochondrial associated proteins, VDAC, Slc25a, and IP3R3, were also identified in the BJ147 pull-down experiments.

These proteins [16,17] along with ATP5A comprise the mitochondria permeability transition (mPT) pore responsible for executing cell death programs during lethal conditions of stress through mitochondrial Ca2+ efflux and are probably activated during neurocytotoxicity [18]. How these molecules figure in the activities of J147 is presently not known, although it would be tempting to hypothesize that J147 may directly inhibit the mPT in cells experiencing neurotoxicity.

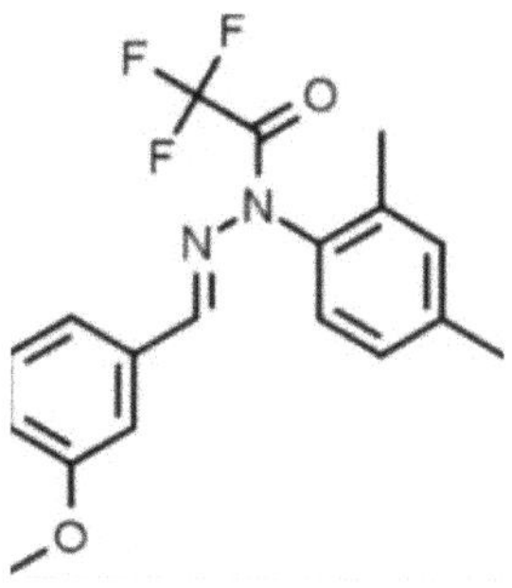

Figure 4.2. Molecular structure of J147

J147 Modulates Mitochondrial Bioenergetics

The mitochondrial membrane potential ($\Delta\psi$m) is a key measure of cellular vitality. Mitochondrial dysfunction characterized by lower $\Delta\psi$m correlates with reduced levels of ATP in aging and Alzheimer's dementia (AD) [19, 20]. Using a cationic dye assay [21].

J147 was shown to increase the $\Delta\psi$m, which is consistent with slower dissipation of the proton gradient by ATP synthase. Similar results were found when ATP5A levels were reduced by specific siRNA treatment. The reduced ATP synthase activity was accompanied by augmented production of superoxide, which typically occurs upstream of ATP synthase (Complex V) at Complexes I and III [14]. These findings are consistent with the "retrograde, ROS-mediated prosurvival response" previously described by Formentini *et al.* [22].

Perhaps most importantly, cellular levels of ATP increased by 4 hours post-treatment with J147 although with maximal effect at a concentration of 100nM [14].

Why do ATP levels increase, when a key component of ATP production is inhibited?

Increased ATP levels are associated with cell survival. Although not discussed by Goldberg et al., one possibility is that another capability of ATP synthase is involved. ATP synthase is fully capable of the hydrolyzing ATP as well as creating ATP. Interestingly, it has been reported that embryonic neuronal cell types, unlike adult neurons, have ATP synthase activity that tends to consume rather than create ATP [23]. In fact, the HT22 cell line used by Goldberg et al. to measure ATP levels is known to be resistant to glutamate induced oxidative stress because of reverse activity of ATP synthase [24]. It should be noted that Goldberg et al. also did observe increase of ATP in drosophila heads treated with J147. The combination of unimpeded ATP production by glycolysis, increased ATP synthesis by AMP-activated protein kinase (AMPK)-related pathways, reduction of ATP hydrolysis by ATP synthase, and cell type specificity may explain the apparent anomaly and raise questions about how generally does J147 increase ATP levels.

J147 Modulates Resting Ca^{2+} Homeostasis to Activate the AMPK/Mammalian Target of Rapamycin Axis

J147 treatment augments cytosolic Ca^{2+} levels with subsequent activation of Ca^{2+}/Calmodulin-mediated activation of CamKinaseKinase 2. This contributes to activation of AMPK in the brain [25] by J147 despite the increased ATP levels, which typically would inhibit AMPK. Studies with inhibitors demonstrate that CA^+ signaling is required for the observed AMPK activation by J147. This calcium flux changes with the mitochondrial membrane potential ($\Delta\psi_m$) that is maintained by the proton flux and activity of the ATP synthase. [26] Goldberg et al. [14] do not understand how J147 inhibition or siRNA knockdown of ATP5A leads to compartmental changes in the observed levels of calcium.

Common Mechanisms: J147, Alpha-Ketoglutarate, and ATP5A Modulate AMPK/Mammalian Target of Rapamycin Signaling

AMPK activation is known to lead to mammalian target of rapamycin (mTOR) inhibition. The mTOR is the catalytic subunit of two structurally distinct complexes: mTORC1 and mTORC2 that integrate both intracellular and extracellular signals of cell metabolism, growth, proliferation, and survival. mTORC1 is composed of mTOR, regulatory-associated protein of mTOR (Raptor), mammalian lethal with SEC13 protein 8 (mLST8), and the noncore components PRAS40 and DEPTOR. This complex functions as a nutrient/energy/redox sensor and controls protein synthesis [27]. The activity of mTORC1 is regulated by insulin, growth factors, phosphatidic acid, certain amino acids, and their derivatives (*e.g.*, l-leucine and β-hydroxy β-methylbutyric acid), mechanical stimuli, and oxidative stress. Rapamycin inhibition of mTORC1 appears to provide most of the beneficial effects of the drug (including life-span extension in animal studies). In contrast, mTORC2 inhibition produces reduced glucose tolerance and insensitivity to insulin.

AMPK is activated through phosphorylation of threonine 172 on the alpha-subunit. This lowers activity of some ATP-consuming pathways while promoting ATP synthesis through others such as fatty acid oxidation. Goldberg *et al.* showed that J147 mediates a time-dependent activation of AMPK followed by increased phosphorylation of raptor at Ser792, known to be critical for inhibition of mTOR. Then evidence was presented that downstream of mTOR/raptor two important lifespan extension pathways were engaged:

1) S6 kinase with reduced protein translation and
2) Acetyl-CoA carboxylase (ACC1) with increased beta- oxidation of fatty acids, which should lead to overall ATP production, and less fatty acid synthesis [14].
3) ATP Synthase Inhibition Is Neuroprotective

Formentini *et al.* generated a conditional mouse model ex- pressing a mutant form of human ATPase inhibitory factor 1 (hIF1). They reported that reduced ATPase activity in these mice protected CNS neurons from excitotoxic damage [28]. Goldberg *et al.* corroborated these results, showing that hIF1- mediated protection in cell culture neurotoxicity assays with the HT22 transfected with a constitutively activated hIF1 and that ATP5A siRNA-mediated knockdown is neuroprotective [14].

Aging: Lifespan Effects

Although it may be counter-intuitive that reduced ATP synthase activity can promote lifespan extension, several studies support this finding. Although complete loss of mitochondrial function is detrimental, partial suppression of the electron transport chain has been shown to extend the lifespan of *C. elegans* [29–32]. Furthermore, Chin *et al.* [33] demonstrated that the tricarboxylic acid (TCA) metabolite alpha-ketoglutarate (α-KG) extends the lifespan of worms by inhibiting the beta subunit of ATP synthase and TOR, the worm equivalent of mTOR, although in their experiments ATP levels decrease, rather than increase, perhaps suggesting that ATP levels are less relevant than what Goldberg *et al.* hypothesize. Goldberg *et al.* show that J147 extended median lifespan of drosophila up to 12.5%, [14] a result similar to that reported by Sun *et al.* for women with normal TOR activity [34]. It should be noted that a 12.5% increase in drosophila lifespan is modest and that lifespan increase was not explored in any other model system, including mice.

Senescence-accelerated mouse-prone 8 (SAMP8) mice are a spontaneous mutant inbred strain that display a phenotype of accelerated aging and AD-like neurological changes with age [35]. The key genetic changes that lead to accelerated aging have not yet been identified in this model. The method of Rangaraju *et al.* [36] measuring transcriptional drift associated with aging in *C. elegans* was used to examine gene expression in the hippocampus of old SAMP8 mice. Patterns suggestive of a youthful genotype were more common in the J147-treated animals, suggesting that J147 may delay or inhibit epigenetic drift. It would be extremely useful to know whether this effect occurs in normal mice and other tissues.

Medical Implications

Because age is the greatest risk factor for development of AD, an intervention that slows aging or extends the health span is expected to delay onset of disease, providing major benefits to patients [37, 38].

Health span and aging are closely linked to metabolism. Dietary restriction (DR) or calorie restriction are the "gold standards" for life extension and delay of age-related diseases across all species studied [39-41]. A limited number of pathways controlling nutrient or energy metabolism also have longevity benefits. [42, 43] Various metabolites can modulate aging [43-45] and the TCA cycle intermediate α-KG (**Figure 4.3**) was recently shown to extend the lifespan of adult *C. elegans* through inhibition of the ATP synthase beta catalytic subunit that seems similar to that described for J147 that inhibits the allosteric regulating alpha subunit [33].

Starvation-activated anaplerotic gluconeogenesis increases glutamate-linked transaminases in the liver to provide carbon derived from amino acid catabolism with elevation of α-KG levels.

α-KG levels are increased upon starvation and additional α-KG does not extend the lifespan of DR animals, indicating that α-KG is a key metabolite that mediates longevity by DR. However, there are subtle differences among these modulators of the ATP synthase. Unlike J147, α-KG inhibition of the ATP synthase leads to reduced ATP content, decreased oxygen consumption, and increased autophagy in both C. *elegans* and mammalian cells. However, α-KG and J147 treatment ultimately inhibits the canonical mTOR pathway.

Recent studies have highlighted a role for ATP synthase in the regulation of mTOR and lifespan extension in flies and worms [33, 34] and inhibition of mTOR/TOR through activation of AMPK is a canonical longevity-associated pathway [46]. It is possible that inhibition of mTOR/TOR by J147 explains the modest increase in lifespan observed in flies and worms.

Shabalina *et al.* describe a mitochondria-targeted super- antioxidant SkQ1 [47]. Dramatic effects on various eye disorders from dry eye to glaucoma and on wound healing are documented with a recent report showing that SkQ1-treated mice live significantly longer (335 vs. 290 days). SkQ1 also delays an AD-like phenotype in a rat model of AD [48]. Shabalina *et al.* achieved anti-aging and apparent neuroprotective effects by delivering a potent antioxidant to the mitochondrial inner space to reduce ROS. In contrast, J147 appears to increase ROS. Together these suggest that ROS may either play a dual role in neuroprotection depending on context.

J147 inhibits the ATP synthase only about 20%, and the superoxide increases do not seem all that great (the measurement appears to be mitochondria specific, as it uses fluorescent indicator MitoSox M36008 from molecular probes). The differences seem modest and the apparent contradiction of inhibiting the synthase while simultaneously increasing ATP levels and in generating more ROS but pre- venting age-related pathologies are not as great as they appear at first glance. Clearly, although J147 is binding to the alpha subunit of ATP synthase, it appears to be doing far more than just inhibiting the synthase. It may not be so much an inhibitor as altering the allosteric activity of the alpha subunit of ATP synthase. Perhaps some of the other J147 targets are important in this regard, such as the three other proteins involved in mTP that Goldberg detected in their pull-down, but not DART assays.

Improvements and Future Directions

Based on the demonstrated neurogenic potential of J147 in mouse models, the Schubert laboratory developed a human neuronal stem cell screening assay to optimize derivatives of J147 for human neurogenesis. The best derivative of J147, CAD-031, maintains the neuroprotective and memory-enhancing properties of J147, yet is more active in the human neural stem cell assays [13]. Which, if any, of these molecules is heading into human clinical trials remains an open question.

A talented Chinese medicinal chemistry group headed by Professor Yuqiang Wang (Jinan University, Guangzhou, PRC) have published and patented a promising compound based on the J147 story. A lead candidate T-006 in which the methoxyphenyl group of J147 was replaced by tetramethylpyrazine has been selected for preclinical development [49].

The ability of J147 to delay epigenic drift, a potentially critical hallmark of aging, is significant and deserves exploration in subsequent experiments. Such studies may lead to greater understanding of the mechanisms that underlie genetic drift.

J147 and related molecules impact many of the pathways contributing to neurodegenerative conditions. For example, Daugherty *et al.* reported that J147 slowed many of the markers of diabetic neuropathy in the streptozotocin-induced mouse model of type 1 diabetes [50]. In any event, significant follow-up in normally aging mice is required to confirm the antiaging of J147 effects in a mammalian system. Although J147 does demonstrate neuroprotective efficacy in a mouse model of AD, several other mouse models of AD should be investigated as well, including tauopathy models, because of the limited ability of mouse AD models to predict efficacy in humans. If such studies are performed, it would be very interesting indeed to compare J147 with its parental compound curcumin simultaneously in the same model system. In general, the multitargeting curcumin tends to inhibit ROS unlike J147, is neuroprotective in AD mouse models, [7] and also extends lifespan in flies, [51-53] and in addition extends *C. elegans* lifespan, [54] which has not yet been reported for J147. Apparently curcumin is not as strongly neuroprotective as J147, [11] although a direct comparison in animal models of AD is warranted. It is important to note that there is opinion suggesting that despite the apparent problems with curcumin, there are enough statistically significant data to not dismiss its potential clinical potential [55]. In any case, translation of this work into human clinical trials for AD is eagerly awaited.

References

1. Baker M. Deceptive curcumin offers cautionary tale for chemists. Nature 2017;541:144-145.
2. Nelson KM, Dahlin JL, Bisson J, Graham J, Pauli GF, Walters MA. The essential medicinal chemistry of curcumin. J Med Chem 2017;60:1620-1637.
3. Baell J, Walters MA. Chemistry: Chemical con artists foil drug discovery. Nature 2014;513:481-483.
4. Bisson J, McAlpine JB, Friesen JB, Chen S-N, Graham J, Pauli GF. Can invalid bioactives undermine natural product- based drug discovery? J Med Chem 2016;59:1671-1690.
5. Burgos-Moron E, Calderon-Montano JM, Salvador J, Robles A, Lopez-La´zaro M. The dark side of curcumin. Int J Cancer 2010;126:1771-1775.
6. Baell JB. Feeling nature's PAINS: Natural products, natural product drugs, and pan assay interference compounds (PAINS). J Nat Prod 2016;79:616-628.
7. Lim GP, Chu T, Yang F, Beech W, Frautschy SA, Cole GM. The curry spice curcumin reduces oxidative damage and amyloid pathology in an Alzheimer transgenic mouse. J Neurosci 2001;21:8370-8377.
8. Yang F, Lim GP, Begum AN, Ubeda OJ, Simmons MR, Ambegaokar SS, *et al.* Curcumin inhibits formation of amyloid beta oligomers and fibrils, binds plaques, and re- duces amyloid *in vivo*. J Biol Chem 2005;280:5892-5901.
9. Liu Y, Dargusch R, Maher P, Schubert D. A broadly neuroprotective derivative of curcumin. J Neurochem 2008; 105:1336-1345.
10. Schubert DR, Liu Y. Methods for protecting cells from amyloid toxicity and for inhibiting amyloid protein production. 2000. US Patent 6472436.
11. Chen Q, Prior M, Dargusch, Roberts A. Riek, R. Eichmann C, *et al.* A novel neurotrophic drug for cognitive enhancement and Alzheimer's disease. PLoS One 2011;6:e27865.
12. Savonenko A, Xu GM, Melnikova T, Morton JL, Gonzales V, Wong MPF, *et al.* Episodic-like memory deficits in the APPswe/PS1dE9 mouse model of Alzheimer's disease: Relationships to beta-amyloid deposition and neurotrans-mitter abnormalities. Neurobiol Dis 2005;18:602-617.
13. Prior M, Dargusch R, Ehren JL, Chiruta C, Schubert D. The neurotrophic compound J147 reverses cognitive impairment in aged Alzheimer's disease mice. Alzheimers Res Ther 2013;5:25.
14. Goldberg J, Currais A, Prior M, Fischer W, Chiruta C, Ratliff E, *et al.* The mitochondrial ATP synthase is a shared drug target for aging and dementia. Aging Cell 2018 [Epub ahead of print]; DOI: 10.1111/acel.12715.
15. Pai MY, Lomenick B, Hwang H, Schiestl R, McBride W, Loo JA, *et al.* Drug affinity responsive target stability (DARTS) for small molecule target identification. Methods Mol Biol 2015;1263:287-298.
16. Baines CP. The molecular composition of the mitochon- drial permeability transition pore. J Mol Cell Cardiol 2009; 46:850-857.

17. Bernardi P, Rasola A, Forte M, Lippe G. The mitochondrial permeability transition pore: Channel formation by F-ATP synthase, integration in signal transduction, and role in pathophysiology. Physiol Rev 2015;95:1111–1155.

18. Rao VK, Carlson EA, Yan SS. Mitochondrial permeability transition pore is a potential drug target for neurodegeneration. Biochim Biophys Acta 2014;1842: 1267–1272.

19. Reddy PH, Tripathi R, Troung Q, Tirumala K, Reddy TP, Anekonda V, et al. Abnormal mitochondrial dynamics and synaptic degeneration as early events in Alzheimer's disease: Implications to mitochondria-targeted antioxidant therapeutics. Biochim Biophys Acta BBA-Mol Basis Dis 2012;1822: 639–649.

20. Zhang C, Rissman RA, Feng J. Characterization of ATP Alternations in an Alzheimer's Transgenic Mouse Model. J Alzheimers Dis JAD 2015;44:375–378.

21. Perry SW, Norman JP, Barbieri J, Brown EB, Gelbard HA. Mitochondrial membrane potential probes and the proton gradient: A practical usage guide. Biotechniques 2011;50: 98–115.

22. Formentini L, Sanchez-Arago M, Sanchez-Cenizo L, Cuezva JM. The mitochondrial ATPase inhibitory factor 1 triggers a ROS-mediated retrograde prosurvival and proliferative response. Mol Cell 2012;45:731–742.

23. Surin AM, Khiroug S, Gorbacheva LR, Khodorov BI, Pinelis VG, Khiroug L. Comparative analysis of cytosolic and mitochondrial ATP synthesis in embryonic and post- natal hippocampal neuronal cultures. Front Mol Neurosci 2013;5:102.

24. Pfeiffer A, Jaeckel M, Lewerenz J, Noack R, Pouya A, Schacht T, et al. Mitochondrial function and energy metabolism in neuronal HT22 cells resistant to oxidative stress. Br J Pharmacol 2014;171:2147–2158.

25. Racioppi L, Means AR. Calcium/calmodulin-dependent Physiology. J Biol Chem 2012;287:31658–31665.

26. Brookes PS, Yoon Y, Robotham JL, Anders MW, Sheu S-S. Calcium, ATP, and ROS: A mitochondrial love-hate triangle.

27. Harrison DE, Strong R, Sharp ZD, Nelson JF, Astle CM, Flurkey K, et al. Rapamycin fed late in life extends lifespan in genetically heterogeneous mice. Nature 2009;460:392– Am J Physiol Cell Physiol 2004;287:C817–C833. 395.

28. Kim D-H, Sarbassov DD, Ali SM, King JE, Latek RR, Erdjument-Bromage H, et al. mTOR interacts with raptor to form a nutrient-sensitive complex that signals to the cell growth machinery. Cell 2002;110:163–175.

29. Formentini L, Pereira MP, Sanchez-Cenizo L, Santa- catterina F, Lucas JJ, Navarro C, et al. in vivo inhibition of the mitochondrial H+-ATP synthase in neurons promotes metabolic preconditioning. EMBO J 2014;33:762–778.

30. Tsang WY, Sayles LC, Grad LI, Pilgrim DB, Lemire BD. Mitochondrial respiratory chain deficiency in Caenorhabditis elegans results in developmental arrest and increased life span. J Biol Chem 2001;276:32240–32246.

31. Dillin A, Hsu A-L, Arantes-Oliveira N, Lehrer-Graiwer J, Hsin H, Fraser AG, et al. Rates of behavior and aging specified by mitochondrial function during development. Science 2002;298:2398–2401.

32. Lee SS, Lee RYN, Fraser AG, Kamath RS, Ahringer J, Ruvkun G. A systematic RNAi screen identifies a critical role for mitochondria in C. elegans longevity. Nat Genet 2003;33:40–48.

33. Curran SP, Ruvkun G. Lifespan regulation by evolutionarily conserved genes essential for viability. PLoS Genet 2007;3:e56.

34. Chin RM, Fu X, Pai MY, Vergnes L, Hwang H, Deng G, et al. The metabolite alpha-ketoglutarate extends lifespan by inhibiting the ATP synthase and TOR. Nature 2014;510: 397–401.

35. Sun X, Wheeler CT, Yolitz J, Laslo M, Alberico T, Sun Y, et al. A mitochondrial ATP synthase subunit interacts with TOR signaling to modulate protein homeostasis and life- span in Drosophila. Cell Rep 2014;8:1781–1792.

36. Butterfield DA, Poon HF. The senescence-accelerated prone mouse (SAMP8): A model of age-related cognitive decline with relevance to alterations of the gene

expression and protein abnormalities in Alzheimer's disease. Exp Gerontol 2005;40:774–783.

37. Rangaraju S, Solis GM, Thompson RC, Gomez-Amaro RL, Kurian L, Encalada SE, *et al.* Suppression of transcriptional drift extends C. elegans lifespan by postponing the onset of mortality. ELife 2015;4:e08833.

38. Lopez-Ot´ınC, Blasco M A, artridge L, Serrano M, Kroemer G. The hallmarks of aging. Cell 2013;153:1194–1217.

39. Currais A. Ageing and inflammation-A central role for mitochondria in brain health and disease. Ageing Res Rev 2015;21:30–42.

40. Colman RJ, Anderson RM, Johnson SC, Kastman EK, Kosmatka KJ, Beasley TM, *et al.* Caloric restriction delays disease onset and mortality in rhesus monkeys. Science 2009;325:201–204.

41. Mattison J, van der Weyden L, Hubbard T, Adams DJ. Cancer gene discovery in mouse and man. Biochim Biophys Acta 2009;1796:140–161.

42. Mattison JA, Colman RJ, Beasley TM, Allison DB, Kemnitz JW, Roth GS, *et al.* Caloric restriction improves health and survival of rhesus monkeys. Nat Commun 2017;8: 14063.

43. Kenyon CJ. The genetics of ageing. Nature 2010;464:504– protein kinase kinase 2: Roles in signaling and patho- 512.

44. Harrison DE, Strong R, Sharp ZD, Nelson JF, Astle CM, Flurkey K, *et al.* Rapamycin fed late in life extends lifespan in genetically heterogeneous mice. Nature 2009;460:392– Am J Physiology Cell Physiology 2004;287:C817–C833. 395.

45. Williams DS, Cash A, Hamadani L, Diemer T. Oxaloacetate supplementation increases lifespan in Caenorhabditis elegans through an AMPK/FOXO-dependent pathway. Aging Cell 2009;8:765–768.

46. Lucanic M, Held JM, Vantipalli MC, Klang IM, Graham JB, Gibson BW, *et al.* N-acylethanolamine signaling me- diates the effect of diet on lifespan in C. elegans. Nature 2011;473:226–229.

47. Johnson SC, Rabinovitch PS, Kaeberlein M. mTOR is a key modulator of ageing and age-related disease. Nature 2013;493:338–345.

48. Shabalina IG, Vyssokikh MY, Gibanova N, Csikasz RI, Edgar D, Hallden-Waldemarson A, *et al.* Improved healthspan and lifespan in mtDNA mutator mice treated with the mitochondrially targeted antioxidant SkQ1. Aging 2017;9: 315–336.

49. Stefanova NA, Muraleva NA, Maksimova KY, Rudnits- kaya EA, Kiseleva E, Telegina DV, *et al.* An antioxidant specifically targeting mitochondria delays progression of Alzheimer's disease-like pathology. Aging 2016;8:2713– 2731.

50. Chen H-Y, Xu D-P, Tan G-L, Cai W, Zhang G-X, Cui W, *et al.* A potent multi-functional neuroprotective derivative of tetramethylpyrazine. J Mol Neurosci 2015;56:977–987.

51. Daugherty DJ, Marquez A, Calcutt NA, Schubert D. A novel curcumin derivative for the treatment of diabetic neuropathy. Neuropharmacology 2018;129:26–35.

52. Shen L-R, Xiao F, Yuan P, Chen Y, Gao Q-K, Parnell LD, *et al.* Curcumin-supplemented diets increase superoxide dismutase activity and mean lifespan in Drosophila. Age 2013;35:1133–1142.

53. Lee K-S, Lee B-S, Semnani S, Avanesian A, Um C-Y, Jeon H-J, *et al.* Curcumin extends life span, improves health span, and modulates the expression of age-associated aging genes in Drosophila melanogaster. Rejuvenation Res 2010; 13:561–570.

54. Soh J-W, Marowsky N, Nichols TJ, Rahman AM, Miah T, Sarao P, *et al.* Curcumin is an early-acting stage-specific inducer of extended functional longevity in Drosophila. Exp Gerontol 2013;48:229–239.

55. Liao VH-C, Yu C-W, Chu Y-J, Li W-H, Hsieh Y-C, Wang T-T. Curcumin-mediated lifespan extension in Caenorhabditis elegans. Mech Ageing Dev 2011;132:480–487.

56. Heger M. Drug screening: Don't discount all curcumin trial data. Nature 2017;543:40.

Chapter 5

Inflammation, Stem Cells and the Aging Hypothalamus

The aging hypothalamus has been hypothesized to play a key role in vertebrate aging. Ectopic brain-specific expression of SIRT1, localized hypothalmic expression of a dominantly acting NF-Kb inhibitor to microglia or to neural stem cells extends lifespan in mice. In the latter case, increased inflammation in microglial cells during aging reduces the number of neural stem cells in the mediobasal region of the hypothalamus. Neural stem cells in the hypothalamus secrete miRNA-containing exosomes and GnRH that oppose the aging-associated neurological and skeletomuscular dysfunction. These results suggest that stem cells are not mere repositories of potential differentiated cells, but can also be active physiological effectors. Development of drugs that target microglial inflammation and neural stem cell maintenance may have significant utility for extending health and life span.

Introduction

The aging hypothalamus has been hypothesized to play a key role in vertebrate aging [1]. The hypothalamus, a small almond-shaped organ in human brains, consists of several sub-regions or clusters of neurons called nuclei that control many homeostatic functions including circadian rhythm, body temperature, hunger, thirst, attachment behaviors, sleep, and fatigue/wakefulness [2]. The hypothalamus is a key component of the neuroendocrine system, a nexus between the nervous and endocrine systems, stimulating endocrine secretions from the pituitary gland. Because of its important role in homeostasis, the hypothalamus has long been hypothesized as a potential master "regulator" of aging (neuroendocrine theories of aging), and recent evidence suggests that indeed aging-associated molecular and cellular changes in the hypothalamus impact systemic homeostasis and lifespan in mammals [3-5]. Regardless of theoretical questions surrounding the existence of aging "master regulators", the hypothalamus' key integrative role in maintaining systemic homeostasis identifies it as a potential key point of organism-wide physiological loss of function.

The most compelling reasons to believe that the hypothalamus plays a key role in aging derives from two reports whereby genetic manipulation of the hypothalamus results in extended lifespan and delayed aging-associated dysfunction. Mice which over express sirtuin SIRT1 in the brain (BRASTO) have a lifespan extension of 16% for females and 9% for males. SIRT1 increases neural activity in the DMH and LH regions of the hypothalamus resulting in increased Ox2r expression, a G-protein receptor that is involved in feeding behavior [5]. Are there any potential artifacts? Food intake was monitored, but the BRASTO mice use the mouse prion (prp) promoter to express SIRT1, which was observed to also express in the kidney and heart as well as in the brain of transgenic mice. Moreover, prp promoter is known to be transcribed in immune cells, which may complicate interpretation of the these data.

In another provocative study, inflammation associated with increased NF-Kb activity was observed with increasing age in the MBH region of the hypothalamus. Ectopic expression of an inhibitor of pro-inflammatory NF-Kb/IKKb signaling in the MBH region of the hypothalamus increased life span in male mice. A dominantly acting IκBα driven by the microglial-specific CD11b promoter using lentiviral vectors injected into the MBH region of the hypothalamus increased lifespan by 23% in male mice and decreased aging-related dysfunction in the nervous system and skeletal muscles: increasing neurogenesis, skin thickness, bone density, while decreasing collagen cross linking. Increased NF-Kb reduced expression endocrine factor GnRH by 2 fold. GnRH treatment attenuated the aging-associated phenotypes [3]. One potential caveat is that female mice were not studied in the lifespan extension studies, but responded similarly phenotypically.

Neural stem cells in the hypothalamus affect the rate of systemic aging by secretion of exosomal miRNAs

In a potentially paradigm-shifting followup study to work that showed that inhibition of NF-KB-mediated neuroinflammation in the hypothalamus results in anti-aging effects, Zhang and colleagues demonstrate that neural stem cells (NSC) in the hypothalamus (htNSC) are lost during aging, but can be preserved by genetic modification to withstand an inflammatory microenvironment, resulting reduction of aging phenotype and lifespan extension. Of particular significance is that these htNSC secrete factors and miRNA-containing exosomes that reduce aging- associated dysfunction[4], and so have an effector cell function independent of their ability to differentiate into neurons or neuroendocrine cells, extending our understanding of what stem cells are capable and the key role that their dysfunction or loss may play in aging.

First, Zhang et al identified NSC in the third ventricle wall of the mediobasal region (MBH) of the hypothalamus in mice by observing co-expression of NSC biomarkers Sox2 and BMI1, as well as other biomarkers that are often expressed in NSCs: nestin, Musashi1, and Cxcr4. All of these biomarkers decreased with age, suggesting that few htNSC remain in old mice. BrdU incorporation, which identifies cells that have undergone DNA replication decreases to almost undetectable levels in old mice [4].

To determine the significance of htNSC to normal physiology and aging, Zhang et al injected cells in the MBH with engineered lentiviral vectors that express the HSV thymidine kinase (TK) gene from the stem cell specific Sox2 promoter. These lentiviruses were used to kill SOX2-expressing NSC by treating middle-aged animals (15-months) with ganclyclovir, which is converted into a toxic product by TK, resulting in a 70% loss of htNSC. Followed over a 3-4 month period, mice with ablated htNSC displayed increased loss of novel object recognition, decreased treadmill performance, endurance and coordination compared to untreated controls. Similar experiments using other engineered lentiviruses dependent on a different cytotoxic mechanisms to kill htNSCs or the Bmi1 promoter instead of the Sox2, yielded similar results ruling out major potential artifacts. Significantly, lifespan was affected by loss of htNSC as well: injecting younger mice (8 month old) with the Sox2-TK lentiviruses resulted in about 10% shorter median and maximum lifespan. Interestingly, the total number of neurons in the MBH was not affected by the elimination of the majority of htNSC [4].

Since it is much easier to reduce biological function to negatively affect health and lifespan, Zhang et al sought to demonstrate the converse by preventing or slowing age-related dysfunction by injecting htNSCs from newborn mice that were genetically engineered to express GFP as a marker into the MBH of middle-aged mice. As might be expected from their earlier work, these neurons did not survive, most likely due to the inflammatory environment already present by middle-age in the MBH. To overcome this problem, Zhang et al engineered NK-Kb inflammation resistant neurons that constitutively express a dominantly acting IKBa, an inhibitor of NF-KB to protect the neurons from pro-inflammatory signals. Two months after injection, about 50% of these IκBα htNSCs survived. As controls. Zhang et al injected GFP labeled mesenchymal stem cells (MSC) or astrocytes into the MBH of similarly middle-aged mice. Only mice that had received the inflammation resistant Iκ Bα - htNSCs showed an approximate 10% increase in median and maximum lifespan, as well as improved locomotion, endurance, coordination, treadmill performance, novel recognition and sociability 3-4 months post injection, suggesting that htNSC play a key role in maintaining systemic homeostasis and viability [4]. This is quite a significant increase in lifespan for a treatment started at late middle age (15 months), but is not as significant as the 23% median/20% maximum lifespan increase observed by the authors previously using a microglia conditional knockout of IKKB [3], a co-factor necessary for NF-Kb function. Perhaps this is not surprising as the IKKB knockout is expected to affect all cells in exposed to the microenvironment including mature neurons and astrocytes as well as htNSCs. Another take home lesson that will be familiar to biomedical scientists is that stem cells are not all alike, MSC's had no effect, although to be fair, neither the MSCs nor astrocytes were treated with equivalent Iκ Bα anti-inflammatory lentiviruses and so would be expected to be subject to pro-inflammatory signals from the microglial cells in the MBH. The authors suggest that their survival, unlike the htNSCs, results from resistance to inflammation [4], but there are numerous examples in the literature of inflammation causing dysfunction rather than cell death. In any case, a local increase in htNSC in the MBH, a relatively small area of the brain, results in a significant anti-aging effect.

To determine the molecular and cellular mechanisms behind the anti-aging effects of the htNSCs, Zhang et al postulated that neurogenesis was unlikely to have made much difference in such a "short" period of 3-4 months [4], although they provide no direct evidence for this. It would have been interesting to inducibly express an inhibitor of cell cycle progression, for example, CDK inhibitor p21, or neural differentiation, to determine the role of cell proliferation and neurogenesis. Instead they postulated that endocrine role of the hypothalamus must be involved. Specifically, they hypothesized that exosomal miRNAs may play a key role. miRNAs have been shown to profoundly effect stem cell function and fate as well as effect aging and fibrosis in the heart [6-8] and exosomes are known to be an efficient method of miRNA intercellular trafficking [9]. Zhang et al used electron microscopy to observe a large number of multivescular bodies, which are precursors to exosomes, in the htNSCs in the MBH, but not in astrocytes from the same body. Interestingly, cultured htNSC produce many times more exosomes, with a 100 fold higher RNA content than cultured MSCs or astrocytes. In comparison with exosomes from hippocampal NSCs, which also extensively produce exosomes, miRNA content in htNSCs is significantly higher with a different pattern of expression. Given that htNSCs are potentially a major source of miRNA containing exosomes and that they decrease with age, Zhang et al observed that miRNA levels of 20 miRNAs associated with htNSCs are substantially decreased in the cerebrospinal fluid (CSF) of middle-aged mice. To demonstrate that the htNSCs in the MBH are responsible, mice were treated with lentiviruses that used shRNA to knock down expression of Rab27a, a protein necessary for exosomal secretion. Young mice treated for one week, showed substantially less miRNA in their CSF, and middle-aged mice injected with the Rab27 shRNA lentiviruses showed some mild impairments after 6 weeks, but clearly not equal to the effect of ablating htNSCs [4].

To demonstrate that exosomal delivery of miRNAs had functional consequences, htNSC-derived exosomes from cells expressing GFP to label the exosomes were injected into middle-aged mice using a cannula placed in the third ventricle of the hypothalamus 3 times a week for 4 months. First, the exosomes helped to maintain htNSCs, and this was likely due to reduced hypothalmic inflammation, suggesting that the miRNA from the exosomes may have anti-inflammatory effects. Second, when exosomes are injected into mice whose htNSCs had been mostly ablated by a Bmi1-TK lentivirus and gancyclivor just before a 4 month course of exosome treatment, in other words the hypothalamus-based accelerated aging model created by this group, multiple phenotypes associated with loss of htNSCs and aging are ameliorated including locomotion, coordination, treadmill capacity, novel object recognition, sociability and spatial memory. Third, in normally aging mice treated with htNSC exosomes, these same aging related phenotypes remain relatively stable over 4 months [4]. Altogether these data demonstrate that htNSC derived exosomal miRNAs as the authors have hypothesized or at least htNSC derived exosomes, play an important role in dysfunction associated with aging, although their role is obviously partial.

It is important to mention that this group previously reported levels of GnRH are diminished in the aging hypothalamus and that treatment with exogenous GnRH increases neurogenesis and also ameliorates the same aging-associated dysfunction in similar assays [3]. Of interest here, is that Zhang et al report that some of the htNSCs stain for GnRH and may be the source of at least some of the GnRH normally found in the hypothalamus. It would be interesting to determine how many of the aging effects resulting from the inflammation of the microglial cells hypothalamus can be reversed by the combination of GnRH and ht-NSC derived miRNAs.

This work connects the aging-associated increased inflammation of the MBH region of the hypothalamus with loss of htNSCs and provides data that htNSCs or their direct progeny play a significant role via a newly discovered aspect of their endocrine function, exosomal miRNAs in maintaining their own homeostasis and opposing aging.

Medical Implications

The medical implications of the two papers from Cao's group are profound, since they suggest that a small region of the relatively small hippocampus can affect lifespan and age-associated loss of neurological and muscular function, as well as collagen-cross linking, skin thickness and bone density and that inflammation-resistant-htNSCs, reduction of microglial inflammation, ht-NSC derived exosomal miRNAs or endocrine hormones such as GnRH can ameliorate many of the aging- associated phenotypes studied. It would interesting to know if any of the other systemic functions controlled by the hippocampus, albeit by different nuclei or regions, such as the suprachiasmatic nucleus which controls circadian rhythms, are affected as well. It is important to note that lifespan extension was only examined and observed for injection of inflammation-resistant-htNSCs in Zhang *et al.* (2017) or treatment with engineered lentiviruses to create inflammation-resistant hippocampal microglia in Zhang (2013) and not for exosomes or GnRH.

Because ht-NSC exosomes appear to require direct introduction into the hypothalamus, they can not be considered a practical therapeutic modality. Introduction into CSF might allow transit to the hypothalamus, but would probably not be practical for anti-aging therapies. However, it is interesting that blood plasma from human umbilical cords have been recently reported to revitalize hippocampus function in old mice [10]. Blood plasma contains a rich set of exosomes, although the effects were attributed to proteins such as Timp2, it is not difficult to believe that exosomes may be a beneficial component of cord blood plasma or even play a significant role in parabiosis experiments. Discovering drugs that stimulate ht-NSC exosome secretion, or better protect, htNSC from their inflammatory microenvironment or even better still, reduce hippocampal microglia inflammation would be potentially useful to maintaining or extending both healthspan and lifespan.

Interestingly it has been recently reported that acarbose (ACA), 17-α-estradiol (17αE2), and nordihydrog-uaiaretic acid (NDGA) reduce hypothalmic inflammation and extend lifespan in male mice. The three drugs reduced several pro- inflammatory parameters including TNF-a secretion as well as the number of activated Iba-1-positive microglia and GFAP-positive astrocytes. Interestingly these drugs had no effects on female mice [11]. This raises a very interesting question about the sex specificity of Zhang *et al,*'s lifespan extension data since they only used male mice in their longevity studies. Significantly, caloric restriction significantly reduced hypothalmic inflammation in both sexes, and is known to extend lifespan in rodents as well many other animals [11]. Perhaps a key target responsible for lifespan extension effects of CR are the hypothalmic microglia and HT-NSC. Ironically, the hypothalamus may play a role in detecting and initiating CR protective effects [12] as well as contributing to obesity and glucose resistance in response to over nutrition [13].

The question remains how CR or these drug reduce hypothalmic inflammation, which begs the question of the origin of hypothalmic inflammation with age in the first place. Multiple mechanisms have been proposed including RNA stress and immune dysfunction due to immunosenescence outside of the brain [14]. Some evidence exists that decreased integrity of the BBB with age [15] may contribute to brain inflammation in general by allowing systemic factors to interact with brain tissue, and this may very will play a key role. And what is the cause of the BBB breakdown? Some evidence exists for vascular cell senescence presumably resulting from mechanical stress or DNA damage playing a role [16]. So if this chain of reasoning is correct will elimination of senescent cells prevent hypothalmic inflammation and downstream systemic effects? Does senescence play a role in hypothalamus inflammation, although senescent neurons, and glial cells have been described in the literature? The answers are unknown at present.

Is there any connection between the htNSC data and data that suggest that enhanced brain-specific SIRT1 activity extend murine lifespan through increased orexin type 2 receptor expression in the DMH and LH regions of the hippocampus? The answer is unknown, but it would be surprising if these research groups did not at least try preliminary experiments to find a connection.

Because the hippocampus plays an integrative, bidirectional role in homeostasis, it is a candidate for helping to synchronize various systemic aging clocks that have been described. For example, the Horvath DNA methylation clock [17] includes tissue-type independence which would seem to require some mechanism of synchronization which could be provided by the hypothalamus. However, despite the existence of the Horvath clock, it remains more than possible that aging of tissues proceeds at different rates. The Horvath clock is really just an integrated large set of aging biomarkers based on epigenetics. Perhaps the decrease of ht-NSC derived exosomes carrying a defined set of miRNA may prove a useful, albeit difficult to obtain, alternative novel biomarker for aging.

Conclusion

An emerging connection between age-associated inflammation in the MBH region of the hypothalamus and loss of stem cells may generalize to other tissues, but given the central role of the hippocampus in homeostasis, its significance may be no where greater. That neural stem cells in the hippocampus may also act as effector cells that communicate through secreted factors, and exosomal miRNA suggest that stem cell biology is more complex than so far appreciated. New pro-regenerative strategies that alter stem cell viability and the stem cell milieu are likely to be developed.

References

1. Bernardis LL, Davis PJ. Aging and the hypothalamus: research perspectives. Physiol Behav 1996;59:523–36.
2. Lechan RM, Toni R. Functional Anatomy of the Hypothalamus and Pituitary. In: De Groot LJ, Chrousos G, Dungan K, Feingold KR, Grossman A, Hershman JM, et al., editors. Endotext, South Dartmouth (MA): MDText.com, Inc.; 2000.
3. Zhang G, Li J, Purkayastha S, Tang Y, Zhang H, Yin Y, et al. Hypothalamic Programming of Systemic Aging Involving IKKβ/NF-κB and GnRH. Nature 2013;497:211–6. doi:10.1038/nature12143.
4. Zhang Y, Kim MS, Jia B, Yan J, Zuniga-Hertz JP, Han C, et al. Hypothalamic stem cells control ageing speed partly through exosomal miRNAs. Nature 2017. doi:10.1038/nature23282.
5. Satoh A, Brace CS, Rensing N, Cliften P, Wozniak DF, Herzog ED, et al. Sirt1 Extends Life Span and Delays Aging in Mice through the Regulation of Nk2 Homeobox 1 in the DMH and LH. Cell Metab 2013;18:416–30. doi:10.1016/ j.cmet.2013.07.013.
6. Shi Y, Zhao X, Hsieh J, Wichterle H, Impey S, Banerjee S, et al. MicroRNA Regulation of Neural Stem Cells and Neurogenesis. J Neurosci 2010;30:14931- doi:10.1523/JNEUROSCI.4280-10.2010.
7. Li Q, Gregory RI. MicroRNA Regulation of Stem Cell Fate. Cell Stem Cell 2008;2:195–6. doi:10.1016/j.stem.2008.02.008.
8. Boon RA, Iekushi K, Lechner S, Seeger T, Fischer A, Heydt S, et al. MicroRNA-34a regulates cardiac ageing and function. Nature 2013;495:107–10. doi:10.1038/nature11919.
9. Zhang J, Li S, Li L, Li M, Guo C, Yao J, et al. Exosome and Exosomal MicroRNA: Trafficking, Sorting, and Function. Genomics Proteomics Bioinformatics 2015;13:17–24. doi:10.1016/j.gpb.2015.02.001.
10. Castellano JM, Mosher KI, Abbey RJ, McBride AA, James ML, Berdnik D, et al. Human umbilical cord plasma proteins revitalize hippocampal function in aged mice. Nature 2017;544:488–92. doi:10.1038/nature22067.
11. Sadagurski M, Cady G, Miller RA. Anti-aging drugs reduce hypothalamic inflammation in a sex-specific manner. Aging Cell 2017;16:652–60. doi:10.1111/acel.12590.
12. Dacks PA, Moreno CL, Kim ES, Marcellino BK, Mobbs CV. Role of the hypothalamus in mediating protective effects of dietary restriction during aging. Front Neuroendocrinol 2013;34:95–106. doi:10.1016/j.yfrne.2012.12.001.
13. Zhang X, Zhang G, Zhang H, Karin M, Bai H, Cai D. Hypothalamic IKKβ/NF-κB and ER Stress Link Overnutrition to Energy Imbalance and Obesity. Cell 2008;135:61–73. doi:10.1016/j.cell.2008.07.043.
14. Tang Y, Purkayastha S, Cai D. Hypothalamic Micro-inflammation: A Common Basis of Metabolic Syndrome and Aging. Trends Neurosci 2015;38:36–44. doi:10.1016/j.tins.2014.10.002.

15. Mooradian AD. Effect of aging on the blood-brain barrier. Neurobiol Aging 1988;9:31–9.

16. Yamazaki Y, Baker DJ, Tachibana M, Liu C-C, Deursen JM van, Brott TG, *et al.* Vascular Cell Senescence Contributes to Blood–Brain Barrier Breakdown. Stroke 2016;47:1068–77. doi:10.1161/STROKEAHA.115.010835.

17. Horvath S. DNA methylation age of human tissues and cell types. Genome Biol 2013;14:3156. doi:10.1186/gb-2013-14-10-r115.

Chapter 6

The NAD+/PARP1/SIRT1 Axis In Aging

NAD+ levels decline with age in diverse animals from *C. elegans* to mice. Raising NAD+ levels by dietary supplementation with NAD+ precursors NR or NMN improves mitochondrial function and muscle, neural and melanocyte stem cell function in mice as well as increasing murine lifespan. Decreased NAD+ levels with age reduces SIRT1 function and reduces the mitochondrial unfolded protein response, which can be overcome by NR supplementation. Decreased NAD+ levels cause NAD+-binding protein DBC1 to form a complex with PARP1, inhibiting PARP catalytic activity. Old mice have increased amounts of DBC1-PARP1 complexes. lower PARP activity, increased DNA damage and reduced non-homologous end joining (NHEJ) and homologous recombination (HR) repair. DBC1-PARP1 complexes in old mice can be broken by increasing NAD+ levels through treatment with NMN, reducing DNA damage and restoring PARP activity to youthful levels. The mechanism of declining NAD+ levels and its fundamental importance to aging are yet to be elucidated. There is a correlation of PARP activity with mammalian lifespan, that suggests that a NAD+/SIRT1/PARP1 may be more significant than the modest effects on lifespan observed for NR supplementation on old mice. A NAD+/PARP1/SIRT1 axis may link NAD+ levels and DNA damage with the apparent epigenomic DNA methylation "clocks" that have been described.

Introduction

NAD+ levels decline with age in diverse animals from *C. elegans* to mice [1-5] and raising NAD+ levels has apparent anti-aging effects [3-5]. Increasing NAD+ levels by dietary supplementation with NAD+ precursors NR or NMN improved mitochondrial function [4], and muscle, neural and melanocyte stem cell function in mice. NR supplementation also increased lifespan modestly in mice [5].

Although the mechanisms of gradual NAD+ decline with age remain unclear, beneficial effects have been linked to mitochondrial rejuvenation via restoration of OXPHOS subunits via sirtuin SIRT1/HIF1a/c-myc pathway [4], and stem cell function via stimulation of the mitochondrial unfolded protein response (UPSmt) [5] and synthesis of prohibitins, a family of mitochondrial stress response proteins linked to senescence of fibroblasts in mammals. Improvement of stem cell function by NAD+ is SIRT1 dependent [5].

NAD+ levels are significant for metabolic homeostasis in that they are important for redox reactions, and as substrates of sirtuins (SIRT1 to SIRT7) and other enzymes including PARPs ([poly(adenosine diphosphate-ribose) polymerases) as well as yet uncharacterized roles through other NAD+ interacting proteins. Sirtuins have been implicated in aging, as well as in a large number of key cellular processes including mitochondrial biogenesis, stress resistance, inflammation, transcription via epigenomic modulation of histones, apoptosis [7, 8] and SIRT1 can even affect circadian clocks [9].

PARPs are NAD-dependent pleiotropic enzymes that play a key role in detecting and responding to single-stranded DNA break repair as well as in inflammation, apoptosis induction and DNA methylation. Increasing PARP activity has been correlated with differential longevity of 13 mammalian species with humans having about 5 fold more PARP activity than rats [10]. Intuitively, increasing PARP activity would seem to be beneficial to organisms and potentially be of benefit to delay aging by maintaining DNA integrity, but PARPs are major consumers of NAD+ and PARP activity can deplete sufficient NAD+ to detrimentally effect mitochondria function. In fact, in apparent contradiction to the species longevity results, PARP1 knockout in mice increases tissue NAD+ levels, enhances mitochondrial function and blocks inflammation [11]. Moreover, ectopic expression of human PARP1 in mice, an enzyme which has about 2 fold more intrinsic PARP activity than mouse PARP1, induces a set of aging related phenotypes including cardiomyopathy, hepatitis, pneumonitis, kyphosis, nephropathy, adiposity, dermatitis, anemia, increased glucose resistance, and increased incidence of carcinomas. Paradoxically human PARP1 transgenic mice even have delayed DNA repair [12]. One possible explanation is that human PARP is consuming more NAD+ in mice than can be compensated for metabolically, causing dysfunction.

Clearly decreased NAD+ levels that have been observed in aging animals could be detrimental by multiple mechanisms, which require careful elucidation.

Decreasing NAD+ levels with aging cause DBC1 to bind and inhibit PARP1 allowing accumulation of DNA damage.

Li *et al.* [13] have recently established that NAD+ levels control protein-protein interactions of two NAD+ binding proteins: DBC1/CCAR2 and PARP1. At low NAD+ levels DBC1 binds to PARP1 and inhibits PARP activity. In aging mice, DBC1 increasingly binds to PARP1 causing the accumulation of DNA damage, linking reduced NAD+ levels directly to DNA damage.

DBC1 was already known to bind to and inhibit SIRT1, as well as histone deacetylase HDAC3 and methyltransferase SUV39H1. Since SIRT1 is regulated by NAD+, Li *et al* explored the hypothesis that DBC1 could also bind and inhibit PARP1, another NAD-dependent enzyme. In HEK293T cells co- immunoprecipitation/Western studies showed that PARP1 and DBC1 physically interact. A catalytically inactive PARP1 also interacted with DBC1 in these studies demonstrating that PARP catalytic activity was not necessary for the interaction with DBC1. However, unlike the DBC1/SIRT1 interaction, the DBC1/PARP1 interaction was sensitive to and broken by NAD+ in the physiological range (100um-500um), while similar doses of nicotinamide or its structural analog 3-AB had no effect. NADH and adenine had only weak effects, suggesting that DBC1/PARP1 interaction requires low levels or the absence of NAD+. A catalytically inactive PARP1 behaved similarly to wild type suggesting that NAD+ cleavage or covalent attachment was not necessary for NAD+ to inhibit the DBC1/PARP1 interaction [13].

In HEK293T, an inhibitor of NAD+ biosynthesis or depleting NAD+ by genotoxic stress increased the DBC1/PARP1 interaction. Various treatments that increased NAD+, decreased DBC1/PARP1 interaction. These data are strong evidence that NAD+ inhibits the formation of the DBC1/PARP1 complex [13].

In order to determine which domains of DBC1 and PARP1 were interacting, Li *et al.* expressed a variety of truncated mutants of DBC1 and PARP1. DBC1 lacking a nudix homology domain (NDH) did not bind to PARP1, but a DBC1 carrying only a NDH domain did bind to PARP1. Moreover, DBC1 interacted with a PARP1 mutant consisting only of a BRCT domain, but not with a PARP1 having only a catalytic domain, suggesting that the NDH domain of DBC1 binds to the BRCT domain of PARP1. Homology modeling based on the known crystal structures of 5 NDH proteins suggested that NAD+ directly binds the DBC1 NHD, and this was confirmed by competition experiments in which radio labeled or biotin labeled NAD+ bound to DBC1-NHD and was then competed off with unlabeled NAD+ [13].

Of significance is that PARP1 activity was inhibited by DBC1 interaction *in vitro* and stimulated in cell culture by siRNA knockdown of DBC1. DBC1 but not DBC1Q391A, a mutant of DBC1 that binds NAD+ poorly and does not interact well with PARP1, reduced PARP1 activity. Reducing DBC1 increased DNA repair after paraquat treatment, as assessed by lower gammaH2AX, reduced DNA fragmentation, increased NHEJ and HR recombination pathway activity and cell viability. NMN. which raises NAD+ levels. had similar effects on these cells. These data support the hypothesis that NAD+ binding to DBC1-NHD regulates two key pathways of DNA repair through controlling PARP1 activity [13].

DNA repair capability decreases with increasing age [14]. Similarly PARP1 activity has been reported to decrease with age [10], suggesting a possible connection between PARP1 activity and overall DNA repair. Li et al hypothesize that increased DBC1/PARP1 binding occurs with reduced NAD+ levels during aging to reduce DNA repair and increase DNA damage. In 22-month old mice, levels of NAD+ were reduced in the liver compared to young mice. Old mice had increased amounts of DBC1-PARP and increased staining for DNA-damage associated gammaH2AX. A week of daily NMN treatment (500 mg/kg) intraperitoneally increased NAD+ levels, reduced the number of DBC1-PARP1 complexes and decreased DNA damage as reported by decreased levels gammaH2AX in old mice. Reduced PARP1 activity in old mice was restored by NMN treatment. To show that repair was affected, old mice were subjected to gamma irradiation. Irradiated mice were observed to have reduced DNA damage when treated with NMN either before irradiation or even one hour after irradiation [13].

These data support the hypothesis that reduced NAD+ with aging causes increased DBC1/PARP1 inhibiting PARP1-mediated repair of DNA damage. The authors reasonably speculate that DBC1 evolved as a buffer to prevent PARP1 from depleting NAD+ levels to cytotoxic levels [15]. They also point out that DBC1 is often mutated or down regulated in cancer and that increased repair capability and protection from radiation are potential mechanisms by which elimination of DBC1 could help cancer cells evade treatment [13]. Another possible mechanism for the tumor suppressor DBC1 is that the known stabilizing interaction of DBC1 with p53 is important [16].

Medical Implications

Evidence is accumulating that diminished NAD+ during aging results in mitochondrial and stem cell dysfunction, as well as reduced DNA repair activity. Supplementation with NMN or especially NR at doses of 100, 300 or 1000 mg can increase NAD+ levels systemically in humans [17] and may counteract NAD+ aging-associated phenotypes, although more preclinical and human studies are needed to establish efficacy of NR or NMN as anti-aging interventions.

A key question arises, if NAD+ levels and in particular PARP activity levels are so important to maintaining homeostasis and contribute to the biological processes called aging, why did treatment with NR, although beneficial to stem cell function, only increase mean and maximum longevity modestly in one study: about a 5% increase when treatment was initiated in very old mice (24 months) [5]. One point is that the intervention was started very late, which may not allow reversal of aging associated damage or loss of epigenomic information. On the other hand, the effect of increasing NAD+ is significantly less than that achieved by rapamycin, for example[18]. The simplest explanation is that decreased NAD+ represents only one of a set of key regulatory changes that result in the effects of aging.

However, it is possible that the role of PARP is more profound. Given the apparent correlation of PARP activity with mammalian longevity for diverse species, it is quite possible that increasing PARP1 expression by genetic or pharmaceutical means in the context of increasing NAD+ through supplementation may have profound effects on aging. One interesting experiment would be to supplement the human PARP1 transgenic mice [12], which express a PARP1 2-fold more active than mouse PARP1, with NR or NMN from birth to overcome the potential detrimental effects of decreased NAD+ levels from the overactive human PARP1. We hypothesize that these mice would not only not be sick, but would thrive and potentially live longer than wild-type animals.

The significance of PARP1 activity to aging is at least somewhat tied to its DNA repair activity. It is controversial whether that the accumulated effects of DNA mutations alone are sufficient to drive aging [19], normal cells apparently accumulate hundreds to a few thousand mutations over a lifetime of cell divisions [20]. Non-dividing cells should possess significantly fewer mutations. While some premature aging syndromes and cancer are driven by increased genome instability, it is unclear that accumulation of ~1000 genetic substitutions would sufficiently degrade cell function. On the other hand, because decreased PARP1 activity is expected to also cause increased chromosomal instability through reduced NHEJ and HR DNA repair, PARP1 activity probably plays a significant role in preventing age-associated cancer.

If PARP1 plays a central role in aging via its role in DNA repair, it could do so indirectly, through effects on the epigenome. PARP1 and other members of the PARP family have been shown to have profound effects on the epigenome through Poly(ADP-ribosyl)ation (PARylation), affecting DNA methylation/demethylation via effects on DNMT1 and CTCF, histone acetylation, histone methylation, and organizing chromatin domains [21]. DNA repair events initiated by single-stranded DNA breaks could change the balance of PARP1 activities changing the epigenome in defined ways. Animals with higher intrinsic PARP1 activity may have less DNA damage and fewer epigenomic alterations over a given amount of chronological time, resulting in a younger biological "age". Superimposed upon the effects of decreased NAD+ levels, it does not escape attention that the NAD+/PARP1/SIRT1 axis could contribute to creating the apparent epigenetic aging "clocks" that are reflected in the tissue-invariant and tissue-specific DNA methylation patterns observed to strongly correlate biological age in humans, chimpanzees and mice [22-24] through modulation of DNA methylation through DNMT1 and CTCF.

References

1. Braidy N, Guillemin GJ, Mansour H, Chan-Ling T, Poljak A, Grant R. Age Related Changes in NAD+ Metabolism Oxidative Stress and Sirt1 Activity in Wistar Rats. PLOS ONE 2011;6:e19194. doi:10.1371/journal.pone.0019194.

2. Yoshino J, Mills KF, Yoon MJ, Imai S. Nicotinamide Mononucleotide, a Key NAD+ Intermediate, Treats the Pathophysiology of Diet- and Age-Induced Diabetes in Mice. Cell Metab 2011;14:528–36. doi:10.1016/j.cmet.2011.08.014.

3. Mouchiroud L, Houtkooper RH, Moullan N, Katsyuba E, Ryu D, Cantó C, et al. The NAD+/Sirtuin Pathway Modulates Longevity through Activation of Mitochondrial UPR and FOXO Signaling. Cell 2013;154:430–41. doi:10.1016/ j.cell.2013.06.016.

4. Gomes AP, Price NL, Ling AJY, Moslehi JJ, Montgomery MK, Rajman L, et al. Declining NAD+ Induces a Pseudohypoxic State Disrupting Nuclear-Mitochondrial Communication during Aging. Cell 2013;155:1624–38. doi:10.1016/j.cell.2013.11.037.

5. Zhang H, Ryu D, Wu Y, Gariani K, Wang X, Luan P, et al. NAD+ repletion improves mitochondrial and stem cell function and enhances life span in mice. Science 2016;352:1436–43. doi:10.1126/science.aaf2693.

6. Bhullar KS, Hubbard BP. Lifespan and healthspan extension by resveratrol. Biochim Biophys Acta BBA - Mol Basis Dis 2015;1852:1209–18. doi:10.1016/j.bbadis.2015.01.012.

7. Grabowska W, Sikora E, Bielak-Zmijewska A. Sirtuins, a promising target in slowing down the ageing process. Biogerontology 2017. doi:10.1007/s10522-017-9685-9.

8. Mei Z, Zhang X, Yi J, Huang J, He J, Tao Y. Sirtuins in metabolism, DNA repair and cancer. J Exp Clin Cancer Res CR 2016;35. doi:10.1186/s13046-016-0461-5.

9. Masri S, Sassone-Corsi P. Sirtuins and the circadian clock: bridging chromatin and metabolism. Sci Signal 2014;7:re6. doi:10.1126/scisignal.2005685.

10. Grube K, Bürkle A. Poly(ADP-ribose) polymerase activity in mononuclear leukocytes of 13 mammalian species correlates with species-specific life span. Proc Natl Acad Sci U S A 1992;89:11759–63.

11. Bai P, Cantó C, Oudart H, Brunyánszki A, Cen Y, Thomas C, et al. PARP-1 Inhibition Increases Mitochondrial Metabolism through SIRT1 Activation. Cell Metab 2011;13:461–8. doi:10.1016/j.cmet.2011.03.004.

12. Mangerich A, Herbach N, Hanf B, Fischbach A, Popp O, Moreno-Villanueva M, et al. Inflammatory and age-related pathologies in mice with ectopic expression of human PARP-1. Mech Ageing Dev 2010;131:389–404. doi:10.1016/j.mad.2010.05.005.

13. Li J, Bonkowski MS, Moniot S, Zhang D, Hubbard BP, Ling AJY, et al. A conserved NAD(+) binding pocket that regulates protein-protein interactions during aging. Science 2017;355:1312–7. doi:10.1126/science.aad8242.

14. Gorbunova V, Seluanov A, Mao Z, Hine C. Changes in DNA repair during aging. Nucleic Acids Res 2007;35:7466–74. doi:10.1093/nar/gkm756.

15. Yang H, Yang T, Baur JA, Perez E, Matsui T, Carmona JJ, et al. Nutrient-Sensitive Mitochondrial NAD+ Levels Dictate Cell Survival. Cell 2007;130:1095–107.

16. Qin B, Minter-Dykhouse K, Yu J, Zhang J, Liu T, Zhang H, et al. DBC1 Functions as a Tumor Suppressor by Regulating p53 Stability. Cell Rep 2015;10:1324–34. doi:10.1016/j.celrep.2015.01.066.

17. Trammell SAJ, Schmidt MS, Weidemann BJ, Redpath P, Jaksch F, Dellinger RW, et al. Nicotinamide riboside is uniquely and orally bioavailable in mice and humans. Nat Commun 2016;7. doi:10.1038/ncomms12948.

18. Harrison DE, Strong R, Sharp ZD, Nelson JF, Astle CM, Flurkey K, et al. Rapamycin fed late in life extends lifespan in genetically heterogeneous mice. Nature 2009;advanced online publication. doi:10.1038/nature08221.

19. López-Otín C, Blasco MA, Partridge L, Serrano M, Kroemer G. The Hallmarks of Aging. Cell 2013;153:1194–217. doi:10.1016/j.cell.2013.05.039.

20. Martincorena I, Campbell PJ. Somatic mutation in cancer and normal cells. Science 2015;349:1483–9. doi:10.1126/science.aab4082.

21. Ciccarone F, Zampieri M, Caiafa P. PARP1 orchestrates epigenetic events setting up chromatin domains. Semin Cell Dev Biol 2017;63:123–34. doi:10.1016/j.semcdb.2016.11.010.

22. Horvath S. DNA methylation age of human tissues and cell types. Genome Biol 2013;14:3156. doi:10.1186/gb-2013-14-10-r115.

23. Hannum G, Guinney J, Zhao L, Zhang L, Hughes G, Sadda S, et al. Genome-wide methylation profiles reveal quantitative views of human aging rates. Mol Cell 2013;49:359–67. doi:10.1016/j.molcel.2012.10.016.

24. Stubbs TM, Bonder MJ, Stark A-K, Krueger F, von Meyenn F, Stegle O, et al. Multi-tissue DNA methylation age predictor in mouse. Genome Biol 2017;18. doi:10.1186/s13059-017-1203-5.

Chapter 7

Pharmaceutical Rejuvenation of Age-Associated Decline in Spatial Memory

Asthma→ spatial memory restoration

Spatial memory and cognition decline during aging. Montelukast, an FDA approved drug for the treatment of asthma can restore spatial memory in old rats to levels similar to those of young animals. Treatment improves three hallmarks of aging in the brain: reducing microglial-mediated neuro-inflammation, brain blood barrier permeability and increasing neurogenesis in the hippocampus although not completely to youthful levels. Other aging-associated parameters, such as reduced synaptic density, are not affected, suggesting that anti-aging therapeutics may be further optimized. Montelukast targets leukotriene receptors GPR17 and CysLTR1 and appears to invert leukotriene signaling, converting an inflammatory signal into an anti-inflammatory signal. This acts as a dominant factor to overcome the dysfunctional effects of aging reportedly mediated in part by blood-borne factors such as beta-2 microglobulin that inhibit neurogenesis in the dentate gyrus of the hippocampus. The key mechanism for cognitive improvement by montelukast may be restoration of BBB integrity, which would presumably decrease the amount of deleterious blood borne factors to enter the brain. Whether or not this hypothesis is true for montelukast, drugs that restore or maintain BBB integrity may be useful in combating age-related loss of cognitive function.

Introduction

Decreased cognitive abilities associated with aging include microglial-based neuroinflammation, reduced integrity of the blood brain barrier (BBB), decreased synapse densities and reduced levels of neurogenesis in the subventricular regions and the dentate gyrus of the hippocampus [1-7]. Heterochronic parabiosis, intertwining the circulatory systems of old and young animals, has been shown to improve cognition, decrease microglia mediated inflammation, and increase neurogenesis in old mice of the pair, while reducing these phenotypes in the young mice 8. These results lead to the idea that young blood contains pro-neurotrophic protective factors that aid cognition and that old blood contains factors that impede brain function and cognition [9.] Specific blood-borne factors that alter neurological function in aging have been identified. A controversial report identified GDF11 as a potential beneficial neurotrophic factor present in greater levels in young blood [10.] Increased blood levels of beta-2 microglobulin (B2M), a component of MHC I [11], and CCL11 (eotaxin) 4 have been identified as potential problematic factors affecting brain function in old individuals.

Because of the connection between inflammation and neurological dysfunction, montelukast an approved anti-asthma drug that inhibits leukotriene and leukotriene-related signaling through CysLTR1 and GPR17 was identified as a candidate therapy to decrease pro-inflammatory cytokine levels and confer protection in ischemia-reperfusion induced neuroinflammation [12-14]. Interestingly, HAMI 3379, a CysLTR2 antagonist, confers even stronger anti-neuroinflammatory activity and protection [14]. Of particular interest to potential regenerative strategies is that montelukast stimulates neurogenesis from neuronal precursor cells in culture [15]. Just because a drug can stimulate neurogenesis in culture or in young animals, doesn't necessarily imply that it can do so in an aged brain. For example, some drugs, such as minocycline, have been reported to stimulate neurogenesis in adults, but not in old animals [16]. Screening for drugs that can overcome age-associated dysfunction may be an efficacious path to treating pathologies of old age, so it is of interest to characterize whether montelukast can stimulate neurogenesis and inhibit neuroinflammation in old animals *in vivo*.

Approved anti-asthma drug montelukast restores hippocampal function in aged rats.

Marschallinger *et al.* extended earlier studies by testing the effects of montelukast on young (4-months-old) and moderately old rats (20-months-old) on performance in spatial navigation and learning tests, such as finding the location of a hidden platform in a water maze. Treatment with oral montelukast for 6 weeks resulted in improved task learning, such that the old rats learned the task in a time similar to that of young rats [17]. Interestingly, montelukast had no effect on the learning time of the young rats, suggesting that montelukast overcomes specific aging-associated dysfunctionality.

To understand the underlying physiology behind the restoration of spatial memory and cognition, Marschallinger *et al* investigated whether there were improvements in three physical parameters of aging-associated cognitive dysfunction in the hippocampus:

1) Inflammatory activity of the microglia
2) Leakiness of the BBB
3) Reduced neurogenesis

The hippocampus is considered a key location for spatial cognition and is one of two sites of neurogenesis in mammalian brains. Investigation of four markers of neuroinflammation, revealed that only two markers, the size of the body (soma) of the microglia and the expression and size of phagocytosis-associated CD68 particles were increased in old animals. The number of proliferating cells, as assessed by PCNA expression, and the expression of IBA1/AIF1, a marker of macrophage activation were unchanged, suggesting only modest neuro-inflammation was present in the microglia. Treatment with montelukast reduced the soma size of microglia and reduced the CD68 particle size in old animals, having no effect in young animals [18]. Thus it is reasonable to conclude that montelukast partially reduced microglial inflammation.

Given that these *in vivo* data were supportive but not conclusive, the BV-2 mouse microglial cell line was treated with leukotriene D4 (LTD4) in combination with montelukast for 24 hours to strengthen the hypothesis that montelukast reduces neuroinflammation. LTD4 treatment alone did indeed increase levels of proinflammatory enzyme NOS2 about 1.5 fold; montelukast alone had no effect, but addition of montelukast to LTD4 reduced NOS2 levels to about 50% of normal, suggesting that montelukast inverts LTD4 mediated inflammation. Interestingly, the combination of proinflammatory LTD4 and montelukast also reduced cytokine CCL2, which has been reported to increase during aging [4], and increased TGF-beta, which is neuroprotective in the brain [19], below and above baseline levels respectively [17]. Interestingly TGF-beta expression is often associated with pro-inflammatory dysfunction in other tissues, such as in muscle, where it can block stem cell function. We find intriguing that montelukast may define a new class of drugs that inverts cell signaling. Unfortunately, the reported cell culture data should be considered as merely suggestive. Similar data *in vivo* would make a stronger case, but was not explored.

Because the BBB is known to become leaky in neuroinflammatory diseases and aging, the extent of BBB integrity was assessed by staining for claudin-5, a tight junction protein that helps maintain the BBB. Claudin-5 expression in old rats was diffuse and weak indicating BBB permeability; but after montelukast treatment, claudin-5 showed stronger, more continuous staining more similar to young rats [17]. Montelukast appears to restore BBB integrity, an intriguing result, not yet investigated in more depth.

Dentate gyrus (DG) neurogenesis has long been associated with spatial learning and memory, although contradictory data showing cause and effect exists. Marschallinger et al observed a three fold decrease in PCNA+ cells in the hippocampi of old rats, which they used as a surrogate for the number of proliferating cells. Montelukast treatment restores the number of PCNA+ cells in the DG to about 50% of that in young animals. However, there was no increase in Sox2+ neural precursor cells which remain at about 50% of youthful numbers.

There was an increase in DCX+ immature neurons, from about 50% found in the young rats to about 70%, suggesting that this population was expanded by the montelukast treatment. These neurons survived for at least four weeks as determined by retention of a short pulse of BRDU into cells in the DG. BRDU labels proliferating cells. Since mature neurons are postmitotic, only proliferating cells, for example those undergoing neurogenesis, will be labeled. By costaining cells that had incorporated BRDU with mature neural specific marker NeuN and astrocyte marker GFAP, newly formed cells were determined to be approximately 60% to 80% neural and 15% glial, as is typically observed. Overall about a 70% increase was observed in newly formed mature neurons in old rats treated with montelukast compared to age-matched controls [9]. Interestingly, montelukast had no effect on and did not restore the reduced synaptic density or expression of c-fos a marker for activated neurons, suggesting that alterations in these are not responsible for the restoration of cognition and also suggesting that an opportunity to further rejuvenate old hippocampi remains [17].

In order to try to differentiate between microglial activation and neurogenesis, correlation analysis was performed on the learning improvement of individual rats with changes in microglial soma size, the number of proliferating cells as determined by PCNA+ cells, and the number of proliferating cells as determined by BRDU incorporation. Interestingly there was no correlation of learning with microglial size, but a modest correlation with proliferation in control, vehicle treated old rats. Treatment of old rats with montelukast increased the correlation of learning with proliferation [17]. Taken together the data suggest that increased neurogenesis by montelukast, rather than decreased microglial activation, is associated with improved learning. It would have been interesting if any correlation existed between the integrity of the BBB of the rats and learning, however this analysis was not performed.

To test that the emerging hypothesis that antagonism of CysLTR1 and GPR17 by montelukast partially restores age-diminished spatial learning, leukotriene signaling in the brain was assessed indirectly by mRNA expression analysis of the key rate-limiting enzyme in leukotriene synthesis, 5-LOX. Consistent with the hypothesis, increased 5-LOX mRNA was found in the two neurogenic areas, the hippocampus and subventricular zone (SVZ), but not in other regions such as the cortex of old rats. At least for the DG, increased 5-LOX protein is also observed, although data concerning the SVZ was not shown. A similar pattern of increased 5-LOX protein with age was observed in the DG region in samples from human brains, comparing subjects less than 35 with those greater than 60-years-old [17]. Overall, these data provide circumstantial evidence that increased leukotriene signaling may play a role in the loss of spatial learning ability with age, but a more direct analysis with for example conditional genetic mutants may be warranted to draw stronger conclusions.

To order to further specify the hypothesis, the expression pattern of montelukast targets CysLTR1 and GPR17 in the DG was explored. Oligodendroglial and early and mature neuronal lineages predominantly expressed GPR17. Astrocytes and neural stem cells did not express GPR17. CysLTR1 was mostly expressed on astrocytes and microglia and was absent from neural stem cells and neuronal lineage cells. The authors hypothesized that this expression pattern was most consistent with the neuronal specific GPR17 being the key target for the beneficial effects of montelukast. Although reasonable, it would require more extensive experiments to rule out indirect effects neuronal cells by microglia or astrocytes. In any case, preliminary experiments with neurospheres, cultured balls of neurons, that were engineered to lack either FoxO1,3,4, which is an upstream regulator of GPR17 necessary for its expression, or lacking GPR17 itself, grew significantly faster than neurospheres derived from wild-type animals and were unresponsive to any increase in growth rate by montelukast [17]. That a FoxO1,3,4 knockout could stimulate neurogenesis is not surprising, since

FoxO1,3,4-/- transgenic mice have previously been reported to have larger brains, increased neurogenesis when very young and eventually decreased neurogenesis as adults due to stem cell exhaustion [20]. By contrast, montelukast stimulated the proliferation of wild-type neurospheres. Although these preliminary data support the proposed hypothesis, more direct *in vivo* experiments are necessary, including experiments which allow selective genetic ablation of CysLTR1 or GPR17 in defined cell types of the DG.

Perhaps the most intriguing aspect of this work is that it appears to present a pharmaceutical intervention to partially reverse the effects of increased levels of factors in the blood of aging animals, such as B2M, which block neurogenesis in old mice [11] and perhaps old people. We believe that a simple unexplored hypothesis may have great explanatory power: that improved cognition observed after montelukast treatment may result from the restoration of BBB integrity, reducing access of blood-borne factors deleterious factors to the brain. That an antagonist to leukotriene signaling can counter the effects of B2M, a component of MHC1 suggests that subtle change in immune-related regulators and cytokines may play profound effects in the function and aging of the brain.

Medical Implications

Montelukast is an FDA approved anti-asthma drug, that has undergone safety testing in humans and is available as a generic drug for potential off-label uses, such as maintenance of spatial memory in old age. However, enthusiasm is limited by the fact that there is no direct evidence that montelukast can provide the same benefit in people as observed in rodents. Clearly, clinical studies to determine its efficacy are needed. It is possible that the extent of benefits may be limited for other types of cognition, such as prospective memory, not associated with the hippocampus, but instead associated with the frontal lobe of the cerebral cortex, but much depends on the actual mechanism of action. For example, restoration of BBB integrity could have beneficial effects throughout the brain.

What about dose in humans and pharmacology? Marchallinger *et al* reanalyzed the original CNS pharmacology data and show that montelukast can penetrate the BBB and enter the brain, contrary to initial conclusions during its development [17]. Moreover, the recommended dose of 10 mg per day for asthma in humans achieves a similar blood and CSF concentration to that observed to be efficacious on the spatial memory of old rats in their study.

Is there room for improvement?

If increased neurogenesis indeed is important to restoration of spatial learning, it's likely that decreased synaptic densities in old rats (and humans) presents a possible additive or synergistic target for development.

Marchallinger *et al* suggest that minocycline may be a potential candidate for such a drug.

What about neurodegenerative diseases?

Treatment with montelukast attenuated behavioural deficits, inflammation and structural defects in various animal models of neurodegenerative diseases, including a kainic acid-induced loss of memory function model [21], a quinolinic acid acute Huntington's disease model [22], a malonic acid injection induced degeneration of striatal neurons, and a beta-amyloid injection model of Alzheimer's disease [23]. However, these studies have not been expanded to the large number of neurodegenerative models available, and it is reasonable to assume that inhibition of leukotriene and other signaling mediated by GPR17 and CysLTR1 may only have an auxiliary effect on this class of diseases given leukotrienes *in vitro* are not toxic to rat cortical neurons [24].

What about effects on neurogenesis in the SVZ?

It is unclear whether the authors looked and found no effect, or just did not perform the needed studies.

Are there any potential downsides?

Singulair (tradename of montelukast), has been linked to suicidal thoughts and neuropsychiatric events in a very small minority of young people, which is under investigation by the FDA. [25] Perhaps even more serious for older patients, montelukast has been linked to increased incidence (>= 5%) of respiratory infections (Merck and Company, Singulair label), which is almost certainly due to attenuation of the early inflammatory response to fighting infection by reduced leukotriene signaling.

Do we understand the mechanism by which montelukast works well enough to develop better drugs?

The precise mechanism by which montelukast improves spatial learning remains to be elucidated. At the molecular level, even if the hypothesis that montelukast acts directly through inhibition of GPR17 is correct, there are molecular details to unravel: GPR17 is a G-protein coupled receptor (GPCR) which may actually bind several ligands other than leukotrienes, such as oxysterols and SDF-126 In fact, it is controversial whether leukotrienes bind GPR7 at all *in vivo* [27, 28]. At the cellular level, the intriguing hypothesis that montelukast restores BBB integrity deserves serious investigation. Although repeated injections of young plasma into old mice restores reduced spatial learning ability in old mice [8], a recent report indicates that the negative effects of factors in old blood can dominate the potential positive effects of young murine blood in a single exchange [29], suggesting that restoring BBB integrity could have significant benefit in protecting sensitive neurons in the brain from potentially neurotoxic systemic factors in the circulation.

Conclusion

Montelukast is a potentially safe drug to maintain and possibly restore spatial memory in old age, if clinical studies confirm the data from rat studies in humans. Montelukast may represent the first in a series of pharmaceuticals that can override deleterious age-associated blood and CSF borne factors that promote age-associated dysfunction.

References

1. Sierra A, Gottfried-Blackmore AC, McEwen BS, Bulloch K. Microglia derived from aging mice exhibit an altered inflammatory profile. Glia 2007;55:412–24.
2. Hefendehl JK. Homeostatic and injury-induced microglia behavior in the aging brain. Aging Cell 2014;13:60–9.
3. Mosher KI, Wyss-Coray T. Microglial dysfunction in brain aging and Alzheimer's disease. Biochem Pharmacol 2014;88:594–604.
4. Villeda SA. The ageing systemic milieu negatively regulates neurogenesis and cognitive function. Nature 2011;477:90–4.
Morrison JH, Baxter MG. The ageing cortical synapse: hallmarks and implications for cognitive decline. Nat Rev Neurosci 2012;13:240–50.
5. Bake S, Sohrabji F. 17beta-estradiol differentially regulates blood-brain barrier permeability in young and aging female rats. Endocrinology 2004;145:5471–5.
6. Kuhn HG, Dickinson-Anson H, Gage FH. Neurogenesis in the dentate gyrus of the adult rat: age- related decrease of neuronal progenitor proliferation. J Neurosci 1996;16:2027–33.
7. Villeda SA. Young blood reverses age-related impairments in cognitive function and synaptic plasticity in mice. Nat Med 2014;20:659–63.
8. Conboy IM, Conboy MJ, Rebo J. Systemic Problems: A perspective on stem cell aging and rejuvenation. Aging 2015;7:754–65.
9. Katsimpardi L, Litterman NK, Schein PA, Miller CM, Loffredo FS, Wojtkiewicz GR, *et al.* Vascular and neurogenic rejuvenation of the aging mouse brain by young systemic factors. Science 2014;344:630–4. doi:10.1126/science.1251141.
10. Smith LK, He Y, Park J-S, Bieri G, Snethlage CE, Lin K, *et al.* β2-microglobulin is a systemic pro-aging factor that impairs cognitive function and neurogenesis. Nat Med 2015;21:932–7. doi:10.1038/nm.3898.
11. Saad MA, Abdelsalam RM, Kenawy SA, Attia AS. Montelukast, a cysteinyl leukotriene receptor- 1 antagonist protects against hippocampal injury induced by transient global cerebral ischemia and reperfusion in rats. Neurochem Res 2015;40:139–50.
12. Lecca D. The recently identified P2Y-like receptor GPR17 is a sensor of brain damage and a new target for brain repair. P Lo One 2008;3:e3579.
13. Zhang XY. HAMI 3379, a CysLT2 receptor antagonist, attenuates ischemia-like neuronal injury by inhibiting microglial activation. J Pharmacol Exp Ther 2013;346:328–41.
14. Huber C. Inhibition of leukotriene receptors boosts neural progenitor proliferation. Cell Physiol Biochem 2011;28:793–804.
15. Kohman RA, Bhattacharya TK, Kilby C, Bucko P, Rhodes JS. Effects of minocycline on spatial learning, hippocampal neurogenesis and microglia in aged and adult mice. Behav Brain Res 2013;242:17–24.

16. Marschallinger J, Schäffner I, Klein B, Gelfert R, Rivera FJ, Illes S, *et al*. Structural and functional rejuvenation of the aged brain by an approved anti-asthmatic drug. Nat Commun
2015;6. doi:10.1038/ncomms9466.

17. Marchesini M, Matocci R, Tasselli L, Cambiaghi V, OrlethOrleth A, Furia L, *et al*. PML is required for telomere stability in non-neoplastic human cells. Oncogene 2015. doi:10.1038/onc.2015.246.

18. Dobolyi A, Vincze C, Pál G, Lovas G. The Neuroprotective Functions of Transforming Growth Factor Beta Proteins. Int J Mol Sci 2012;13:8219–58. doi:10.3390/ijms13078219.

19. Paik JH. FoxOs cooperatively regulate diverse pathways governing neural stem cell homeostasis. Cell Stem Cell 2009;5:540–53.

20. Kumar A, Prakash A, Pahwa D, Mishra J. Montelukast potentiates the protective effect of rofecoxib against kainic acid-induced cognitive dysfunction in rats. Pharmacol Biochem Behavior 2012;103:43–52.

21. Kalonia H, Kumar P, Kumar A, Nehru B. Protective effect of montelukast against quinolinic acid/malonic acid induced neurotoxicity: possible behavioral, biochemical, mitochondrial and tumor necrosis factor-alpha level alterations in rats. Neuroscience 2010;171:284–99.

22. Lai J. Montelukast rescues primary neurons against Abeta1-42-induced toxicity through inhibiting CysLT1R-mediated NF-kappaB signaling. Neurochem Int 2014;75:26–31.

23. Yagami T, Yamamoto Y Kohma H. Leukotriene receptor antagonists, LY293111 and ONO-1078, protect neurons from the sPLA2-IB-induced neuronal cell death independently of blocking their receptors. Neurochem Int 2013;63:163–71.

24. Aldea Perona A, García-Sáiz M, Sanz Álvarez E. Psychiatric Disorders and Montelukast in Children: A Disproportionality Analysis of the VigiBase(®). Drug Saf 2016;39:69–78. doi:10.1007/s40264-015-0360-2.

25. Parravicini C, Daniele S, Palazzolo L, Trincavelli ML, Martini C, Zaratin P, *et al*. A promiscuous recognition mechanism between GPR17 and SDF-1: Molecular insights. Cell Signal 2016; 28:631–42. doi:10.1016/j.cellsig.2016.03.001.

26. Qi AD, Harden TK, Nicholas RA. Is GPR17 a P2Y/leukotriene receptor? examination of uracil nucleotides, nucleotide sugars, and cysteinyl leukotrienes as agonists of GPR17. J Pharmacol Exp Ther 2013;347:38–46.

27. Hennen S. Decoding signaling and function of the orphan G protein-coupled receptor GPR17 with a small-molecule agonist. Sci Signal 2013;6:ra93.

28. Rebo J, Mehdipour M, Gathwala R, Causey K, Liu Y, Conboy MJ, *et al*. A single heterochronic blood exchange reveals rapid inhibition of multiple tissues by old blood. Nat Commun 2016;7:13363. doi:10.1038/ncomms13363.

Chapter 8

Reversal of Aged Muscle Stem Cell Dysfunction

The loss of muscle stem cell (MuSC) numbers and function in the elderly results in a dramatic delay or incomplete repair of muscle following injury or surgery. Prolonged immobility can exacerbate the loss of muscle mass with increased morbidity of affected patients. Stem cells and their niche cooperate to regulate the activation, self-renewal, differentiation and return to quiescence of MuSCs. Extracellular matrix fibronectin and MuSC β1-integrin have been identified as critical factors in the dysfunction of aging muscle. Reduced amounts and/or function of β1-integrin and fibronectin are critical factors in the decline in muscle stem cell regeneration and homeostasis with aging. Replacement of fibronectin and/or stimulation of β1-integrin may provide a novel means to augment the decline in MuSC function with age.

Introduction

Muscle stem cells (MuSC) (a.k.a. myosatellite cells or satellite cells) are small multi-potent cells found in mature muscle [1]. Under normal circumstances MuSC are quiescent, lying between the basement membrane and the sarcolemma of muscle fibers in grooves parallel or transverse to the longitudinal axis of the fiber (see **Figure 8.1**).

Figure 8.1: Regenerative cycle of muscle stem cells. Following mechanical strain or direct injury, quiescent MuSC broach the basement membrane, and become activated.

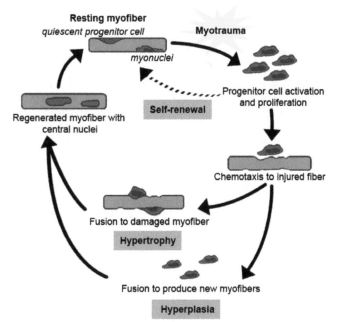

Activated MuSC initially proliferate as myoblasts prior to myogenic differentiation to form new post-mitotic myotubes (**Figure 8.2**).

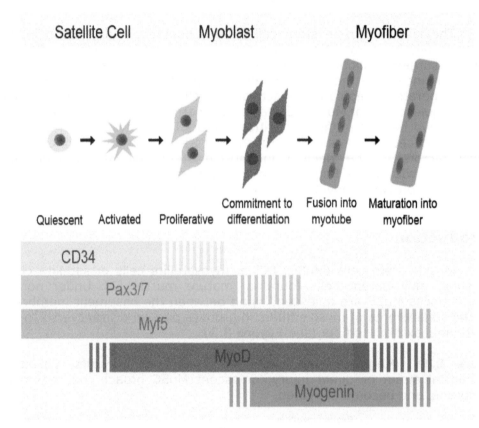

Figure 8.2: Markers of muscle stem cell myogenesis. MuSCs remain quiescent in normal adult muscle. Activation follows strain or damage. Upon activation MuSCs divide to produce myoblasts that further proliferate, before differentiation and fusion to form myotubes. These then mature into myofibers (Self-renewal of MuSCs are depicted in **Figure 8.2**). CD34 and Pax3/7 are expressed in quiescent satellite cells. Satellite cell activation is marked by the rapid onset of MyoD expression, whereas myogenin later marks the commitment to differentiation. Adapted from Zammit, 2006.

In addition the MuSC can fuse with existing myofibers to facilitate growth and repair. This process of muscle regeneration involves considerable changes to the extracellular matrix (ECM) and the expression of distinctive genetic markers and second messenger pathways. For example, most MuSC express PAX3 and PAX 7 [2].

Impaired muscle healing in the elderly is a major clinical problem [3, 4]. Aging, diabetes, obesity and cancer cachexia cause a loss of MuSC function with concomitant decline in the regenerative capacity of skeletal muscle tissue [4-9]. The loss of MuSC numbers and function in the elderly results in a dramatic delay or incomplete healing of muscle (**Figure 8.3**) following injury or surgery which prolongs immobility that in turn exacerbates the loss of muscle mass that accompanies aging [10, 3].

Figure 8.3: Aging of Muscle Stem Cells and Niche. Balance of lineage commitment and self-renewal is maintained during regeneration in young muscle by adequate levels of extracellular matrix fibronectin and MuSC-expressed β1-integrin. Aged muscles show increased lineage commitment (solid arrows) to myogenic progenitors (green cells) and a lack of self-renewal (dashed arrows), resulting in impaired regeneration and slow exhaustion of the MuSC reserve (blue cells). MuSC from very old ('geriatric') muscles enter senescence and lose their ability to re-enter the cell cycle.

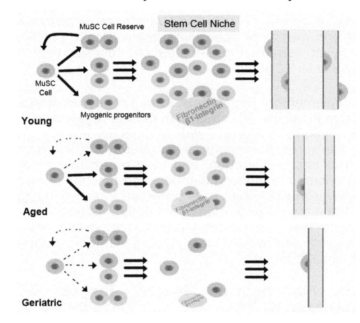

Conboy *et al.* [11] suggested that circulating factors were the primary mediators of the dysfunction of aged MuSC. While more recent reports corroborated the "humoral" factors observed in the initial parabiosis studies [12], questions remain regarding whether an alteration in the systemic environment acts directly on stem cells or perhaps the milieu supporting MuSCs becomes dysfunctional with age.

Extrinsic signals from the stem cell niche, critically regulate MuSCs. After injury, the muscle stem cell niche is subject to the coordinated entry of various cell types that release regulatory growth factors, modify the ECM, and interact directly with MuSCs. The activation, self-renewal, differentiation and re-entry into quiescence of MuSCs, is regulated by these complex interactions. The physical composition of the niche, for example, tissue stiffness, can determine the fate of MuSCs [13-15]. Furthermore, ECM molecules such as collagen VI and fibronectin (FN) provide signals necessary for MuSC self-renewal during adult muscle regeneration [15-17]. Pathways constitutively activated in aged MuSC include: the fibroblast growth factor (FGF)–ERK MAP kinase cascade, the p38 mitogen-activated protein (MAP) kinase and the Janus kinase (JAK)–STAT transcription factor pathway [18-22]. Attenuation of signaling via these pathways restores self-renewal of MuSC to promote muscle healing in aged mice. Beneficial exercise triggers release of various growth factors such as hepatocyte growth factor (HGF), insulin growth factor-1 (IGF-1) and fibroblast factor (FGF) that activate and enhance proliferation of MuSC.

Two recent papers advance our understanding of the fundamental molecular basis of aging MuSC, suggesting that changes in the stem cell niche leads to an upstream modification of these signaling cascades. Lukjanenko *et al.* [23] demonstrate that loss of FN in ECM from old regenerating muscle decreases MuSC function by reducing integrin signaling via protein tyrosine kinase 2 (PTK2)/FAK/MAP kinase pathways. Restoration of the levels of FN in muscle of aged mice rescues MuSC function to improve healing. They hypothesize that loss of stem cell adhesion to niche-derived FN is a major cause of MuSC aging.

In a complementary paper, Rozo *et al.* [24] demonstrate a key roll for another adhesion molecule, β1-integrin, in muscle regeneration. Muscle stem cells utilize β1-integrin to interact with fibronectin, among possible targets [25]. Muscle stem cell β1-integrin is absolutely crucial for the cycle of dormancy, activation, proliferation, and then return to dormancy. Reduced β1-integrin contributes to reduced numbers and function of muscle stem cell function and fewer muscle stem cells observed in aging. Restoration of β1-integrin activation by a monoclonal antibody restored the regenerative capacity of aged MuSC to youthful levels. The strong link between β1-integrin, fibronectin, and muscle stem cell regeneration suggests some very promising therapeutic targets.

ACT ONE: Fibronectin: Major Target within the Extracellular Matrix
1. Fibronectin is reduced in aged muscle.

To evaluate the hypothesis that the composition of the extra-cellular matrix (ECM) is affected by aging [23] Lukjanenko *et al.* used a variety of ECM-protein-specific slow-off-rate-modified aptamers [26] to identify ECM molecules present in muscle of control (uninjured) versus various times post-injury of young (9-weeks) and old (24-months) mice. Young regenerating muscle exhibited a sharp increase in FN levels post-injury, a response that was significantly blunted in aged muscle.

Differential expression of FN was determined in MuSCs, lineage-positive (Lin+) cells, which include immune, hematopoietic and endothelial cells and fibroadipogenic progenitors (FAPs). Lin+ cells were the primary producers of FN and this cell population was lost in regenerating muscle of aged mice. Studies of young FN-knockout mice exhibiting a 90% reduction in FN transcripts revealed a loss of MuSCs similar to aged control mice.

Together these studies demonstrated that fibronectin is essential for the maintenance of MuSCs during muscle regeneration.

1.2. Fibronectin is the preferred ECM binding substrate for mouse and human muscle progenitors.

Integrins (more on this below) and the syndecan-4-frizzled-7 (Sdc4-Fzd7) co-receptor complex mediate adhesion of MuSCs to FN [23-27] examined binding of MuSC to an array of 36 different ECM conditions spotted onto a layered hydrogel [29, 30]. Human and mouse myoblasts showed a pronounced preference for binding to FN alone or in combination with other components of the ECM. Furthermore, aged MuSC demonstrated a lower adhesive capacity vs. young controls.

1.3. Aging of muscle stem cells is modulated by adhesion to fibronectin.

Expression from mouse MuSC-derived myoblasts grown on FN for 72 h versus cells grown on collagen I, commonly used to culture primary myoblasts was compared using an antibody array having 1,318 site-specific antibodies covering a wide range of signaling molecules. 64 proteins were changed more than 10% in their phosphorylation levels on the FN substrate. Most apparent were the cell matrix receptor β1-integrin and several components of the ERK and p38 mitogen-activated protein kinase (MAPK) pathways and cell cycle control pathways, these are all known to be altered in old MuSCs.

1.4. Aged MuSC are more prone to anchorage-dependent programmed cell death (anoikis): fibronectin overcomes age-related defects of aged MuSCs.

Compared to laminin or collagen, FN is the preferred adhesion substrate in the ECM for MuSCs. However, the concentration of FN is decreased in old regenerative niches, leading to increased anoikis and reduced FAK signaling. Indeed, FN significantly improved the attachment of freshly isolated aged MuSCs.

Young MuSCs showed a similar preference for FN over collagen or laminin. Growth on FN also reduced the number of TUNEL+ aged cells (a measure of cell death) and led to a slightly higher number of proliferating cells that incorporated EdU. Defective FAK signaling observed in aged MuSC was also reversed. Taken together these data indicate that FN can overcome multiple age-related defects of MuSCs, including reduced proliferative capacity, impaired adhesion capacity, and tendency to undergo anoikis.

1.5. *In vivo* proof-of-concept: Fibronectin improves muscle rejuvenation.

Aged and young control mice were injected with purified murine FN to directly demonstrate a therapeutic benefit. The tibial is anterior muscles of 9 week old (young) and 24-month-old (aged) mice were injured with a 50 uL injection of 20 uM cardiotoxin solution. Two and 5 days post-injury 0.5 mg/mL mouse FN or vehicle (pH 7.5 50 mM Triss-aline) was injected. No significant changes were observed in the young mice. However, treatment with FN restored the number of MyoD1 myogenic commitment marker positive cells and devMHC+ fibers (a marker of the earliest stage of muscle fiber formation) and FAK signaling. Perhaps most importantly, FN injection of the aged mice accelerated muscle regeneration with significantly larger muscle fibers at 7 days post-injection. Thus restoration of FN to levels observed in young animals rescues the niche-dependent loss of MuSC function associated with aging.

ACT II: β1 Integrin: A Connection to the Extracellular Matrix

2.1. MuSCs without β1-Integrin cannot maintain quiescence.

To define the function of β1-integrin in adult MuSCs, Rozo *et al.*, (2016) generated a tamoxifen (tmx)-inducible Itgb1 conditional allele (Itgb1f) in MuSCs. The number of Itgb1−/− MuSCs was unchanged for 7 d after the tmx treatment, as compared to that in control cells. However, MuSC were reduced approximately 50% relative to control cells 21 d after tmx administration. The number of Itgb1−/− MuSCs continued to decline over time, but the number of MuSCs was greatly reduced 180 days after tmx treatment. Using lineage-labeled myofibers, the authors suggest that the number of mutant MuSCs decreased due to terminal differentiation and fusion into muscle fibers. Because cadherin 15 (Cdh15), a cell polarity protein, and par-3 family cell polarity regulator (Pard3) were not localized appropriately in Itgb1−/−MuSCs the authors concluded that β1-integrin senses the quiescent MuSC niche, maintaining correct polarity and preventing accidental activation or differentiation.

2.2. MuSCs without β1-integrin cannot sustain proliferation after injury.

Next, to determine whether Itgb1−/− MuSCs can support regeneration, muscle-injury was induced with cardiotoxin (CTX), at 3 d after tmx treatment. Regeneration was significantly reduced at 5, 10 and 30 d after cardiotoxin-mediated muscle injury. Furthermore, labeling studies of MuSC with EdU confirmed that β1-integrin is required for MuSC proliferation and self-renewal to drive muscle regeneration.

2.3. β1-integrin cross-talks with FGF signaling in muscle stem cells.

Previous studies implicated integrin-ECM cross-talk with receptor tyrosine kinases (RTKs), including FGF receptors and Fgf2 was known to stimulate myoblast proliferation via ERK/MAP kinases ([38]. Responsiveness of the Itgb1−/− myoblasts to FGF along with fibronectin was measured by measuring the levels of phosphorylation of FGF and integrin downstream signaling effectors, Erk and Akt (pErk1, pErk2 and pAkt). The Itgb1−/− MuSCs showed a compromised response to Fgf-2 that can be partially restored by exogenous Fgf-2. Thus β1-integrin cooperates with fibroblast growth factor 2 (Fgf2), a potent growth factor for MuSCs, to synergistically activate their common downstream effectors, mitogen-activated protein (MAP) kinase Erk and protein kinase B (Akt).

2.4. Aged MuSCs are defective in integrin activity.

The β1-deficient MuSCs (Itgb1−/−) share several features with MuSC in aged individuals: a) gradual loss from the niche during aging [19] b) reduced capacity for proliferation [11], c) a commitment to differentiation [20] and d) defective self-renewal [18]. To test the hypothesis that β1-integrin activity is aberrant in aged cells, thereby desensitizing aged MuSCs to Fgf2, Rozo et al. [24] utilized 9EG7, an antibody that targets the 'high-affinity' ligand-bound active β1-integrin [39, 40]. The aged MuSCs demonstrated abnormal antibody localization as well as a dysregulation of overall integrin activity.

2.5. Activating β1-integrin in aged MuSCs enhances FGF signaling to promote expansion of MuSCs.

To test the hypothesis that dysregulated integrin signaling underlies the dysfunction of aged MuSCs, Rozo et al. [24] utilized β1-integrin-activating antibody TS2/16 [41]. High levels of regeneration in young animals was not improved, however antibody treatment improved regeneration in aged mice to levels comparable to the young mice. Treatment with TS2/16 did not rescue regeneration of Itgb1−/− muscle indicating a requirement for expression of functional β1-integrin. Together, TS2/16 and Fgf2 treatment increased the number of fiber-associated myogenic cells, the ratio of Pax7+ cells, and the fraction of MuSCs expressing polarized pp38. It is possible that muscle damage causes enough Fgf2 to be released to cooperate with TS2/16-activated β1-integrin in old MuSC, because treatment with TS2/16 alone is sufficient to improve aged muscle regeneration in vivo, s. TS2/16 treatment increased the fraction of aged MuSCs on myofibers, relative to that after treatment with control IgG. Together TS2/16 and Fgf2 treatment stimulated pFGFR in most of the aged MuSCs consistent with requirement for both to enhance expansion of old MuSCs. In summary, anti-β1-integrin antibody TS2/16 acts to enhance FGF signaling and restore responsiveness of aged MuSCs to injury.

2.6. Activating β1-integrin improves dystrophic muscles.

Mdx mice do not express dystrophin because of a nonsense mutation in the Dmd gene [42]. Muscle in the mdx mouse has a disorganized ECM, and mdx MuSCs are associated with myofibers having abnormal patterns of active β1-integrin. A single dose of TS2/16 injected into the tibial is anterior (TA) muscle of mdx mice promoted myogenic cell expansion, as evidenced by increased EdU incorporation 3 d after treatment. When TS2/16 treatment was extended to four weekly injections the myofiber lamina was reduced, reflecting an improvement in MuSC–niche interaction. Mdx muscles treated with TS2/16 had deceased cross-sectional areas, compared to IgG-treated mdx and mdx muscles. An apparent reversal from the typical observed hypertrophy. TS2/16-treated muscles showed improved strength, using a variety of techniques. Therefore, development of therapeutics to activate β1-integrin may be a rational way to restore muscle repair and function in patients wtih pathological muscle-injury and dystrophy.

Medical Implications

Following identification of novel targets on opposing sides of the "synapse" of the MuSC with its milieu, the most preliminary mouse proof-of-concept studies have been reported (Lukjanenko *et al.* [23] and Rozo *et al*. [24]. On the one hand, extracellular matrix protein fibronectin injected into injured muscle improved MuSC function and myogenesis, on the other hand an anti-β1 integrin monoclonal antibody binding to the target MuSCs augmented muscle repair with improved myogenesis in a murine model of muscular dystrophy.

Although fibronectin and β1-integrins functionally interact, for example in partnering with Fgf2 to stimulate the MAP kinase signaling pathway, there is more to the story than dysregulation of these two biomolecules. Given that numerous manipulations reverse age-associated muscle dysfunction including parabiosis between young and old animals [11], a TGF-β receptor I kinase (Alk5) inhibitor [43], and p38 kinase inhibitors [20], among others, it is reasonable to think that age-associated dysregulation occurs at multiple levels, but that enough redundancy in satellite cell maintenance exists so that a functional phenotype can be restored by stimulation of downstream or parallel interacting signaling networks. On the other hand, changes to the ECM, such as loss of fibronectin, offer a ready explanation for why young cells transplanted to the old host do worse than in their native environment [10]. That the ECM changes may be due to a loss of support cells in skeletal muscle, begs the question of what drives the tissue remodeling with age: again a multifactorial cause is likely.

While this work is a leap forward in our understanding of muscle stem cell biology, much work remains to be carried out prior to clinical translation. Perhaps most importantly, the targets will need to be validated with human cells and tissue. No mention is made of potential toxicities. What will be the best molecules for use in humans? What will be the optimal dose, dose schedule, pharmacokinetics? Can the proteins/antibodies be given by a parenteral route, or must they be directly injected into the muscles? Are biomarkers available to optimize the human translational work? Finally, while sarcomas or other tumors of muscle are rare, will this type of intervention increase the chances of abnormal muscle growth and/or repair?

But before biotechnology entrepreneurs become too excited, it should be remembered that small molecule inhibitors also can rejuvenate MuSC, so it is not all clear that therapy should be based on targeting β1-integrin or fibronectin with expensive biologicals. The promise of a plasma-based recapitulation of the pro-myogenic effects of parabiosis has captured the imagination of many. Deciphering the precise mechanisms by which the expression of these key proteins are altered and how for example, support cells cell migrate, die or senesce would be critical. Moreover, these changes occur in old, but not geriatric animals, where there is evidence of more significant dysfunction including senescence of the MuSC themselves.

With regard to Duchenne's muscular dystrophy, loss of sarcolemmal dystrophin and the dystrophin-associated glycoprotein (DAG) complex promotes muscle fiber damage during muscle contraction. This mechanism causes an efflux of creatine kinase (CK), an influx of calcium ions, and the recruitment of immune cells, (T cells, macrophages, and mast cells) to the damaged muscle, causing progressive myofiber fibrosis and necrosis. Much research has focused on the restoration of dystrophin or proteins that are analogous to dystrophin, such as utrophin, via cell therapy, gene therapy, gene correction, and in recent years CRISPR/Cas9 technology. Presently no therapies slow the progression of any of the muscular dystrophies. Thus the results of Rozo *et al.* [24] in the mdx model provide hope for an alternative approach to these devastating diseases.

Conclusion

Reduced functions and/or amounts of β1-integrin and fibronectin are critical factors in the decline in muscle stem cell regeneration and homeostasis with aging. Replacement of fibronectin and/or stimulation of β1-integrin may provide a novel means to augment the decline in MuSC function with age.

References

1. Birbrair A, Delbono O. Pericytes are Essential for Skeletal Muscle Formation. Stem Cell Rev 2015;11:547–8. doi:10.1007/s12015-015-9588-6.
2. Relaix F, Rocancourt D, Mansouri A, Buckingham M. A Pax3/Pax7-dependent population of skeletal muscle progenitor cells. Nature 2005;435:948–53. doi:10.1038/nature 03594.
3. Blau HM, Cosgrove BD, Ho ATV. The central role of muscle stem cells in regenerative failure with aging. Nat Med 2015;21:854–62. doi:10.1038/nm.3918.

4. Sousa-Victor P, García-Prat L, Serrano AL, Perdiguero E, Muñoz-Cánoves P. Muscle stem cell aging: regulation and rejuvenation. Trends Endocrinol Metab TEM 2015;26:287–96. doi:10.1016/j.tem.2015.03.006.

5. D'Souza DM, Trajcevski KE, Al- Sajee D, Wang DC, Thomas M, Anderson JE, et al. Diet-induced obesity impairs muscle satellite cell activation and muscle repair through alterations in hepatocyte growth factor signaling. Physiol Rep 2015;3:e12506. doi:10.14814/phy2.12506.

6. He WA, Berardi E, Cardillo VM, Acharyya S, Aulino P, Thomas-Ahner J, et al. NF-κB–mediated Pax7 dysregulation in the muscle microenvironment promotes cancer cachexia. J Clin Invest 2013;123:4821–35. doi:10.1172/JCI68523.

7. Fujimaki S, Wakabayashi T, Takemasa T, Asashima M, Kuwabara T. Diabetes and Stem Cell Function. BioMed Res Int 2015;2015. doi:10.1155/2015/592915.

8. Watters JM, Clancey SM, Moulton SB, Briere KM, Zhu JM. Impaired recovery of strength in older patients after major abdominal surgery. Ann Surg 1993;218:380–90; discussion 390–3.

9. Müller M, Tohtz S, Dewey M, Springer I, Perka C. Age-related appearance of muscle trauma in primary total hip arthroplasty and the benefit of a minimally invasive approach for patients older than 70 years. Int Orthop 2011;35:165–71. doi:10.1007/s00264-010-1166-6.

10. Carlson ME, Suetta C, Conboy MJ, Aagaard P, Mackey A, Kjaer M, et al. Molecular aging and rejuvenation of human muscle stem cells. EMBO Mol Med 2009;1:381–91. doi:10.1002/emmm.200900045.

11. Conboy IM, Conboy MJ, Wagers AJ, Girma ER, Weissman IL, Rando TA. Rejuvenation of aged progenitor cells by exposure to a young systemic environment. Nature 2005;433:760–4. doi:10.1038/nature03260.

12. McCullagh KJ. Can a young muscle's stem cell secretome prolong our lives? Stem Cell Res Ther 2012;3:19. doi:10.1186/scrt110.

13. Gilbert P, Havenstrite K, Magnusson K, Sacco A, Leonardi N, Kraft P, et al. Substrate elasticity regulates skeletal muscle stem cell self-renewal in culture. Science 2010;329:1078–81. doi:10.1126/science.1191035.

14. Lv H, Li L, Sun M, Zhang Y, Chen L, Rong Y, et al. Mechanism of regulation of stem cell differentiation by matrix stiffness. Stem Cell Res Ther 2015;6. doi:10.1186/s13287-015-0083-4.

15. Bonaldo P, Braghetta P, Zanetti M, Piccolo S, Volpin D, Bressan GM. Collagen VI deficiency induces early onset myopathy in the mouse: an animal model for Bethlem myopathy. Hum Mol Genet 1998;7:2135–40.

16. Urciuolo A, Quarta M, Morbidoni V, Gattazzo F, Molon S, Grumati P, et al. Collagen VI regulates satellite cell self-renewal and muscle regeneration. Nat Commun 2013;4:1964. doi:10.1038/ncomms2964.

17. Tierney MT, Gromova A, Sesillo FB, Sala D, Spenlé C, Orend G, et al. Autonomous Extracellular Matrix Remodeling Controls a Progressive Adaptation in Muscle Stem Cell Regenerative Capacity during Development. Cell Rep 2016;14:1940–52. doi:10.1016/j.celrep.2016.01.072.

18. Bernet JD, Doles JD, Hall JK, Kelly-Tanaka K, Carter TA, Olwin BB. P38 MAPK signaling underlies a cell autonomous loss of stem cell self-renewal in aged skeletal muscle. Nat Med 2014;20:265–71. doi:10.1038/nm. 3465.

19. Chakkalakal JV, Jones KM, Basson MA, Brack AS. The aged niche disrupts muscle stem cell quiescence. Nature 2012;490:355–60. doi:10.1038/nature11438.

20. Cosgrove BD, Gilbert PM, Porpiglia E, Mourkioti F, Lee SP, Corbel SY, et al. Rejuvenation of the muscle stem cell population restores strength to injured aged muscles. Nat Med 2014;20:255– 64. doi:10.1038/nm.3464.

21. Price FD, von Maltzahn J, Bentzinger CF, Dumont NA, Yin H, Chang NC, et al. Inhibition of JAK/STAT signaling stimulates adult satellite cell function. Nat Med 2014;20:1174–81. doi:10.1038/nm.3655.

22. Tierney MT, Aydogdu T, Sala D, Malecova B, Gatto S, Puri PL, *et al.* STAT3 signaling controls satellite cell expansion and skeletal muscle repair. Nat Med 2014;20:1182–6. doi:10.1038/nm.3656.

24. Lukjanenko L, Jung MJ, Hegde N, Perruisseau-Carrier C, Migliavacca E, Rozo M, *et al.* Loss of fibronectin from the aged stem cell niche affects the regenerative capacity of skeletal muscle in mice. Nat Med 2016;22:897–905. doi:10.1038/nm.4126.

25. Lozo M, Li L, Fan C-M. Targeting β1-integrin signaling enhances regeneration in aged and dystrophic muscle in mice. Nat Med 2016;22:889–96. doi:10.1038/nm.4116.

26. Tanentzapf G, Devenport D, Godt D, Brown NH. integrin-dependent anchoring of a stem cell niche. Nat Cell Biol 2007;9:1413–8. doi:10.1038/ncb1660.

27. Gold L, Ayers D, Bertino J, Bock C, Bock A, Brody EN, *et al.* Aptamer-Based Multiplexed Proteomic Technology for Biomarker Discovery. PLOS ONE 2010;5:e15004. doi:10.1371/journal.pone.0015004.

28. Bentzinger CF, Wang YX, von Maltzahn J, Soleimani VD, Yin H, Rudnicki MA. Fibronectin Regulates Wnt7a Signaling and Satellite Cell Expansion. Cell Stem Cell 2013;12:75–87. doi:10.1016/j.stem.2012.09.015.

29. Siegel AL, Atchison K, Fisher KE, Davis GE, Cornelison DDW. 3D timelapse analysis of muscle satellite cell motility. Stem Cells Dayt Ohio 2009;27:2527–38. doi:10.1002/stem.178.

30. Brafman DA, Shah KD, Fellner T, Chien S, Willert K. Defining long-term maintenance conditions of human embryonic stem cells with arrayed cellular microenvironment technology. Stem Cells Dev 2009;18:1141–54. doi:10.1089/scd.2008.0410.

31. Brafman DA, de Minicis S, Seki E, Shah KD, Teng D, Brenner D, *et al.* Investigating the role of the extracellular environment in modulating hepatic stellate cell biology with arrayed combinatorial micro environments. Integr Biol Quant Biosci Nano Macro 2009;1:513–24. doi:10.1039/b912926j.

32. Sousa-Victor P, Gutarra S, García-Prat L, Rodriguez-Ubreva J, Ortet L, Ruiz-Bonilla V, *et al.* Geriatric muscle stem cells switch reversible quiescence into senescence. Nature 2014;506:316–21. doi:10.1038/nature13013.

33. Mori S, Takada Y. Crosstalk between Fibroblast Growth Factor (FGF) Receptor and Integrin through Direct Integrin Binding to FGF and Resulting Integrin-FGF-FGFR Ternary Complex Formation. Med Sci 2013;1:20–36. doi:10.3390/medsci1010020.

34. Assoian RK, Schwartz MA. Coordinate signaling by integrins and receptor tyrosine kinases in the regulation of G1 phase cell-cycle progression. Curr Opin Genet Dev 2001;11:48–53.

35. Jones NC, Fedorov YV, Rosenthal RS, Olwin BB. ERK1/2 is required for myoblast proliferation but is dispensable for muscle gene expression and cell fusion. J Cell Physiol 2001;186:104–15. doi:10.1002/1097-4652(200101)186:1<104::AID-JCP1015>3.0.CO;2-0.

36. Roovers K, Davey G, Zhu X, Bottazzi ME, Assoian RK. α5β1 Integrin Controls Cyclin D1 Expression by Sustaining Mitogen-activated Protein Kinase Activity in Growth Factor-treated Cells. Mol Biol Cell 1999;10:3197–204. doi:10.1091/mbc.10.10.3197.

37. Polanska UM, Fernig DG, Kinnunen T. Extracellular interactome of the FGF receptor-ligand system: complexities and the relative simplicity of the worm. Dev Dyn Off Publ Am Assoc Anat 2009;238:277–93. doi:10.1002/dvdy.21757.

38. Murakami M, Elfenbein A, Simons M. Non-canonical fibroblast growth factor signalling in angiogenesis. Cardiovasc Res 2008;78:223–31. doi:10.1093/cvr/cvm086.

39. Miyamoto S, Teramoto H, Gutkind JS, Yamada KM. Integrins can collaborate with growth factors for phosphorylation of receptor tyrosine kinases and MAP kinase activation: roles of integrin aggregation and occupancy of receptors. J Cell Biol 1996;135:1633–42.

40. Bazzoni G, Shih DT, Buck CA, Hemler ME. Monoclonal antibody 9EG7 defines a novel beta 1 integrin epitope induced by soluble ligand and manganese, but inhibited by calcium. J Biol Chem 1995;270:25570–7.

41. Takagi J, Springer TA. Integrin activation and structural rearrangement. Immunol Rev 2002;186:141–63.

42. Hintermann E, Bilban M, Sharabi A, Quaranta V. Inhibitory Role of α6β4-Associated Erbb-2 and Phosphoinositide 3-Kinase in Keratinocyte Haptotactic Migration Dependent on α3β1 Integrin. J Cell Biol 2001;153:465–78.

43. Bulfield G, Siller WG, Wight PA, Moore KJ. X chromosome-linked muscular dystrophy (mdx) in the mouse. Proc Natl Acad Sci U S A 1984;81:1189–92.

44. Yousef H, Conboy MJ, Morgenthaler A, Schlesinger C, Bugaj L, Paliwal P, et al. Systemic attenuation of the TGF-β pathway by a single drug simultaneously rejuvenates hippocampal neurogenesis and myogenesis in the same old mammal. Oncotarget 2015;6:11959–78.

Chapter 9

Preclinical Reversal of Atherosclerosis by FDA-Approved Compound that Transforms Cholesterol into an Anti-Inflammatory "Prodrug"

Although atherosclerosis is treatable with lipid-lowering drugs, not all patients respond. Hydroxypropyl-beta-cyclodextrin (CD) is an FDA-approved compound for solubilizing, capturing, and delivering lipophilic drugs in humans. Zimmer *et al.* report that CD mediates regression of atherosclerotic plaques in two mouse models by solubilizing cholesterol crystals (CCs), and promoting metabolism of CCs into water-soluble 27-hydroxy-cholesterol, which, in turn, activates anti-inflammatory LXR receptor target genes, promotes active and passive efflux of cholesterol from macrophages, and increases metabolic processing of cholesterol. In effect, CD inverts the role of its cargo, cholesterol, from inflammatory to anti-inflammatory by converting cholesterol into a "prodrug" that when modified to 27-hydroxycholesterol reduces atherosclerosis. This mechanism defines a new class of pharmaceuticals, "inverters": compounds that cause innate biomolecules to act opposite to their normal function. However, chronic CD treatment in animal models damages auditory cells, which must be addressed before CD can be developed as a systemic drug for atherosclerosis.

Introduction

Atherosclerosis is a disease of arterial wall remodel- ing, in which lipids accumulate in the subendothelial layer, leading to an inflammatory response that stimulates further pathogenic changes [1]. Atherosclerosis underlies cardiovascular disease, leading to heart attacks and strokes, which are common causes of death. Atherosclerosis is a progressive disease that is often associated with aging.

In atherosclerosis, lipid deposition leads to the formation of cholesterol crystals (CCs), which stimulate inflammation by inducing innate immunity pathways, complement activation, neutrophil extracellular trap formation, and trans- formation of macrophages into foam cells. Targeting CC formation has been a successful therapeutic approach with lipid-lowering drugs considered a first-line treatment to block progression of atherosclerosis. Although existing lipid- lowering drugs that target low density lipoprotein (LDL) levels can slow or sometimes halt progression of atherosclerosis, they often do not reverse the pathogenesis of atherosclerosis and are ineffective in some patients [2–4].

One simple idea is to attempt to solubilize cholesterol in atherosclerotic plaques to promote its clearance and catabolism. A possible agent to solubilize cholesterol is 2-hydroxypropyl-beta-cyclodextrin (CD), an FDA-approved compound for solubilizing, capturing, and delivering lipophilic drugs in humans. [5,6] Preliminary reports suggest that in cultured cells, CD can solubilize cholesterol, increasing solubility in aqueous solution 150,000, stimulate cholesterol efflux from foam cells, and reduce inflammation [7, 8].

Cholesterol-Solubilizing Compound Reverses Atherosclerosis

In a potentially groundbreaking preclinical study, Zimmer *et al.* show that CD treatment inhibits and partially reverses atherosclerosis in several mouse models of atherosclerosis [9]. In an initial experiment, mice deficient in apolipoprotein E (ApoE-/-) were fed a cholesterol-rich diet simultaneously with twice weekly subcutaneous injections of CD for 8 weeks. CD reduced plaque area relative to untreated animals (60% - 35%) and CC density (0.28–0.18) in the aortic root, as well as greater than 50% reductions in reactive oxygen species, and inflammatory cytokines TNF-alpha, IL-6, and IL-8. Beyond the change in CCs, plaque composition was unchanged as were serum cholesterol levels. General physiological parameters such as weight and blood pressure were also unchanged [9]. This experiment demonstrated that CD could inhibit atherosclerosis.

To determine whether CD could actually reverse atherosclerosis, ApoE-/- mice were fed a cholesterol-rich diet for 8 weeks to induce robust plaque formation and then switched to a normal chow diet or maintained on the cholesterol-rich diet. CD treatment resulted in a 45% regression of plaque size (to values similar to that seen in the simultaneous dosing study) for both diets, suggesting that CD can regress pre-existing plaques to a similar extent that it can prevent plaque formation. Furthermore, CC formation was reduced to similar levels seen for simultaneous CD treatment for mice continuing on the cholesterol-rich diet and to almost 50% lower levels when switched to the normal chow, suggesting that the beneficial effect of CD can be enhanced by lowering lipids, which might imply potential synergy with pre-existing drugs such as statins that lower cholesterol. These results were confirmed in the LDL-R-/- mouse model of atherosclerosis as well (see hereunder) [9].

As expected, CD increased solubility of CCs *in vitro*, where 10 mM CD was capable of almost completely solubilizing 1 mg of CCs. At a dose of 2 g/kg, and assuming a 25g mouse has 1.6mL of blood, the maximum blood concentration of CD in these animals is about 30mM. In contrast, CD probably does not achieve the maximum calculated concentration in the blood and it will bind other lipids as well, but the high CD dosage used in Zimmer *et al.*'s experiments could potentially solubilize deposited CCs. Because CCs are often intracellular, Zimmer *et al.* treated macrophages in culture with fluorescently labeled cholesterol and then determined that 10 mM CD could dissolve 50% of the intracellular Ccs [9].

To determine whether the observed anti-atherosclerotic effects went beyond mere solubilization of CCs and involved increased metabolism of cholesterol, Zimmer *et al.* loaded macrophages with CCs composed of cholesterol labeled with six deuterium atoms (D6-cholesterol) so that the metabolites could be identified by gas chromatography– mass spectrometry-selective ion monitoring (GC-MS-SIM). A significant amount of cholesterol esters was observed after CD treatment. Cholesterol esters, formed by the action of acetyl CoA acetyltransferase (ACAT1), are less cytotoxic than cholesterol and are typically stored in lipid droplets. Also, the total cellular pool of D6-cholesterol was reduced by efflux of the labeled cholesterol to the medium. It is likely that active transport through the ABCA1 and ABCG1 reverse cholesterol transport (RCT) is involved, given that CD increased ABCA1 and ABCG1 expression beyond the levels associated with CCs treatment [9]. However, the importance of active transport was not clearly established in this experiment.

ABCA1 and ABCG1 transporters are positively regulated by oxysterols through LXR/RXR receptors. Zimmer *et al.* determined that production of 27-hydroxycholesterol, a freely diffusible oxysterol, was increased 15-fold by CD in CC- treated macrophages. Interestingly, CYP27a1 the enzyme that catalyzes the formation and secretion of 27-hydroxycholesterol was not upregulated. Furthermore, 27-hydroxycholesterol levels increased even in control macrophages grown in medium with normal levels of cholesterol [9]. Apparently, increased levels of 27-hydroxycholesterol are due to the solubilization of CCs into free cholesterol so that it is avail- able as a substrate for CYP27a1.

Consistent with the activation of LXR genes, genome- wide mRNA profiling indicated that LXR target gene expression, [10, 11] including ABCA1 and ABCG1, was increased by CCs and even further increased by CD after CCs. Moreover, CD was sufficient to induce LXR target gene expression even without prior CC treatment. As expected, expression of genes known to be down regulated by LXR activation, such as proinflammatory cytokines IL-1B, IL6, and TNF-alpha, was reduced. To prove the point, macrophages engineered to lack LXR function (LXRa-/LXRb-) do not induce LXR target gene expression under any of these treatments [9]. These results are not entirely unexpected as previous work has shown that CD can not only mobilize cholesterol that is trapped in the lysosomes by a mutation in the NPC1 trans-porter in Niemann-Pick Disease Type C (NPC) but also activate LXR-regulated genes [11, 12].

To test whether CD stimulated active transport of CCs *in vivo*, bone marrow-derived macrophages from wild-type (WT) or LXRa/LXRb mice were loaded with D6-CCs *in vitro* and then injected into the peritoneum of WT mice. CD stimulated the excretion of D6-cholesterol into the feces, which suggests the involvement of active transport, and into the urine, which suggests that CD also stimulates passive transport through cholesterol solubilization. These results were extended to humans in an experiment with three NPC patients. Intravenous injection of CD resulted in increased urinary cholesterol excretion over 10 hours, suggesting CD solubilizes cholesterol in humans and that CD- mediated passive cholesterol efflux occurs in both mice and humans [9].

To further determine whether CD might also reverse atherosclerosis in humans, human carotid artery biopsies containing plaques were cultured for

24 hours with or without CD. Again CD promoted the transfer of cholesterol from plaques to supernatant and the production of LXR activator 27-hydroxycholesterol. Simultaneous global gene expression experiments were similar to those from the mice experiments: LXR-regulated target genes were increased and genes involved in regulation of inflammatory response were decreased, including the inflammasome sensor NLRP3, as was observed for the mice [9].

Using the LDL-R-/- mouse model of atherosclerosis, Zimmer *et al.* confirmed that macrophages possessing functional LXR are necessary for atherosclerotic plaque regression by irradiating the mice to destroy their immune systems and then transplanting bone marrow from LXRa/ LXRb or WT mice to reconstitute their immune systems. Unlike using transplants from WT mice, no plaque reduction was found in mice with macrophages lacking LXR. Interestingly, similar experiments with macrophages lacking the ABCA1 and ABCG1 transporters *did* show plaque reduction, which suggests that active transport RCT is not necessary for plaque regression [9]. One possible explanation is that the anti-inflammatory effects promoted by CD perhaps through 27-hydroxycholesterol synthesis are of paramount importance.

The mechanism of CD in atherosclerosis is novel. CD interacts with cholesterol and CCs in such a way as to invert their role from promoting to inhibiting inflammation. Increasing cholesterol's enzymatic conversion to 27-hydroxycholesterol essentially makes the cholesterol/CD complex a "prodrug." *CD defines a new kind of pharmaceutical, an "inverter": a compound that causes innate biomolecules to act inversely to their function.* This is possible because there is a feedback mechanism that controls the extent to which cholesterol increases inflammation.

The proinflammatory signaling associated with excess cholesterol or CCs induces an anti-inflammatory braking mechanism through modification to 27-hydroxycholesterol. Pathology arises when too much cholesterol is present in CCs and can be reversed by increasing the amount of 27-hydroxycholesterol.

Medical Implications

These preliminary studies suggest that CD may be a useful therapeutic to potentially reverse atherosclerosis. How- ever, there are caveats. The mouse models used in these studies are imperfect [13]. For example, ApoE mice can be manipulated to show significant plaque reduction by feeding a reduced cholesterol diet. In humans, it is typically more difficult to reverse atherosclerosis, although dietary changes and statin drug therapy are often sufficient to halt or slow progression. Certainly the CD studies would have to be replicated and then appropriate randomized clinical trials performed.

A key issue may be unwanted side effects. Even though CD (a) is considered safe, (b) has a very high LD50, (c) is commonly used in drug formulations, and (d) is in clinical trials for NPC1 (NCT02534844), the compound is not without problems. Chronic treatment of NPC1 cats with CD significantly extends lifespan, inhibits neurological symptoms, and blocks cerebellar dysfunction and Purkinje cell death. However, these benefits are accompanied by hearing loss [14] by removing cholesterol from prestin in sensory cells [15]. This problem may have solutions. Should CD be developed for treating atherosclerosis in humans, perhaps treatment could be intermittent to limit or prevent irreversible damage to hearing. In that scenario, after regression of plaques, lipid-lowering therapies could be employed to maintain healthy arteries. Alternatively, perhaps it might be possible to use cholesterol-containing ear drops to supplement the sensory hairs sufficiently to afford protection.

Questions remain with regard to viability of commercial development of CD. Although Vitesse, Inc. may have been granted orphan drug status for CD to treat NPC1, atherosclerosis is not an orphan disease and CD is probably not patentable for this application, making development through a traditional pharmaceutical model difficult. Coupled with the potential damage to the auditory system, it is very unlikely that CD will be developed for atherosclerosis unless a government or nonprofit organization with deep pockets steps in.

One obvious question arising from this work is why not just target LXR, since Zimmer *et al.* and earlier studies point to this potentially very effective drug target for atherosclerosis? The answer is that LXR has been targeted. LXR agonists do show significant benefit in preclinical studies, but these drugs showed liver toxicity and lipogenic effects, [16-19] unlike CD.

Conclusion

The idea of melting away atherosclerotic plaques is an appealing one. CD, considered generally safe by the FDA, is a relatively benign substance representing a potentially significant and inexpensive molecule to treat atherosclerosis. However, beyond confirmatory preclinical studies, which are likely to succeed, the potential chronic side effects on hearing need to be addressed.

References

1. Yurdagul A, Finney AC, Woolard MD, Orr AW. The ar- terial microenvironment: The where and why of athero- sclerosis. Biochem J 2016;473:1281–1295.
2. Task Force Members, Montalescot G, Sechtem U, Achen- bach S, Andreotti F, Arden C, et al. 2013 ESC guidelines on the management of stable coronary artery disease: The Task Force on the management of stable coronary artery disease of the European Society of Cardiology. Eur Heart J 2013;34:2949–3003.
3. Sabatine MS, Giugliano RP, Wiviott SD, Raal FJ, Blom DJ, Robinson J, et al. Efficacy and safety of evolocumab in reducing lipids and cardiovascular events. N Engl J Med 2015;372:1500–1509.
4. Robinson JG, Farnier M, Krempf M, Bergeron J, Luc G, Averna M, et al. Efficacy and safety of alirocumab in re- ducing lipids and cardiovascular events. N Engl J Med 2015;372:1489–1499.

5. Gould S, Scott RC. 2-Hydroxypropyl-beta-cyclodextrin (HP-beta-CD): A toxicology review. Food Chem Tox- icol Int J Publ Br Ind Biol Res Assoc 2005;43:1451– 1459.

6. Loftsson T, Jarho P, Ma´sson M, Ja¨rvinen T. Cyclodextrins in drug delivery. Expert Opin Drug Deliv 2005;2:335-351.

7. Liu SM, Cogny A, Kockx M, Dean RT, Gaus K, Jessup W, *et al.* Cyclodextrins differentially mobilize free and esteri- fied cholesterol from primary human foam cell macro- phages. J Lipid Res 2003;44:1156–1166.

8. Atger VM, de la Llera Moya M, Stoudt GW, Rodrigueza WV, Phillips MC, Rothblat GH. Cyclodextrins as catalysts for the removal of cholesterol from macrophage foam cells. J Clin Invest 1997;99:773–780.

9. Zimmer S, Grebe A, Bakke SS, Bode N, Halvorsen B, Ulas T, *et al.* Cyclodextrin promotes atherosclerosis regression via macrophage reprogramming. Sci Transl Med 2016;8: 333ra50–333ra50.

10. Janowski BA, Willy PJ, Devi TR, Falck JR, Mangelsdorf DJ. An oxysterol signalling pathway mediated by the nu- clear receptor LXR alpha. Nature 1996;383:728–731.

11. Repa JJ, Turley SD, Lobaccaro JA, Medina J, Li L, Lustig K, *et al.* Regulation of absorption and ABC1-mediated ef- flux of cholesterol by RXR heterodimers. Science 2000; 289:1524–1529.

12. Taylor AM, Liu B, Mari Y, Liu B, Repa JJ. Cyclodextrin mediates rapid changes in lipid balance in Npc1-/- mice without carrying cholesterol through the bloodstream. J Lipid Res 2012;53:2331–2342.

13. Getz GS, Reardon CA. Use of mouse models in athero-sclerosis research. Methods Mol Biol Clifton NJ 2015; 1339:1

14. Vite CH, Bagel JH, Swain GP, Prociuk M, Sikora TU, Stein VM, *et al.* Intracisternal cyclodextrin prevents cerebellar dysfunction and Purkinje cell death in feline Niemann-Pick type C1 disease. Sci Transl Med 2015;7: 276ra26–276ra26.

15. Takahashi S, Homma K, Zhou Y, Nishimura S, Duan C, Chen J, *et al.* Susceptibility of outer hair cells to cholesterol chelator 2-hydroxypropyl-b-cyclodextrine is prestin-dependent. Sci Rep 2016;6:21973.

16. Joseph SB, McKilligin E, Pei L, Watson MA, Collins AR, Laffitte BA, *et al.* Synthetic LXR ligand inhibits the de- velopment of atherosclerosis in mice. Proc Natl Acad Sci U S A 2002;99:7604–7609.

17. Feig JE, Pineda-Torra I, Sanson M, Bradley MN, Ven- grenyuk Y, Bogunovic D, *et al.* LXR promotes the maximal egress of monocyte-derived cells from mouse aortic plaques during atherosclerosis regression. J Clin Invest 2010; 120:4415–4424.

18. Li X, Yeh V, Molteni V. Liver X receptor modulators: A review of recently patented compounds (2007–2009). Ex- pert Opin Ther Pat 2010;20:535–562.

19. Loren J, Huang Z, Laffitte BA, Molteni V. Liver X receptor modulators: A review of recently patented compounds (2009–2012). Expert Opin Ther Pat 2013;23: 1317–1335.

Chapter 10

Systemic Factors Mediate Reversible Age-Associated Brain Dysfunction

Brain function declines in aging mammals. Recent work has identified dysregulation of key blood-borne factors whose altered expression during aging diminishes brain function in mice. Increased C-C motif chemokine 11 (CCL11) expression with aging is detrimental to brain function. On the other hand, plasma levels of the trophic factor growth/differentiation factor 11 (GDF11) decrease with aging. Restoration of youthful levels of GDF11 by injection partially restores brain function and neurogenesis by improving endothelial cell function and vasculature. Moreover, GDF11 has a rejuvenative effect on cardiac and skeletal muscle. Decreased type II interferon (IFN-II) and increased type I interferon (IFN-I) signaling during aging at the choroid plexus (CP), which constitutes the brain–cerebrospinal fluid barrier (B-CSF-B), negatively effects brain function. Blood from young mice contains factors that restore IFN-II levels. IFN-II is required for maintenance of the CP, and low IFN-II levels are associated with decreased cognitive abilities. IFN-I levels appear to drive increased CCL11 expression through the CSF. Blood from young animals does not restore IFN-I levels.

However, injecting anti-interferon-α/β receptor (IFNAR) antibodies into the CSF inhibits downstream IFN-I gene and protein expression and decreases expression of CCL11, partially restoring neurogenesis and cognitive function. These results suggest that IFN-I plays a critical role in increasing CCL11 during aging of the brain. An emerging theme is that aging-associated loss of function in mammals may involve a set of defined, potentially reversible changes in many tissues and organs, including the brain, permitting development of potential rejuvenative therapies.

Introduction

Aging-associated loss of function in mammals seems to involve a set of defined, potentially reversible changes in many tissues and organs, including the brain. Cognitive function/memory and neurogenesis in the sub-ventricular zone (SVZ) of the lateral vesicles and sub-granular zones (SGZ) of the hippocampus diminish with increasing age. So-called "heterochronic parabiosis," in which the circulatory systems of old and young mice are interconnected, have been used to demonstrate several key factors whose altered expression leads to diminished cognitive function with age.

The most important identified brain factors so far include C-C motif chemokine 11 (CCL11) and growth/differentiation factor 11 (GDF11). CCL11 increases in the plasma and cerebrospinal fluid (CSF) of aging mice and humans and causes impaired learning and memory, at least in young mice—likely a conserved effect. [1] The plasma concentration of GDF11 decreases with age, and treatment of old mice with GDF11, known to promote endothelial cell function and vasculature integrity, [2] increases cognition and neurogenesis in old mice. So far these two key effectors appear to exert their effects on the brain by affecting supportive or auxiliary tissue. CCL11 is an immune/inflammatory regulator, and GDF11 maintains the cerebral vasculature. Interestingly, GDF11 has also been shown to play a potential rejuvenative role in heart [3,4] and skeletal muscle [5]. Other unknown plasma-borne factors in young blood lead to phosphorylation and activation of the cAMP response element-binding protein (CREB), which contributes to partial rejuvenation of cognitive activity in old mice [6]. An emerging theme emerges from this pioneering work—supporting tissue, such as blood vessels and the immune system, plays a key role in the aging of diverse organs.

Type I Interferon Genes Are Induced in the Choroid Plexus of Old Mice and People, Adversely Impacting Cognitive Function

In an important paper that extends understanding of the connection between the immune and central nervous systems, Baruch *et al.* show that abnormal induction of type I interferon (IFN-I) signaling in the choroid plexus (CP) is linked to diminished cognition and reduced neurogenesis. [7] IFN-I signaling is mediated by IFNs-α and –βbeta. The CP, a mono- layer of epithelial cells, produces the CSF and forms the brain–CSF barrier (B-CSF-B). The B-CSF-B integrates signals from the brain and circulation by controlling translocation of macromolecules between the circulation and the brain.

Baruch *et al.* used RNA sequencing to investigate differences between organs and tissues from young (3-months-old) and old (22-months-old) mice. All tissues examined showed aging-related changes, but only the CP showed an increase in genes corresponding to IFN-I signaling (*irf7, ifn-beta, ifit1*). [7] One interpretation of this result might be that the old mice have had chronic viral brain infections, because IFN-I is known to be induced by viral infection. However, the authors hypothesize that the increased IFN-I gene expression levels are associated with aging. To support this idea, they showed that different groups of mice in different animal centers all show the increased IFN-I response. At the same time, further investigation revealed a decrease in expression of genes involved in the type II interferon (IFN-II) response (*icaml, cxcl10, ccl17*). These data argue against a localized viral infection inducing IFN-I just in the investigators' mice, but by themselves do not rule out the possibility that older mice could have a greater propensity for viral infections in the brain and CP. To strengthen their argument, Baruch *et al.* also stained brain sections from humans, who died without apparent brain disease, for expression of IFN-I proteins. They observed an increase in an IFN-I–associated protein expression pattern in the CP of old people [7].

To test whether factors in the circulation were involved in the altered expression of IFN-I and IFN-II, heterochronic parabiosis experiments, in which the circulatory systems of old and young mice were surgically joined, were performed. Such experiments have shown previously that the blood of young mice increases cognition and neurogenesis of old partners, and that the blood of old mice reduces neurogenesis and cognition in young parabionts

[1,2,6]. Here, the blood of old mice did not increase IFN-I signaling in the CP of young mice, suggesting that factors that increase IFN-I signaling are not present in the circulation. However, the blood from the old mice did diminish expression of IFN-II genes (mediated primarily by IFN-c), which resulted in increased expression of CCL11, a chemokine whose expression has been reported to impair neuronal plasticity. Consistent with the possibility that the blood of young mice has factors to maintain IFN-II levels is that blood from young parabionts restored IFN-II levels in old partners with one exception. Young blood did not reduce increased levels of IFN-II–associated CCL11 expression in old parabionts. These data suggest that there is more to increased CCL11 expression in old animals than the simple proposed model [8] wherein CCL11 is induced by IL-4 in the absence of significant levels of IFN-γ.

Young blood did not reduce IFN-I expression to normal levels. Moreover, induction of IFN-I is unlikely to be mediated by blood-borne factors. To test the possibility that IFN-I induction is dependent on factors in the CSF, primary cultures of CP cells were exposed to CSF from old and young mice. Only CSF from old mice induced IFN-I–dependent genes, suggesting that CSF-borne factors were responsible [7].

The authors propose the simple idea that in old mice, in- creased IFN-I levels, especially IFN-β, induced by CSF-borne factors, causes reduced IFN-II expression levels, resulting in increased CCL11 expression and subsequent reduced neurogenesis and cognition (**Figure 10.1**).

They promote this model because it is known that chronic IFN-I signaling can interfere with IFN-II-mediated inflammation resolution in infection [9–11]. However, the parabiosis experiments in which IFN-II is regulated independently of IFN-I in aged animals suggests that this model is too simple. Nevertheless, Baruch *et al.* demonstrate the importance of IFN-II expression by showing that mutant mice with deficient IFN-II signaling, both via a IFN-γ receptor knockout or Tbx21 null mice (which are deficient in CD4+ cell–derived IFN-γ) have memory and spatial learning defects as well as reduced neurogenesis. IFN-γ has been re- ported to be a trophic factor for the CP,12 and mice deficient in IFN-II signaling also had reduced CP function, including reduced leukocyte trafficking.

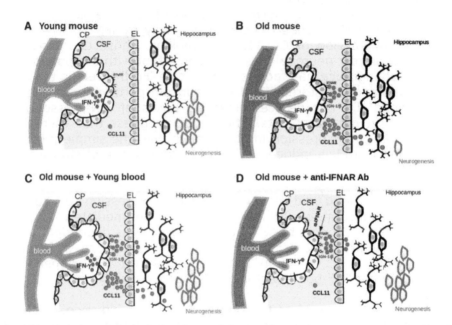

Figure 10.1 Young blood and anti-interferon receptor antibody partially restore cognition and neurogenesis in old mice. (A) In young mice, factors in young blood and stromal interferon-γ (IFN-γ) help maintain choroid plexus (CP) function. (B) During aging, type I interferon (IFN-I) gene expression increases, type II interferon (IFN-II) decreases, and the CP produces C-C motif chemokine 11 (CCL11), which results in reduced leukocyte trafficking, affecting brain function. Both neurogenesis and cognitive abilities decline. (C) In heterochronic parabiosis, young blood (red) from the young parabiont partially restores cognition and neurogenesis. IFN-II signaling is also restored. However, CCL11 and IFN-I expression remain elevated. (D) In old mice, injection with an antibody to interferon-a/b receptor (IFNAR) in the cerebrospinal fluid (CSF), blocked IFN-I signaling, reduced CCL11 levels to normal, and partially restored CP function and brain plasticity, resulting in increased neurogenesis and cognitive ability. Red, young blood; brown, old blood; dark red, CCL11; magenta, IFN-I signal regulators; blue, IFN-γ; CP, choroid plexus; CSF, cerebrospinal fluid; EL, ependymal cell layer; IFNAR, interferona/β receptor; α-IFNAR; IGN-1/β.

Regardless of their model for IFN-I/II interaction in the CP of old animals, it is possible that IFN-I itself may have detrimental effects on brain function and neurogenesis. In- deed, exposure of CP epithelial cells in culture decreased expression of the neurotrophic factors insulin-like growth factor 1 (IGF-1) and bone-derived neurotrophic factor (BDNF). Furthermore, when an inhibitory anti-interferon receptor antibody (interferon-α/β receptor [α-IFNAR]) is injected into the CSF of mice, levels of IGF-I and BDNF are increased and CCL11 levels are decreased to normal levels.

Baruch *et al.* then investigated effects on cognition and neurogenesis. However, they report experiments in which they were forced to select cognitively impaired mice. Apparently many mice were actually cognitively normal when tested with a novel location recognition task, wherein an object is moved and the amount of time spent with the moved object is evaluated 24 hours later (increased time indicates better memory and cognition). As hypothesized the anti-α-IFNAR antibody raised scores on the task and increased neurogenesis. As might be expected increased expression of interleukin-10 (IL-10), an anti-inflammatory cytokine, was observed as well as reduced inflammation/ damage of astrocytes and microglia [7]. These results are consistent with a detrimental role for chronic IFN-I signaling on CP function and on brain function. It would have been interesting to compare the IFN-I and IFN-II expression levels in the cognitively normal old mice with the cognitively challenged mice to help prove a possible association. Also, Baruch *et al.* did not show that inhibiting IFN-I signaling restored normal IFN-II signaling, with the exception of CCL11 levels, which given the data in Baurch *et al.* are clearly not dependent on IFN-II alone.

It is important to recognize that the source of inflammatory IFN-I signaling in the CSF has not been identified. Discovery of the source of chronic signaling should be a priority. Moreover, there is a formal possibility that the increased IFN-I in old mice and people results from old mammals being more prone to chronic low-level viral infection in the brain/CSF than younger mammals. Perhaps the heterogeneity in cognitive ability in the old genetically identical mouse population is due to infection status rather than aging *per se*. The role of endogenous retroviruses should also be studied given recent work connecting these agent to autoimmune processes [13]. Of related interest is that retrotransposon activation, which might be expected to activate IFN-I response, has been reported to be associated with aging in several systems, including mice [14-18].

Medical Implications

Although Baruch *et al.* did not completely succeed in completely linking reciprocal IFN-I and IFN-II dysregulation to each other during aging, they make a strong case that both IFN-II and IFN-I signaling plays a role in diminished CP function and cognitive decline in aging. That each effect is reversible increases the possibility that successful rejuvenation may be achieved by simultaneously addressing each defect. That IFN-I plays a significant role in brain dysfunction might be predicted from genetic neurological diseases associated with elevated IFN-a expression, such as Aicardi-Goutieres syndrome (AGS) [19].

The work of Baruch *et al.* needs to verified and extended and more carefully combined with studies that have identified other non-immune factors that affect the aging brain, such as GDF11, which effects brain vasculature. Perhaps there are analogous factors to GDF11 that affect the structural integrity of the ventricular system and the subarachnoid space.

IFN-I dysfunction and CCL11 over expression are not affected by the blood of young parabionts. An interesting implication is that factors from young blood will be not enough to achieve full rejuvenation of the brain, even after identification and purification, because other factors from other reservoirs must also be modulated. However, at least one biotech startup is pursuing anti-aging therapeutics based on injection of factors from the blood of young humans. Even if IFN-I dysregulation is shown to be a major source of age-associated brain dysfunction, it is unlikely that anti-α-IFNAR will be investigated or approved as an anti-aging treatment, given the problematic regulatory and industry environment for anti-aging therapies.

Conclusion

Increased IFN-I and decreased IFN-II signaling at the CP decrease function of the B-CSF-B, which in turn negatively affects brain function. Such dysregulation is exemplary of a class of aging-associated bio-molecular changes that are potentially reversible. Dysregulation in the form of over- or under-expression of cytokines, growth factors, hormones, and metabolites in the blood and fluids, as well as altered expression of other signaling molecules on cell surfaces critical for cell–cell interactions, may be responsible for many detrimental changes associated with aging. Aging-associated changes in cells that play a supporting role in tissue/organ function seem to be especially prominent. Each dysregulated biomolecule presents a potential target for rejuvenation.

References

1. Villeda SA, Luo J, Mosher KI, Zou B, Britschgi M, Bieri G, Stan TM, Fainberg N, Ding Z, Eggel A, Lucin KM, Czirr E, Park J-S, Couillard-Despre´s S, Aigner L, Li G, Peskind ER, Kaye JA, Quinn JF, Galasko DR, Xie XS, Rando TA, Wyss-Coray T. The ageing systemic milieu negatively reg- ulates neurogenesis and cognitive function. Nature 2011;477: 90–94.

2. Katsimpardi L, Litterman NK, Schein PA, Miller CM, Loffredo FS, Wojtkiewicz GR, Chen JW, Lee RT, Wagers AJ, Rubin LL. Vascular and neurogenic rejuvenation of the aging mouse brain by young systemic factors. Science 2014;344:630–634.

3. Loffredo FS, Steinhauser ML, Jay SM, Gannon J, Pancoast JR, Yalamanchi P, Sinha M, Dall'Osso C, Khong D, Sha- drach JL, Miller CM, Singer BS, Stewart A, Psychogios N, Gerszten RE, Hartigan AJ, Kim MJ, Serwold T, Wagers AJ, Lee RT. Growth differentiation factor 11 is a circulating factor that reverses age-related cardiac hypertrophy. Cell 2013;153:828–839.

4. Mendelsohn AR, Larrick JW. Rejuvenation of aging hearts. Rejuvenation Res 2013;16:330–332.

5. Sinha M, Jang YC, Oh J, Khong D, Wu EY, Manohar R, Miller C, Regalado SG, Loffredo FS, Pancoast JR, Hirsh- man MF, Lebowitz J, Shadrach JL, Cerletti M, Kim MJ, Serwold T, Goodyear LJ, Rosner B, Lee RT, Wagers AJ. Restoring systemic GDF11 levels reverses age-related dysfunction in mouse skeletal muscle. Science 2014;344: 649–652.

6. Villeda SA, Plambeck KE, Middeldorp J, Castellano JM, Mosher KI, Luo J, Smith LK, Bieri G, Lin K, Berdnik D, Wabl R, Udeochu J, Wheatley EG, Zou B, Simmons DA, Xie XS, Longo FM, Wyss-Coray T. Young blood reverses age-related impairments in cognitive function and synaptic plasticity in mice. Nat Med 2014;20:659–663.

7. Baruch K, Deczkowska A, David E, Castellano JM, Miller O, Kertser A, Berkutzki T, Barnett-Itzhaki Z, Bezalel D, Wyss-Coray T, Amit I, Schwartz M. Aging. Aging-induced

type I interferon response at the choroid plexus negatively affects brain function. Science 2014;346:89–93.

8. Baruch K, Ron-Harel N, Gal H, Deczkowska A, Shifrut E, Ndifon W, Mirlas-Neisberg N, Cardon M, Vaknin I, Ca- halon L, Berkutzki T, Mattson MP, Gomez-Pinilla F, Friedman N, Schwartz M. CNS-specific immunity at the choroid plexus shifts toward destructive Th2 inflammation in brain aging. Proc Natl Acad Sci USA 2013;110:2264– 2269.

9. Wilson EB, Yamada DH, Elsaesser H, Herskovitz J, Deng J, Cheng G, Aronow BJ, Karp CL, Brooks DG. Blockade of chronic type I interferon signaling to control persistent LCMV infection. Science 2013;340:202–207.

10. Teles RMB, Graeber TG, Krutzik SR, Montoya D, Schenk M, Lee DJ, Komisopoulou E, Kelly-Scumpia K, Chun R, Iyer SS, Sarno EN, Rea TH, Hewison M, Adams JS, Popper SJ, Relman DA, Stenger S, Bloom BR, Cheng G, Modlin RL. Type I interferon suppresses type II interferon-trig- gered human anti-mycobacterial responses. Science 2013; 339:1448–1453.

11. Teijaro JR, Ng C, Lee AM, Sullivan BM, Sheehan KCF, Welch M, Schreiber RD, de la Torre JC, Oldstone MB. Persistent LCMV infection is controlled by blockade of type 1 interferon signaling. Science 2013;340:207–211.

12. Kunis G, Baruch K, Rosenzweig N, Kertser A, Miller O, Berkutzki T, Schwartz M. IFN-c-dependent activation of the brain's choroid plexus for CNS immune surveillance and repair. Brain 2013;136:3427–3440.

13. Tugnet N, Rylance P, Roden D, Trela M, Nelson P. Human endogenous retroviruses (HERVs) and autoimmune rheu- matic disease: Is there a link? Open Rheumatol J 2013;7: 13–21.

14. Sedivy JM, Kreiling JA, Neretti N, De Cecco M, Criscione SW, Hofmann JW, Zhao X, Ito T, Peterson AL. Death by transposition—the enemy within? BioEssays News Rev Mol Cell Dev Biol 2013;35:1035–1043.

15. De Cecco M, Criscione SW, Peckham EJ, Hillenmeyer S, Hamm EA, Manivannan J, Peterson AL, Kreiling JA, Neretti N, Sedivy JM. Genomes of replicatively senescent cells undergo global epigenetic changes leading to gene silencing and activation of transposable elements. Aging Cell 2013;12:247–256.

16. Maxwell PH, Burhans WC, Curcio MJ. Retrotransposition is associated with genome instability during chronological aging. Proc Natl Acad Sci USA 2011;108:20376–20381.

17. Li W, Prazak L, Chatterjee N, Gruninger S, Krug L, Theodorou D, Dubnau J. Activation of transposable ele- ments during aging and neuronal decline in Drosophila. Nat Neurosci 2013;16.

18. Barbot W, Dupressoir A, Lazar V, Heidmann T. Epigenetic regulation of an IAP retrotransposon in the aging mouse: Pro- gressive demethylation and de-silencing of the element by its repetitive induction. Nucleic Acids Res 2002;30:2365–2373.

19. Hofer MJ, Campbell IL. Type I interferon in neurological disease-the devil from within. Cytokine Growth Factor Rev 2013;24:257–267.

Chapter 11

Prolonged Fasting/Re-feeding Promotes Hematopoietic Stem Cell Regeneration and Rejuvenation

The sensitivity of hematopoietic stem cells (HSCs) to toxic effects of cancer chemotherapy is one of the major roadblocks in cancer therapy. Moreover, the loss of HSC function in the elderly ("immunosenescence") is a major source of morbidity and mortality. Until recently, it was believed that HSCs were irreversibly damaged by the aging process. Recent work in mice shows that cycles of prolonged fasting (PF) of greater than 72 hr followed by re-feeding can protect HSCs from the toxicity associated with chemotherapy and stimulate the proliferation of and rejuvenate old HSCs. A preliminary phase I trial in humans suggests that PF may confer benefit to people undergoing chemotherapy. These effects are at least partially mediated by lowered insulin-like growth factor-1 levels in the blood and stem cell microenvironment, which leads to lowered protein kinase A (PKA) activity. Reducing PKA levels or activity can replicate at least some of the effects of PF on HSCs. Shorter periods of fasting were not effective. PF represents a potentially profound, low-tech means to enhance cancer treatment and reverse aging of the immune system in the elderly. Because PF is likely to be stressful to the old and fragile, the development of PF mimetics may be warranted.

Introduction

Cancer chemotherapy is often limited by toxicity that can lead to substantial morbidity and mortality. Chemotherapeutic drug dosage needs to be carefully maintained within tolerable limits. Many of the detrimental effects of chemotherapy and radiation result from damage to the immune system. Hematopoietic stem cells (HSCs), which are the population of cells from which all immune cells originate, are particularly sensitive to chemotherapy because they proliferate both to maintain themselves and to populate the immune system by differentiation into progenitors and terminally differentiated cells, which include lymphocytes and myeloid cells. Immunosuppression from chemotherapy is a major medical problem [1, 2].

Immunosenescence, associated with aging of the immune system, shares many of the characteristics of immunosuppression resulting from chemotherapy. These include fewer numbers of lymphocytes, a bias toward myeloid cells, and reduced regenerative capacity of old HSCs [3]. Old HSCs were believed to be irreversibly damaged by insults associated with aging, including DNA damage from increased reactive oxygen species (ROS); however, recent work has suggested that it is possible to rejuvenate HSCs, for example, by altering gene expression of sirtui 3 (SIRT3), reducing ROS, or inhibiting the mechanistic target of rapamycin (mTOR) [4]. These results suggest that other ways may exist to rejuvenate HSCs.

Prolonged fasting (PF) (of greater than 72 hours) before and during chemotherapy has been reported to reduce toxicity due to chemotherapy in mice by Longo's group at the University of Southern California (USC) by a mechanism that involved lowering insulin-like growth factor-1 (IGF-1). However, the mechanisms and critical cell types remained uncharacterized. A recent report by this group extends these results and uncovers PF as a general way to potentially effect rejuvenation of the immune system [7].

PF/Re-feeding Restores Normal HSC Function and Protects HSCs from Chemotherapy

In a potentially very important paper, Cheng *et al.* [7] report that multiple cycles of PF (greater than 72 hr) followed by re-feeding reduce IGF-1 levels and protein kinase A (PKA) activity to protect HSCs from the detrimental effects of chemotherapy in mice [7]. These results may translate to humans because PF appeared to protect people from chemo- toxicity in a small phase I clinical trial. Moreover, PF eliminated the old age–associated differentiation bias of HSCs toward the myeloid lineage.

Drugs used in cancer chemotherapy, such as doxorubicin, etoposide, or cyclophosphamide (CP), induce DNA damage in proliferating cells, preferentially killing them [8]. Such drugs are often effective against rapidly proliferating cancer cells, but they also damage normal dividing cells. It had been previously observed by the same research group that PF protected normal cells and mice from cell death [8, 9]. In this report, these researchers focus on HSCs. One of the consequences of chemotherapy is immunosuppressive toxicity, which results from damage to HSCs and their progeny. After six rounds of fasting (3 days), treatment with CP, followed by feeding (11 days), bone marrow–derived HSCs separated by fluorescence-activated cell sorting (FACS) on the basis of characteristic cell-surface markers showed diminished apoptosis by terminal deoxynucleotidyl transferase dUTP nick end labeling (TUNEL) (which detects double-stranded breaks) and annexin V assays (which detect repositioning of annexin V to the extracellular face of the plasma membrane during apoptosis) than well-fed (*ad libitum*) controls treated with CP at the same time intervals. Interestingly, short-term fasting of 24 hr had no protective effect. PF effectively blocked HSC cell death associated with chemotherapy [7].

Analysis of hematological profiles showed that white blood cell (WBC) counts, especially of lymphocytes, initially dropped after each dose of CP, suggesting that proliferating WBCs were killed by the chemotherapy, regardless of PF. However, by the fourth cycle of chemotherapy, animals receiving PF had higher numbers of lymphocytes than the *ad libitum*–fed mice. By the sixth cycle of chemotherapy and PF, animals undergoing PF had normal levels of lymphocytes and normal ratios of lymphocytes to myeloid cells, unlike *ad libitum*–fed mice, which showed no recovery of lymphocytes with an abnormally low ratio of lymphocytes to myeloid cells (L/M). Self-renewing long- term HSCs (LT-HSCs), which are Lin-Sca-1+ -c-Kit+, CD48-,

CD150+, can be distinguished from short-term HSCs (ST-HSC), which are Lin-Sca-1 + -c-Kit+, CD48-, CD150-, by differential expression of cell-surface proteins, in this case CD150. FACS analysis indicated that numbers of LT-HSCs and ST-HSCs were better preserved in the animals receiving PF. To confirm that the HSCs retained function, similar numbers of bone marrow cells from mice receiving CP with and without PF were transplanted into mice immunocompromised by irradiation with competing bone marrow cells from mice that did not receive chemotherapy. Cells from the experimental donors and competitors were marked genetically with different CD45 alleles. Cells from mice treated with PF competed effectively with the cells from mice that had not received chemotherapy, whereas cells that were fed *ad libitum* did not compete well. The PF-derived HSCs had higher regeneration capacity than the ad libitum–fed mice, and hematological profile analysis showed that PF HSCs reconstituted the immune system with a normal L/M cell ratio [7].

Cheng *et al.* investigated whether PF affected HSC function more generally than just protection from chemotoxicity. PF resulted in a six-fold increase in the number of HSCs that completed DNA replication by measuring incorporation of the nucleotide analog bromodeoxyuridine (BrdU) into DNA. These correlated with increased numbers of LT-HSCs, ST-HSCs, and multipotent progenitors (MPPs) observed by FACS. Interestingly, PF did not result in increased numbers of total bone marrow cells, nor of the total number of progenitor cells, for example, common myeloid or common lymphoid progenitors. FACS-based cell cycle analysis was consistent with the idea that PF stimulated LT- HSCs, ST-HSCs, and MPPs to enter the cell cycle. Apoptotic cell death rates, which are low for HSCs, were reduced even further by PF. The conclusion is that PF stimulates cell cycle entry and subsequent proliferation of HSCs to effect self-renewal [7].

Old animals have reduced immune function ("immunosenescence") that is thought to result from irreversible damage to DNA. However, recent work has shown that it is possible to rejuvenate old HSCs by ectopic expression of SIRT3 or treatment with the antioxidant N-acetylcysteine (NAC) [4, 5]. HSCs from old mice have limited regenerative ability and become myeloid biased, resulting in fewer lymphoid cells, more myeloid cells, and overall fewer white blood cells. Relatively old mice (18-months) were subjected to numerous cycles of PF and re-feeding. After eight cycles of PF, myeloid bias was eliminated, and the L/M ratio was similar to that of young animals fed ad libitum. Moreover, total WBCs were restored to levels of young animals. Repeated PF appears to rejuvenate old HSCs [7]. Unfortunately, Cheng *et al.* did not measure the regenerative capacity of the rejuvenated HSCs, which would have been helpful to assess the extent of the rejuvenation.

Previous work by this group showed that PF reduces IGF-1 levels and that low IGF-1 levels protect mice from chemo-toxicity [9]. To model conditions of reduced IGF-1, Cheng *et al.* used growth hormone knockout mice (GHRKO), which express low levels of IGF-1 in the serum and bone marrow. CP-induced apoptosis was reduced in GHRKO mice similar to levels seen by PF treatment in wild-type mice. HSC number was preserved in

GHRKO mice after chemotherapy. Similar to PF mice, old GHRKO mice had higher numbers of HSCs than wild-type mice and no myeloid bias, suggesting that IGF-1 signaling plays a key role in PF-mediated chemo-protecton and rejuvenation [7]. Stronger proof of the role of IGF-1 in PF could have been established using either antibodies or conditional genetic inactivation to block IGF-1 in adult mice using similar kinetic to the PF experiments. However, Cheng *et al.* did perform the reverse experiment of adding exogenous IGF-1 during PF treatment. In animals not undergoing chemotherapy, IGF-1 blunted both the PF-induced increase of HSCs and the enhanced regenerative capacity of PF-treated HSCs in young animals [7]. IGF-1 clearly plays an important role in PF chemo- protection and rejuvenation.

To assess whether the stem cell microenvironment was involved, bone marrow stromal niche cells (Lin-CD45 -) from PF or ad libitum–fed mice were isolated and co- cultured with LT-HSCs from PF or ad libitum–fed mice. PF-treated niche cells promoted the survival and proliferation of LT-HSCs from both PF-treated and *ad libitum*–fed mice, suggesting that PF changes to the stem cell microenvironment are sufficient to alter HSC function [7].

Analysis of their previously published microarray data [10,11] led Cheng *et al.* to identify PKA catalytic subunit a (PKACα) as reduced in all tested tissue of PF mice. PKA phosphorylates the transcription factor cAMP response element-binding protein (CREB) at Ser-133 to form active p-CREB. Western blots showed that PF reduces p-CREB levels, whereas IGF receptor (IGF-1R) expression was unaffected, suggesting that PKA activity was reduced by PF [7]. PKA is known to have a conserved pro-aging activity [12,13]. Inhibition of PKA protects yeast and mammalian cells from peroxide-induced oxidative stress [14].

PKA positively regulates CREB and G9a, which promote hematopoietic lineage commitment and differentiation, [15,16] and negatively regulates transcription factor Foxo1, which promotes HSC self-renewal and stress resistance [17,18] (**Figure 11.1**).

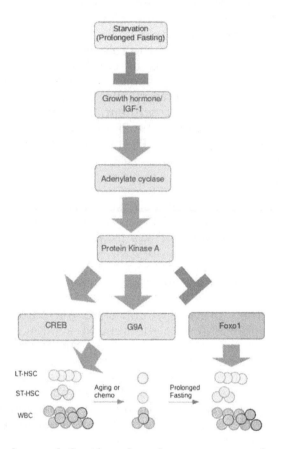

Figure 11.1. Prolonged fasting involves suppression of insulin-like growth factor-1 (IGF-1) signaling and stimulation of FOXO1. Prolonged fasting reduces IGF-1 levels, which in turn lower activity of adneylate cyclase, protein kinase A (PKA), and its downstream effectors cAMP response element-binding protein (CREB) and G9a (G9A). Reduced PKA activity relieves repression of transcription factor FOXO1, which helps stimulate self-renewal of long-term hematopoietic stem cells (LT-HSCs) and short-term hematopoietic stem cells (ST-HSCs) and restoration of youthful white blood cells (WBCs).

G9a H3 Lys-9 methyltransferase is an epigenome modifier. PF reduced IGF-1/pAKT and PKA/pCREB signaling, resulting in increased Foxo1 and reduced G9a expression. Because inhibition of mTOR is also known to increase HSC maintenance and self-renewal,6 and caloric restriction results in reduced mTOR activity, the effects of mTOR inhibition by rapamycin were explored. Contrary to previous studies, rapamycin did not induce HSC proliferation, [19, 20] possibly due to the shorter time period of the experiment. However, in cultured HSCs, rapamycin potentiated the ability of RNA knockdown of PKA to stimulate proliferation of ST-HSC and MPPs. Interestingly, rapamycin and RNA knockdown (using small interfering RNA [siRNA]) of PKA did not result in the increase of LT-HSC, which are induced by either PF or by anti-PKA siRNA. Knockdown of the IGF-1 receptor IGF-1R also increased ST-HSCs and MPPs, but not LT-HSCs. PF should reduce mTOR activity, which was not measured, thus these results suggest that the effect of PF is actually more complex than the model pro- posed by Cheng *et al.* PF is clearly causing an effect that is at least partially dependent on reduced IGF-1 and PKA activity, but other as yet uncharacterized changes are likely significant. On the other hand, treating HSCs with siRNA targeting IGF-1R or PKA resulted in increased bone marrow regenerative capacity in the competition bone marrow re- constitution assay similar to that seen with PF. The in- creased regenerative capacity of HSCs by PF can be at least partially reproduced by more focused alterations relating to IGF-1 signaling.

The question of whether these results translate to humans is paramount. Preliminary results on the chemo-protective ability of PF in a phase I clinical trial indicate that 72 hr of PF, but not short-term fasting of 24hr, correlate with maintenance of normal lymphocyte counts and lineage balance. While encouraging, the effects of PF on preventing chemo-toxicity need to be performed on larger numbers of people. A phase II clinical trial is in progress. Exploration of whether PF can alter immunosenescence associated with aging in humans would be of great interest as well.

The results of Cheng *et al.* are potentially of great significance both as a means to prevent toxicity seen with chemotherapy and to the rejuvenation of immune system function in old people. However, much work remains to be performed. These results are surprising, even in light of the conserved roles for PKA and IGF-1/pAKT in stress protection and earlier studies linking dietary restriction to maintenance of a young phenotype in murine HSCs [21]. Not only does nutrient deprivation actually stimulate proliferation, but given that CP damages DNA and kills proliferating cells, the stimulation of HSC proliferation might have been expected to kill the stimulated HSCs. If the reported proliferative effect is confirmed by others, then the benefit of PF probably extends beyond mere stimulation of proliferation to induction of protective mechanisms. Moreover, given that CP kills proliferating cells, the timing of the PF relative to the CP treatment (72 hours after initiating PF and then switching to ad libitum feeding) is probably critical to the success of PF. Perhaps only 24 hours of fasting does not protect against CP because cells are replicating DNA at too high levels at that time point.

Medical Implications

The medical implications of rejuvenation of immune function in the elderly and chemo-protection by PF are potentially profound. However, these results are in need of replication by other groups. Applicability to humans needs to be more firmly established. Fortunately, at least one phase II trial is ongoing to evaluate PF in chemo-protection.

It is important to recognize that PF is different from caloric restriction and alternate-day fasting. Because both have been reported to lower IGF-1 levels, [22] they may be beneficial to maintaining HSC function. Dietary restriction had previously been reported to maintain HSCs in mice [21]. However, neither has been reported to rejuvenate the immune system or

HSCs, and Cheng *et al.* suggest that a 24-hour fasting period (such as that used in alternate-day fasting) is insufficient for rejuvenation or chemo-protection. The role and kinetics of re-feeding need to be established. It is interesting that both the stem cell niche cells and the HSCs appear capable of at least some rejuvenating effects. The mechanisms underlying the rejuvenative/chemo-protective effects of PF need to be elucidated further. For example, is expression of growth differentiation factor-11 (GDF11), a factor known to promote rejuvenation in the heart, skeletal muscle, and the brain, [23–25] increased?

Of great interest to human aging are questions relating to the extent of rejuvenation of immunosenescent HSCs. Do HSCs from old animals subjected to eight or more cycles of PF have increased regenerative capacity? This experiment should be relatively easy to perform, and the results telling. Will this rejuvenation effect carry over to humans? What effect does rejuvenation have on telomere length? Is telomerase activated?

If not, functional rejuvenation could lead to telomere-based replicative senescence as they shorten with each round of proliferation. How many other stem cell populations respond similarly to increase proliferation and maintain stem cell populations? Most mammalian tissues, excluding the brain, are known to shrink in response to fasting, then repopulate after feeding. Are stem cell numbers actually increasing as overall numbers of differentiated cells decrease? Are any tissues negatively impacted by PF?

The safety of PF needs to be investigated. PF should probably be avoided by diabetics and the very old, even though they might be among those who could benefit most. One potential problem is that fasting may reinforce cachexia. Moreover, there is a fundamental question that needs to be answered. Will PF select for survival of cancer stem cells that are capable of quiescence and contribute to in- creased number of dormant cancer cells? It appears that conventional tumor cells can be negatively impacted by fasting, [11] but dormant cancer stem cells have been associated in some cases with poor prognoses [26, 27]. If so, PF might accelerate the progression of some cancers, especially those that appear to generate cancer stem cells capable of quiescence.

Chemotherapy can be mutagenic. Increased numbers of cancer stem cells can be problematic because they are almost completely resistant to currently available therapeutics. The effects of prolonged fasting cannot be estimated because cancer dormancy and the role of quiescence in cancer stem cell physiology are poorly understood. Protection from the harmful side effects of radiotherapy should be investigated as well.

Conclusion

PF represents a potentially powerful means to protect against the ravages of chemotherapy, perhaps even allowing higher doses of drugs. PF appears to be a way to rejuvenate the immune systems of the elderly. Immune dysfunction in old age often leads to significant morbidity and mortality. If the ability of PF to rejuvenate immunosenesced HSCs is confirmed in humans, great utility could result. Furthermore, elucidation of the mechanisms that underlie HSC chemo-protection and rejuvenation could lead to the development of drugs that would be more suitable for the treatment of fragile, elderly individuals than 72 hours of fasting. Major questions remain concerning how general the effects of PF are and whether there are any detrimental effects. The development of rejuvenative therapies is in their infancy, but these results suggest that a large number of interventions may be developed in the near future.

References

1. Bedford P, Berger MR, Eisenbrand G, Schmahl D. The level of DNA interstrand crosslinking in bone marrow parallels the extent of myelosuppression in mice treated with four chloroethylnitrosoureas. J Cancer Res Clin Oncol 1984;108:141–147.
2. Yahata T, Takanashi T, Muguruma Y, Ibrahim AA, Mat- suzawa H, Uno T, Sheng Y, Onizuka M, Ito M, Kato S, Ando K. Accumulation of oxidative DNA damage restricts the self-renewal capacity of human hematopoietic stem cells. Blood 2011;118:2941–2950.
3. Fulop T, Le Page A, Fortin C, Witkowski JM, Dupuis G, Larbi A. Cellular signaling in the aging immune system. Curr Opin Immunol 2014;29C:105–111.
4. Brown K, Xie S, Qiu X, Mohrin M, Shin J, Liu Y, Zhang D, Scadden DT, Chen D. SIRT3 reverses aging-associated degeneration. Cell Rep 2013;3:319–327.
5. Mendelsohn AR, Larrick JW. Rejuvenation of adult stem cells: Is age-associated dysfunction epigenetic? Rejuvenation Res 2013;16:152–157.
6. Chen C, Liu Y, Liu Y, Zheng P. mTOR regulation and therapeutic rejuvenation of aging hematopoietic stem cells. Sci Signal 2009;2:ra75.
7. Cheng C-W, Adams GB, Perin L, Wei M, Zhou X, Lam BS, Da Sacco S, Mirisola M, Quinn DI, Dorff TB, Kopchick JJ, Longo VD. Prolonged fasting reduces IGF-1/PKA to promote hematopoietic-stem-cell-based regeneration and reverse immunosuppression. Cell Stem Cell 2014;14:810– 823.
8. Raffaghello L, Lee C, Safdie FM, Wei M, Madia F, Bianchi G, Longo VD. Starvation-dependent differential stress resistance protects normal but not cancer cells against high- dose chemotherapy. Proc Natl Acad Sci USA 2008; 105: 8215–8220.
9. Lee C, Safdie FM, Raffaghello L, Wei M, Madia F, Parrella E, Hwang D, Cohen P, Bianchi G, Longo VD. Reduced levels of IGF-I mediate differential protection of normal and cancer cells in response to fasting and improve chemotherapeutic index. Cancer Res 2010; 70:1564–1572.
10. Guevara-Aguirre J, Balasubramanian P, Guevara-Aguirre M, Wei M, Madia F, Cheng C-W, Hwang D, Martin- Montalvo A, Saavedra J, Ingles S, de Cabo R, Cohen P, Longo VD. Growth hormone receptor deficiency is associated with a major reduction in pro-aging signaling, cancer, and diabetes in humans. Sci Transl Med 2011; 3: 70ra13–70ra13.
11. Lee C, Raffaghello L, Brandhorst S, Safdie FM, Bianchi G, 21. Martin-Montalvo A, Pistoia V, Wei M, Hwang S, MerlinoA, Emionite L, de Cabo R, Longo VD. Fasting cycles retard growth of tumors and sensitize a range of cancer cell types 22. to chemotherapy. Sci Transl Med 2012; 4:124ra27.

12. Fabrizio P, Pozza F, Pletcher SD, Gendron CM, Longo VD. Regulation of longevity and stress resistance by Sch 9 in 23. Science 2001; 292:288–290.

13. Rinaldi J, Wu J, Yang J, Ralston CY, Sankaran B, Moreno S, Taylor SS. Structure of yeast regulatory subunit: A glimpse into the evolution of PKA signaling. Struct Lond Engl 1993 2010;18:1471-1482.

14. Yan L, Vatner DE, O'Connor JP, Ivessa A, Ge H, Chen W, Hirotani S, Ishikawa Y, Sadoshima J, Vatner SF. Type 5 24. adenylyl cyclase disruption increases longevity and protects against stress. Cell 2007; 130:247–258.

15. Yamamizu K, Matsunaga T, Katayama S, Kataoka H, Takayama N, Eto K, Nishikawa S, Yamashita JK. PKA/CREB signaling triggers initiation of endothelial and hematopoietic cell differentiation via Etv2 induction. Stem Cells 2012; 30:687–696.

16. Chen X, Skutt-Kakaria K, Davison J, Ou Y-L, Choi E, Malik P, Loeb K, Wood B, Georges G, Torok-Storb B, Paddison PJ. G9a/GLP-dependent histone H3K9me2 patterning during human hematopoietic stem cell lineage commitment. Genes Dev 2012; 26:2499–2511.

17. Tothova Z, Kollipara R, Huntly BJ, Lee BH, Castrillon DH, Cullen DE, McDowell EP, Lazo-Kallanian S, Williams IR, Sears C, ArmstrongSA, Passegue E, DePinhoRA, Gilliland DG. FoxOs are critical mediators of hematopoietic stem cell resistance to physiologic oxidative stress. Cell 2007; 128:325–339.

18. Zhang X, Yalcin S, Lee D-F, Yeh T-YJ, Lee S-M, Su J, Mungamuri SK, Rimmele´ P, Kennedy M, Sellers R, Landthaler M, Tuschl T, Chi NW, Lemischka I, Keller G, Ghaffari S. FOXO1 is an essential regulator of pluripotency in human embryonic stem cells. Nat Cell Biol 2011; 13: 1092–1099.

19. Nakada D, Saunders TL, Morrison SJ. Lkb1 regulates cell cycle and energy metabolism in haematopoietic stem cells. Nature 2010 ;468:653–658.

20. Yilmaz OH, Katajisto P, Lamming DW, Gultekin Y, Bauer- Rowe KE, Sengupta S, Birsoy K, Dursun A, Yilmaz VO, Selig M, Nielsen GP, Mino-Kenudson M, Zukerberg LR, Bhan AK, Deshpande V, Sabatini DM.

21. Paneth cell niche couples intestinal stem cell function to calorie intake. Nature 2012; 486:490–495.

22. Ertl RP, Chen J, Astle CM, Duffy TM, Harrison DE. Effects of dietary restriction on hematopoietic stem-cell aging are genetically regulated. Blood 2008;111:1709–1716. Anisimov VN, Bartke A. The key role of growth hormone- insulin-IGF-1 signaling in aging and cancer. Crit Rev Oncol Hematol 2013; 87:201–223.

23. Loffredo FS, Steinhauser ML, Jay SM, Gannon J, Pancoast JR, Yalamanchi P, Sinha M, Dall'Osso C, Khong D, Shadrach JL, Miller CM, Singer BS, Stewart A, Psychogios N, Gerszten RE, Hartigan AJ, Kim MJ, Serwold T, Wagers AJ, Lee RT. Growth differentiation factor 11 is a circulating factor that reverses age-related cardiac hypertrophy. Cell 2013;153:828–839.

24. Sinha M, Jang YC, Oh J, Khong D, Wu EY, Manohar R, Miller C, Regalado SG, Loffredo FS, Pancoast JR, Hirsh- man MF, Lebowitz J, Shadrach JL, Cerletti M, Kim MJ, Serwold T, Goodyear LJ, Rosner B, Lee RT, Wagers AJ. Restoring systemic GDF11 levels reverses age-related dysfunction in mouse skeletal muscle. Science 2014; 344: 649–652.

25. Katsimpardi L, Litterman NK, Schein PA, Miller CM, Loffredo FS, Wojtkiewicz GR, Chen JW, Lee RT, Wagers AJ, Rubin LL. Vascular and neurogenic rejuvenation of the aging mouse brain by young systemic factors. Science 2014; 344: 630–634.

26. Facompre N, Nakagawa H, Herlyn M, Basu D. Stem-like cells and therapy resistance in squamous cell carcinomas. Adv Pharmacol San Diego, Calif 2012; 65:235–265.

27. Ichihara E, Kaneda K, Saito Y, Yamakawa N, Morishita K. Angiopoietin1 contributes to the maintenance of cell qui- escence in EVI1(high) leukemia cells. Biochem Biophys Res Commun 2011; 416:239–245.

Chapter 12

Paradoxical Effects Of Antioxidants On Cancer

Antioxidants have had a checkered history concerning their reported ability to prevent or treat cancer. Early studies showing ascorbate had benefit in cancer were followed by more definitive studies that demonstrated no benefit. Recent work suggests that biological context may be key to predicting whether antioxidants impede or even promote tumorigenesis.

In a recent report, antioxidants n-acetylcysteine and Vitamin-E accelerated tumorigenesis of lung cancer in mice. Antioxidants decrease ROS levels, which paradoxically increase the proliferation rate of the lung cancer cells, resulting in greater tumor burdens and reduced survival. Increased proliferation rates result from decreased expression of the genomic watchdog protein p53. In mice lacking p53, neither antioxidant affects tumor growth.

But antioxidants can be used to kill cancer, at least in rodents. High concentrations of "antioxidant" ascorbate, achievable only by injection *in vivo*, result in the production of ascorbate radicals and hydrogen peroxide in the extracellular fluid that kill cancer, but not normal cells. In preliminary human trials, ascorbate reduced toxicity of chemotherapy, but showed no statistical benefit on disease progression. Vitamin C is beneficial, but when it acts as an oxidant.

These studies are consistent with others that suggest that even tumor suppressor genes, such as Nrf2, which stimulate innate cellular stress protection pathways that reduce ROS, can promote cancer progression. Nrf2 is required for the cancer preventive effects of compounds such as sulphoraphane, but Nrf2 can help maintain an aggressive tumor phenotype, by stimulating proliferation and offering protection from chemotherapy.

Context determines whether a specific gene is a tumor enhancer or a suppressor. Such paradoxical behavior creates difficult problems for the development of conventional therapeutics to fight cancer. Personal genomic analysis may provide the means to identify context to avoid the paradoxes and obtain a successful outcome. However, cancer prevention may be more difficult than previously thought.

Introduction

There is a tendency for researchers to view specific biomolecules and drugs as health-promoting, health-neutral, or health-damaging. Unfortunately this perspective is a gross simplification. For example, treatments that initially may help prevent or slow cancer can actually promote the creation or selection of more aggressive cancer cells at later stages of the illness.

Antioxidants are a particularly apt example of a class of substances that are thought to be beneficial. Antioxidants are believed by many to slow aging or the diseases associated with aging such as cancer. It has been widely believed that antioxidants could block reactive oxygen species (ROS)-mediated DNA damage that may contribute to cancer initiation or progression. However, there is limited evidence to support this idea. Studies have shown that antioxidants have, at best, no effect. Beta carotene was actually associated with a small increased risk of lung cancer [1]. At the molecular level, it has been known that ectopic over-expression of oncogenic proteins such as RASV12 mutants cause increased ROS levels. Increased ROS was thought to not only increase a transformed cell's rate of mutation, but drive proliferation. However, at least one group reports that oncogenic RAS only increases ROS levels when over-expressed, but actually decreases ROS when expressed at physiological levels. There has been a large body of work accumulating that suggests that in the correct context, significant ROS levels actually protect animals from cancer and conversely antioxidants support cancer growth (Watson, 2013).

Antioxidants can promote tumor-genesis

In an enlightening paper, Sayin *et al.* [2] show that treatment with antioxidants can actually accelerate lung cancer progression in mice. Their results stand in contrast to some earlier experiments that suggested that high ROS levels play a key role in tumorigenesis. For example, the antioxidant N-acetyl cysteine (NAC) prevented lymphomas in mice in which genome integrity master regulator p53 had been knocked out [3]. By contrast, other data show that stimulation of ROS levels by pro-oxidants or agents that stimulate ROS such as elesclomol, inhibit or kill tumors [4]. Expression of activated oncogenes KRAS, B-RAF or Myc at physiological levels increase expression of anti-oxidant master regulator Nrf2, which lowers ROS levels. Reduction of Nrf2 inhibits KRAS-induced proliferation and tumorigenesis in mice [5].

Savin *et al.* use mice which have been genetically engineered to express the [G12D] Kras oncogene when infected with adenovirus expressing the site-specific recombinase Cre by rearranging the DNA so that the Kras2 [G12D] transcriptional promoter. Within one week, mice develop a range of tumors from mild epithelial hyperplasia to aggressive adenocarcinoma. Treatment with water-soluble NAC or fat-soluble Vitamin E resulted in ~2.8 fold higher tumor burden (% tumor area per lung area) than untreated controls. To determine whether the pro-cancer effect of the antioxidants was coding region is juxtaposed with a limited to tumors triggered by mutant KRAS, a similar experiment was performed in mice with a Cre-inducible B-RAF [V600E] mutation. B-RAF mice develop a greater number of tumors than the Kras [G12D] mice, although the tumors are less aggressive. Treatment with NAC or Vitamin E increased tumor burden ~3.4 fold in the B-RAF [V600E] mice and survival time was reduced 50-60% [2]. Keep in mind that the KRAS and BRAF signaling pathways are linked and are known to interact with each other in a variety of epithelial-derived cancers. Therefore, these models are not as independent as the authors suggest.

As expected, treatment with NAC or Vitamin E reduced ROS in the lungs of the Kras [G12D] and B-RAF [V600E] mice, as determined by the fluorescent redox-sensitive probe CM-H DCFDA. Of interest is that the ROS levels in the lungs were already reduced by about 30% in the mutant mice compared to wild-type control mice, an example of decreased oxidative stress associated with tumorigenesis. Consistent with the reduced ROS, increased ratios of reduced to oxidized glutathione were observed. Reduced amounts of DNA containing 8-oxoguanine, which typically results from oxidative damage, meant that antioxidant-treated Kras [G12D] and B-RAF mice had less DNA damage in their lung cells than untreated animals. Interestingly, wild-type animals had more DNA damage in their lung cells than either of the oncogene mutant mice. In tumor extracts, levels of phosphorylated H2AXSer139 and ATMSer1981, which correlate with DNA damage, were also decreased after antioxidant treatment. Of particular interest, is that cell proliferation increased in the lungs of both strains of mutant mice treated with the antioxidants, as assessed by staining for BRDU incorporation (DNA replication) or phosphorylated histone H3 levels (mitosis). Removing antioxidants one week before assaying proliferation reduced DNA proliferation levels to close to that seen in the untreated mutant mice. In primary fibroblasts cultured from the mice expressing either activated RAS or BRAF, treatment with NAC or a water soluble Vitamin E (Trolox) resulted in increased cell proliferation with no change in apoptosis [2]. In summary, antioxidant treatment resulted in increased proliferation despite reduced ROS and DNA damage levels.

The authors hypothesized that the activity of p53, a key regulator of genomic integrity and cell proliferation, which is known to be activated by ROS, might be reduced. Indeed, p53 protein levels were reduced in extracts from cultured fibroblasts or lung tumors treated with antioxidants.

To more rigorously test their hypothesis, mice with either cre-activatible Kras [G12D] or B-RAF [V600E] were crossed with mice with cre-conditional p53 knockout alleles. After simultaneously activating either KRAS or BRAF and inactivating p53, the antioxidants (NAC or Trolox) no longer affected the degree of cell proliferation in culture or *in vivo*. In a preliminary attempt to demonstrate that p53 plays a similar role in human tumors, antioxidants were observed to increased proliferation in p53+ human lung cancer cell lines. When p53 expression was knocked down using shRNA, antioxidants no longer had any effect on cell proliferation. These experiments link p53 to the tumor promoting activity of antioxidants and support a simple model by the authors that reduction of oxidative stress, reduces DNA damage in turn reducing p53. With decreased p53 surveillance, tumor cell proliferation increases [2]. Although DNA damage was reduced, it would be interesting to examine genomic stability in these lung tumors, as lack of p53 is known to result in increased risk of chromosomal instability.

Treatment with 'antioxidant" ascorbate sensitizes tumors to chemotherapy

Ascorbate, a.k.a. Vitamin C, is an antioxidant with a long history of claims touting health benefits among them fighting cancer. Nobel Prize winning chemist Linus Pauling and his medical colleague Cameron reported anti-cancer effects of high doses of ascorbate delivered both intravenously or orally. However, larger clinical trials with oral ascorbate failed to confirm the earlier studies. Later, there have been several reported case histories describing potential benefit of high doses of intravenous vitamin C in patients with terminal cancer diagnoses [6-11]. Unfortunately, uncontrolled case reports, while interesting are of limited utility in determining *bona fide* efficacy.

Fortuitously, Mark Levine's group recently reported that ascorbate kills cancer cells *in vitro* and in mice by acting as a pro-oxidant through generation of hydrogen peroxide [12]. In a recent phase I/IIa clinical trial that was not designed to show efficacy, high dose intravenous ascorbate treatment reduced toxicity associated with chemotherapy. Ma *et al.* [12] hypothesized that failures of vitamin C in the large clinical trials in the late 1970s were caused by the route of delivery. It turns out that oral supplementation of ascorbate can not achieve plasma concentrations greater than 200 uM due to limited adsorption, transport, and excretion by the kidneys. On the other hand, intravenous delivery of Vitamin C can achieve a peak 10 mM plasma concentration in humans for several hours. This is 50-fold higher than oral delivery [13, 14]. In several earlier papers, Levine and colleagues showed that injection of sufficient ascorbate to attain mM plasma levels, leads to the formation of ascorbate radicals and hydrogen peroxide in extracellular spaces, but not in whole blood of rats and mice [15-17]. Ten mM levels of ascorbate appear to have selective toxicity for several different kinds of cancer cell lines in culture, and slow the growth of xenografts of human glioblastoma, ovarian and pancreatic cancer in mice [17].

Ma *et al.* show that [7] cultured ovarian cell lines were sensitive to 0.3-3.5 mM ascorbate (at least 99% loss of viability), while HIO-80, an immortal non-tumorigenic ovarian epithelial cell line, was nearly insensitive (about 25% loss of viability at 3.5 mM ascorbate, almost no loss of viability at lower concentrations).

Ascorbate-mediated production of hydrogen peroxide is necessary for cell death, as addition of peroxide-scavenging enzyme catalase abrogated cytotoxicity. In at least one ovarian cancer cell line (SHIN3), ascorbate induced significant DNA damage as assessed by increased levels of phosphorylated histone H2AX, which binds to DNA with double-stranded breaks, and the Comet assay, a electrophoresis- based method to detect fragmented DNA [12]. Presumably DNA damage directly or indirectly is due to the hydrogen peroxide.

DNA damage could be increased in an ovarian cell line by treatment with both ascorbate and DNA alkylating agent carboplatin. An even greater amount of DNA damage could be induced by using olaparib to block DNA repair via inhibition of poly-ADP ribose polymerase (PARP), an enzyme that plays a key role in repair of single-stranded DNA breaks. Adding catalase prevented DNA damage by ascorbate, demonstrating that hydrogen peroxide is necessary for ascorbate-mediated cancer killing.

Alone carboplatin or olaparib induced only minor DNA damage at the same experimental concentrations where they cooperated with ascorbate to effectively kill cancer cells [12].

Although the results from the Comet assay might suggest tumor cells die via an apoptotic process, previous work suggests that caspases are not involved, and death is by necrosis and associated with increased autophagy [18-20].

Although, Ma *et al.* did not assess caspase activation in this latest work, they did observe a sharp (60%) drop in ATP levels in the tumor cell line compared to a smaller drop (20%) in the non-transformed ovarian cell line, which is consistent with autophagy playing a role in the tumor-specific death. The authors speculate that the tendency of tumor cells to rely on glycolysis for ATP production, i.e., the Warburg effect, may sensitize the tumor cells to ascorbate by reducing ATP production. Glycolysis is far less efficient at ATP production than oxidative phosphorylation. Low ATP levels can cause metabolic stress and indeed biochemical analysis of key stress and growth regulatory factors ATM, AMPK and mTOR suggest that the cancer cell line, but not the normal cell line is metabolically stressed. Ascorbate treatment results in phosphorylation and activation of ATM within 15 minutes. Downstream AMPK is phosphorylated and thereby activated by ATM, which in turn results in decreased expression of mTOR and phosphorylated mTOR, possibly through activation of TSC2. Decreased expression of mTOR is known to increase autophagy [21, 22].

It should be pointed out that there are significant unknowns in the proposed mechanism of action for high ascorbate acting as a pro-oxidant. The most glaring problem is the lack of identification of a specific mechanism by which high levels of ascorbate lead to formation of the ascorbate radicals and in turn produce hydrogen peroxide in cultured cells and in the extracellular fluid. It is important to understand that intracellular levels of ascorbate are tightly controlled by transporters, so the generation of free radicals takes place outside of the cells. The absence of ascorbate radicals and peroxide in the blood is likely due to the presence of reducing enzymes in red blood cells. Furthermore, the mechanism of cell death is somewhat murky, as the relative roles of DNA damage and ATP depletion have not been determined. For example, Ma *et al.* did not try to increase intracellular ATP during ascorbate treatment to untangle the relative contributions of these effects. Also, the percentage of cells with DNA damage in culture was only about 30% with ascorbate, and 40% with the combination of ascorbate, olaparib, and carboplatin.

A drug combination study was performed in culture using constant ratio design analysis [23] which allows determination of synergism, additivity or antagonism between multiple drugs at constant ratios of drugs. In two ovarian cell lines (OVCAR5 and SHIN3), an additive to synergistic effect was shown for ascorbate and carboplatin at all combination ratios, and at a high ascorbate ratio in the third cell line. Carboplatin did affect normal cells, but independently of ascorbate. Together, this suggests that adding ascorbate to carboplatin allows reduction of carboplatin doses to achieve a similar amount of killing.

In a xenograft model, ascorbate reduced tumor burden. The combination of ascorbate and carboplatin reduced tumor burden more than either alone. The combination of ascorbate and paclitaxel, an anticancer drug that targets microtubules also reduced tumor burden more than the individual compounds. The best combination was ascorbate/paclitaxel/carboplatin, which reduced tumor burden by 94 percent. Paclitaxel and carboplatin are frequently used in combination as standard therapy, so if ascorbate had similar effects in humans, it could augment current standard therapy. At the doses used in this study, none of the drug combinations, nor ascorbate alone demonstrated any toxicity to the liver, kidney or spleen [12].

In a phase 1/2a clinical trial lasting 5 years, 12 patients received paclitaxel and carboplatin and 13 patients received that combination with intravenous ascorbate. Toxicity is graded on a scale from 1 to 5 where 5 is death. The addition of ascorbate reduced Grade 1 and 2 toxicities. There was a statistically insignificant trend toward improvement of survival with mean time of progression increased by 8.5 months. However, this study was too statistically underpowered to truly test for efficacy. The authors suggest that a larger clinical trial designed to test efficacy be undertaken, and we believe that would be a good idea, especially in the context of reducing toxicity of conventional chemotherapy, the mechanism of which remains unidentified [12]. Nevertheless, every clinical trial using intravenous Vitamin C so far has failed to show significant clinical effect compared to preclinical rodent models [24].

There are various potential problems: the short half-life ascorbate in the body, development of resistance by cancer cells, and differences between rodents and people.

Medical Implications

There is no evidence that demonstrates that anti-oxidant supplementation extends lifespan or prevents cancer, at least in studies of large populations (Bjalekvic, 2009). In fact, there are a few studies suggesting that some antioxidants are associated with a small increased risk for cancer.

That Vitamin E or N-acetyl cysteine could spur lung tumor progression, even in an animal model raises an alarm bell. That Vitamin C may have anti-cancer activity, but not as an antioxidant but rather as a pro-oxidant at pharmacological concentrations in extracellular fluids, does not diminish the possibility that antioxidants could play a malignant role in some cancers [26]. However, it is important to recognize that the antioxidant lung cancer story is based only on one study in murine models. Only two antioxidants were examined-- it would be useful to confirm the results using other antioxidants. Unfortunately, direct confirmation in humans will be difficult, and require an indirect epidemiological approach.

More importantly, these studies shed light on the potential paradoxical behavior of drugs and genes in cancer cells, and the difficult problem faced in developing conventional therapeutics to fight cancer. For cancer cells, biological context becomes supremely important. In some situations, genes that
are known to be tumor suppressors can actually promote tumor growth. Nrf2, a master regulator of the oxidative stress protection program, is a tumor suppressor gene, which controls a set of antioxidant enzymes that protect cells from ROS, called "phase II detoxifying enzymes," which may play a role in protecting cells from aging-associated oxidative damage. For example. these Nrf2 stimulated enzymes are known to inhibit the action of carcinogens like benzopyrene which can cause stomach cancer. Mice lacking Nrf2 have a greater incidence of cancer after treatment with benzopyrene (stomach cancer) [27] or N-nitrosobutyl (4-hydroxybutyl)amine (BBN) (bladder cancer) [28]. Agents that protect mice from such cancers, such as oltipraz and sulforaphane require Nrf2 to function. So it appears Nrf2 expression is beneficial, however alternately Nrf2 is strongly activated in many cancers and actually plays a critical role in their tumorigenicity. Expression of physiological levels of oncogenic forms of KRAS, B-RAF, or Myc induces Nrf2, resulting in lowered ROS levels [5]. In a mouse model of pancreatic cancer, genetic inactivation of the Nrf2 pathway inhibits K-Ras [G12D] induced proliferation and tumorigenesis *in vivo*. In pancreatic cancer, Nrf2 has the potential to promote cancer [5]. It has been hypothesized that increased levels of phase II detoxifying enzymes may help confer resistance to chemotherapy associated with pancreatic cancer. So context may be of great importance. Even the ultimate tumor suppressor p53 may sometimes act to help cancer cells resist treatment [29]. Paradoxically, w.t. p53 is sometimes associated with worse outcome in breast cancer [30]. Some breast cancer cells carrying w.t. p53 temporarily stop dividing after treatment with DNA damaging drugs such as doxorubicin, protecting them from death via mitotic catastrophe [31]. In lung cancer, w.t. p53 can help protect cancer cells from metabolic stress induced by inhibition of glycolysis by 2-deoxy-glucose [32]. Paradoxically, p53 protects some cancer cells by making them somewhat more normal allowing them to evade therapy.

Analogous to Nrf2, it is quite possible that antioxidants may suppress early stages of cancer initiation, but then promote tumor growth after cancer cells appear; at least in some situations. On the other hand, the presence of exogenous antioxidants has been reported to decrease ROS after exercise [33]: since decreased ROS down regulates stress protective pathways, Nrf2 expression is likely reduced. In the case of antioxidants, it's possible that we have the worst of both worlds: less oxidative damage protection from the potentially more effective phase II detoxifying enzymes with subsequent tumor promotion due to p53 down- regulation.

There are also examples where a beneficial anti-cancer drug can increase tumorigenesis. For example, the BRAF [V600] inhibitors vemurafenib and dabrafenib have been successful in treating melanoma bearing BRAF [V600] mutations. However, these drugs have the ability to paradoxically activate the MAPK pathway through dimerization of wild-type BRAF and there are reports of secondary malignancies in other tissues such as the colon resulting from the treatment [34] (Holderfield, 2014). Even the anti-diabetic drug metformin which is associated with a 40% decreased incidence of cancer in diabetic patients and has significant anti-cancer activity in a variety of preclinical systems may act paradoxically on some cancers. For example, metformin has been reported to promote new blood vessel formation in the ERalpha Negative MDA-MB-435 Breast Cancer Model [35] and increase VEGF-A in several human and mouse melanoma cell lines [36].

The bottom line is that distinguishing between beneficial and detrimental agents in order to prevent cancer may be a difficult task that will strongly depend on genetic predilections. Personal genomic analysis and personalized cancer genome sequencing may provide the means to obtain context to avoid the paradoxes and obtain a successful outcome. However, with these recent data, rationale cancer prevention has become more difficult.

Conclusion

Antioxidants have shown little ability to protect people from cancer. Recent work suggests that antioxidants may even support tumorigenesis in a mouse model of lung cancer. However, much work needs to be done to substantiate and generalize these results. The paradox that potentially helpful agents that prevent damage could actually be harmful in some contexts likely applies to many drugs and specific biomolecules/cellular regulators. Perhaps it is time that we recognize that biomolecules and therapeutics are in some sense beyond good and evil.

References

1. Omenn GS, Goodman GE, Thornquist MD, Balmes J, Cullen MR, Glass A, *et al.* Risk factors for lung cancer and for intervention effects in CARET, the Beta-Carotene and Retinol Efficacy Trial. J Natl Cancer Inst 1996;88:1550–9.
2. Sayin VI, Ibrahim MX, Larsson E, Nilsson JA, Lindahl P, Bergo MO. Antioxidants accelerate lung cancer progression in mice. Sci Transl Med 2014;6:221ra15.
3. Sablina AA, Budanov AV, Ilyinskaya GV, Agapova LS, Kravchenko JE, Chumakov PM. The antioxidant function of the p53 tumor suppressor. Nat Med 2005;11:1306–13.
4. Kirshner JR, He S, Balasubramanyam V, Kepros J, Yang C-Y, Zhang M, *et al.* Elesclomol induces cancer cell apoptosis through oxidative stress. Mol Cancer Ther 2008;7:2319–27.

5. DeNicola GM, Karreth FA, Humpton TJ, Gopinathan A, Wei C, Frese K, et al. Oncogene-induced Nrf2 transcription promotes ROS detoxification and tumorigenesis. Nature 2011;475:106–9.

6. Cameron E, Pauling L. Supplemental ascorbate in the supportive treatment of cancer: Prolongation of survival times in terminal human cancer. Proc Natl Acad Sci U S A 1976;73:3685–9.

7. Cameron E, Pauling L. Supplemental ascorbate in the supportive treatment of cancer: Reevaluation of prolongation of survival times in terminal human cancer*. Proc Natl Acad Sci U S A 1978;75:4538–42.

8. Creagan ET, Moertel CG, O'Fallon JR, Schutt AJ, O'Connell MJ, Rubin J, et al. Failure of high- dose vitamin C (ascorbic acid) therapy to benefit patients with advanced cancer. A controlled trial. N Engl J Med 1979;301:687–90.

9. Moertel CG, Fleming TR, Creagan ET, Rubin J, O'Connell MJ, Ames MM. High-dose vitamin C versus placebo in the treatment of patients with advanced cancer who have had no prior chemotherapy. A randomized double-blind comparison. N Engl J Med 1985;312:137–41.

10. Padayatty SJ, Riordan HD, Hewitt SM, Katz A, Hoffer LJ, Levine M. Intravenously administered vitamin C as cancer therapy: three cases. CMAJ Can Med Assoc J 2006;174:937–42.

11. Drisko JA, Chapman J, Hunter VJ. The use of antioxidants with first-line chemotherapy in two cases of ovarian cancer. J Am Coll Nutr 2003;22:118–23.

12. Ma Y, Chapman J, Levine M, Polireddy K, Drisko J, Chen Q. High-dose parenteral ascorbate enhanced chemosensitivity of ovarian cancer and reduced toxicity of chemotherapy. Sci Transl Med 2014;6:222ra18.

13. Levine M, Conry-Cantilena C, Wang Y, Welch RW, Washko PW, Dhariwal KR, et al. Vitamin C pharmacokinetics in healthy volunteers: evidence for a recommended dietary allowance. Proc Natl Acad Sci U S A 1996;93:3704–9.

14. Padayatty SJ, Sun H, Wang Y, Riordan HD, Hewitt SM, Katz A, et al. Vitamin C pharmacokinetics: implications for oral and intravenous use. Ann Intern Med 2004;140:533–7.

15. Chen Q, Espey MG, Krishna MC, Mitchell JB, Corpe CP, Buettner GR, et al. Pharmacologic ascorbic acid concentrations selectively kill cancer cells: Action as a pro-drug to deliver hydrogen peroxide to tissues. Proc Natl Acad Sci U S A 2005;102:13604–9.

16. Chen Q, Espey MG, Sun AY, Lee J-H, Krishna MC, Shacter E, et al. Ascorbate in pharmacologic concentrations selectively generates ascorbate radical and hydrogen peroxide in extracellular fluid in vivo. Proc Natl Acad Sci 2007;104:8749–54.

17. Chen Q, Espey MG, Sun AY, Pooput C, Kirk KL, Krishna MC, et al. Pharmacologic doses of ascorbate act as a prooxidant and decrease growth of aggressive tumor xenografts in mice. Proc Natl Acad Sci 2008;105:11105–9.

18. Du J, Martin SM, Levine M, Wagner BA, Buettner GR, Wang S, et al. Mechanisms of Ascorbate-Induced Cytotoxicity in Pancreatic Cancer. Clin Cancer Res 2010;16:509–20.

19. Verrax J, Delvaux M, Beghein N, Taper H, Gallez B, Buc Calderon P. Enhancement of quinone redox cycling by ascorbate induces a caspase-3 independent cell death in human leukaemia cells. An in vitro comparative study. Free Radic Res 2005;39:649–57.

20. Chen P, Yu J, Chalmers B, Drisko J, Yang J, Li B, et al. Pharmacological ascorbate induces cytotoxicity in prostate cancer cells through ATP depletion and induction of autophagy. Anticancer Drugs 2012;23:437–44.

21. Alexander A, Cai S-L, Kim J, Nanez A, Sahin M, MacLean KH, et al. ATM signals to TSC2 in the cytoplasm to regulate mTORC1 in response to ROS. Proc Natl Acad Sci 2010;107:4153–8.

22. Alexander A, Kim J, Walker CL. ATM engages the TSC2/mTORC1 signaling node to regulate autophagy. Autophagy 2010;6:672–3.

23. Chou T-C. Theoretical Basis, Experimental Design, and Computerized Simulation of Synergism and Antagonism in Drug Combination Studies. Pharmacol Rev 2006;58:621–81.

24. Stephenson CM, Levin RD, Spector T, Lis CG. Phase I clinical trial to evaluate the safety, olerability, and pharmacokinetics of high-dose intravenous ascorbic acid in patients with advanced cancer. Cancer Chemother Pharmacol 2013;72:139–46.

25. Hoffer LJ, Levine M, Assouline S, Melnychuk D, Padayatty SJ, Rosadiuk K, et al. Phase I clinical trial of i.v. ascorbic acid in advanced malignancy. Ann Oncol 2008;19:1969–74.

26. Watson J. Oxidants, antioxidants and the current incurability of metastatic cancers. Open Biol 2013;3:120144.

28. Ramos-Gomez M, Kwak M-K, Dolan PM, Itoh K, Yamamoto M, Talalay P, et al. Sensitivity to carcinogenesis is increased and chemoprotective efficacy of enzyme inducers is lost in nrf2 transcription factor-deficient mice. Proc Natl Acad Sci 2001;98:3410–5.

29. Iida K, Itoh K, Kumagai Y, Oyasu R, Hattori K, Kawai K, et al. Nrf2 Is Essential for the Chemopreventive Efficacy of Oltipraz against Urinary Bladder Carcinogenesis. Cancer Res 2004;64:6424–31.

30. Rotblat B, Melino G, Knight RA. NRF2 and p53: Januses in cancer? Oncotarget 2012;3:1272.

31. Bertheau P, Turpin E, Rickman DS, EspiéM, de Reyniès A, Feugeas J-P, et al. Exquisite Sensitivity of TP53 Mutant and Basal Breast Cancers to a Dose-Dense Epirubicin−Cyclophosphamide Regimen. PLoS Med 2007;4:e90.

32. Jackson JG, Pant V, Li Q, Chang LL, Quintás-Cardama A, Garza D, et al. p53-Mediated Senescence Impairs the Apoptotic Response to Chemotherapy and Clinical Outcome in Breast Cancer. Cancer Cell 2012;21:793–806.

33. Sinthupibulyakit C, Ittarat W, St Clair WH, St Clair DK. p53 Protects lung cancer cells against metabolic stress. Int J Oncol 2010;37:1575–81.

34. Ristow M, Zarse K, Oberbach A, Klöting N, Birringer M, Kiehntopf M, et al. Antioxidants prevent health-promoting effects of physical exercise in humans. Proc Natl Acad Sci U S A 2009;106:8665–70.

35. Gibney GT, Messina JL, Fedorenko IV, Sondak VK, Smalley KSM. Paradoxical oncogenesis and the long term consequences of BRAF inhibition in melanoma. Nat Rev Clin Oncol 2013;10:390–9.

36. Phoenix KN, Vumbaca F, Claffey KP. Therapeutic Metformin/AMPK Activation Promotes the Angiogenic Phenotype in the ER? Negative MDA-MB-435 Breast Cancer Model. Breast Cancer Res Treat 2009;113:101–11.

37. Martin MJ, Hayward R, Viros A, Marais R. Metformin accelerates the growth of BRAFV600E- driven melanoma by upregulating VEGF-A. Cancer Discov 2012;2:344–55.

Chapter 13

Partial Reversal of Skeletal Muscle Aging by Restoration of Normal NAD$^+$ Levels

That some aging-associated phenotypes may be reversible is an emerging theme in contemporary aging re- search. Gomes *et al.* report that age-associated oxidative phosphorylation (OXPHOS) defects in murine skeletal muscle are biphasic. In the first phase, OXPHOS is decreased because of reduced expression of mitochondrially encoded genes. Treatment of moderately old mice (first-phase OXPHOS defects) with nicotinamide adenine dinucleotide (NAD+) precursor nicotinamide mononucleotide (NMN) for 1 week restores oxidative phosphorylation activity and other markers of mitochondrial function in skeletal muscle. However, muscle strength is not restored. In very old animals (second-phase OXPHOS defects), expression of OXPHOS genes from both the nucleus and mitochondria is reduced and mitochondrial DNA integrity is diminished. Gomes *et al.* propose a model linking decreased NAD+ to loss of nuclear SIRT1 activity to stabilization of the hypoxia-associated transcription factor hypoxia-inducible factor 1-alpha (HIF-1α). HIF-1α promotes an hypoxic-like (Warburg effect) state in the cell. The HIF-1a protein interacts with c-Myc, decreasing c-Myc–regulated transcription of the key mitochondrial regulator mitochondrial transcription factor A (TFAM). Low levels of TFAM lead to first-phase OXPHOS dysfunction. The transition to irreversible phase 2 dysfunction remains to be characterized, but may be related to increased reactive oxygen species (ROS) production. This model suggests that intervention in mitochondrial aging may be possible using appropriate NAD+ precursors such as nicotinamide riboside. Restoring NAD+ levels may be beneficial throughout the organism. For example, aging-associated disturbances in circadian rhythm are linked to diminished SIRT1 activity, and loss of hematopoietic stem cell function to reduced SIRT3. Work to elucidate other biphasic aging mechanisms is strongly encouraged.

Introduction

That some aging-associated phenotypes may be reversible, is an emerging theme in contemporary aging research [1–9] (for review, see Mendelsohn and Larrick). Age-related dysfunction may be operationally classified by two stages—an early stage that is reversible and a later stage that is not. The irreversible stage is associated with permanent damage, such as critical DNA mutations or deletions, or cell death. A critical question is to define the transition point between these states.

Mitochondrial damage has long been associated with metabolic dysfunctions of aging [11]. In animals, mitochondrial aging is characterized by diminished oxidative phosphorylation (reduced adenosine triphosphate [ATP] production), mitochondrial membrane potential, fewer mitochondria resulting in less total mitochondrial DNA (mtDNA), induction of reactive oxygen species (ROS), and loss of mtDNA integrity. Of these changes, only reduced mtDNA integrity is necessarily irreversible, but typically these phenotypes are believed to be interconnected.

Nicotinamide adenine dinucleotide (NAD) is an important player in the metabolism of mitochondria and aging. NAD is an oxidoreductive/redox co-factor that participates in many important metabolic pathways, including beta oxidation, glycolysis, and the citric acid cycle [12, 13]. The reduced form, NADH, is transported from the cytoplasm to the mitochondria and oxidized to NAD+ by the electron transport chain. NADH participates not only in catabolic reactions, but also in diverse reactions, among them anabolic pathways like gluconeogenesis. For example, NAD+ is used as a substrate in adenosine diphosphate (ADP)- ribosylation reactions, as a precursor of calcium signaling regulator cyclic ADP-ribose, by DNA ligases, and as an extracellular signal transducer [13].

One of NAD+'s most important roles in signaling stems from its interaction with sirtuins. Sirtuin family members regulate several key cell processes, including chromatin structure by deacetylating histones, stress responses, and integration of metabolism. Of special relevance to mitochondria and aging, the nuclear-localized sirtuin SIRT1 can activate the mitochondrial biogenesis master regulator peroxisome proliferator-activated receptor c co-activator 1 (PCG-1α) to initiate mitochondrial growth. SIRT1 is a homolog of canonical sirtuin SIR2, which has been shown to be necessary for the increased longevity associated with caloric restriction in yeast. When over-expressed, SIR2 homologs extended life span in a variety of invertebrates including Caenorhabditis elegans. In mice, over-expression of SIRT1 confers some of the phenotypes associated with caloric restriction, such as reduction of insulin and fasting glucose, but this does not extend life span [14,15] unless expression of SIRT1 is limited to the brain, stimulating neural activity in the dorsomedial and lateral hypothalamic nuclei [16]. Like most sirtuins, SIRT1 activity is dependent on the availability of sufficient NAD+, and its activity is regulated by NAD+ levels.

Decreased NAD1 Levels Reversibly Disrupt Nuclear-Mitochondrial Communication During Aging in Skeletal Muscle

In a recent, provocative report, Gomes *et al.* have uncovered new mechanisms to explain how mitochondrial function in skeletal muscle declines with age [17]. Consistent with a large set of previous reports, oxidative phosphorylation (OXPHOS), the process by which electron transport generates ATP, declines in mice. Gomes *et al.* show that mitochondrial decline is a two-step process in which mitochondria first exhibit reduced OXPHOS in 22-month "moderately" old mice and then even lower OXPHOS in 30-month "very old" mice. Of interest is that the Gomes and co-workers report that the integrity of mitochondrial DNA is intact in the moderately old mice, but not in the very old mice, suggesting that mitochondrial DNA loss is secondary to the metabolic changes observed in OXPHOS [17].

Gomes *et al.* then show that the decline in OXPHOS at 22 months is associated with a decline in the activity and expression of mitochondrial-encoded OXPHOS mRNAs (e.g., ND1, Cytb, COX1, ATP6) compared to young 6-month-old mice, but not nuclear-encoded OXPHOS mRNAs (e.g., NDUFS8, SDHb, Uqcrc1, COX5, ATP5a). These data are consistent with earlier work showing that the activity of mitochondrial-encoded OXPHOS complexes I, III, and IV decline with age, but that the activity of the nuclear-encoded OXPHOS complex II does not [18]. At 30-months, all OXPHOS mRNAs levels declined and mtDNA integrity was reduced, suggesting that mitochondrial dysfunction in very old mice is qualitatively different from that in moderately old animals and that aging-associated mitochondrial dysfunction is biphasic [17].

The mammalian sirtuin SIRT1 activates the mitochondria master regulator PGC-1a by deacetylation to maintain or increase mitochondrial mass [19]. SIRT1 has been hypothesized to play a key role in aging in yeast, invertebrates, and possibly mammals, although its precise role is unclear. Gomes *et al.* hypothesized that SIRT1 might play a role in mediating the differential decrease in OXPHOS component expression. In an adult SIRT1 inducible knockout (iKO) mouse, all [13] mitochondrially encoded OXPHOS genes and two ribosomal RNAs were down-regulated at 2-6 months after induction of the knockout. Expression of nuclear-encoded OXPHOS components was unaltered, similar to what is observed in wild-type mice at 22-months. Moreover, mitochondrial mass was unaffected by SIRT1 knockout, raising the possibility that SIRT1 regulates mitochondrial mass independently of PGC-1α. Indeed, in primary myotubes from PGC-1α/b knockout mice, or PGC-1α muscle- specific null mice, over-expression of SIRT1 induced mitochondrial-encoded OXPHOS genes. These results appear to suggest a model whereby loss of SIRT1 activity during aging might be responsible for the differential loss of mitochondrial OXPHOS expression. Furthermore, similar to the *in vivo* aging data, iKO myoblasts exhibit a biphasic loss of OXPHOS capability. At 12 hour, only expression of mitochondrially encoded OXPHOS genes decreases. mtDNA content and membrane potential also decline, but mitochondrial mtDNA integrity (mass) and nuclear-encoded OXPHOS mRNAs are unaffected. At 48 hr, a second stage is observed: mRNA levels decrease from both nuclear and mitochondrial-encoded OXPHOS genes and mtDNA integrity/mass is reduced as well. On the basis of these data, Gomes *et al.* make the implicit basic assumption that the inducible inactivation of SIRT1 in cultured myoblasts accurately models the biphasic OXPHOS dysfunction ob- served *in vivo* during aging [17].

Not so fast! SIRT1 protein levels do not change with aging. Thus arises the obvious hypothesis that perhaps NAD+ levels decline with age, thereby compromising SIRT1 activity. In primary myoblasts, small hairpin (sh) RNA knockdown experiments to lower NAD+ levels by reducing expression of cell compartment–specific isoforms of nicotinamide mononucleotide adenylyltransferase (NMNAT) revealed that only knockdown of the nuclear isoform (NMNAT1), but not the Golgi or mitochondrial-specific isoforms, resulted in a specific reduction of mitochondrially encoded OXPHOS genes. The hypothesis is extended: If nuclear NAD+ levels decline compromising SIRT1 activity, then this results in reduced mitochondrial OXPHOS gene expression and activity. Consistent with this idea, Gomes *et al.* found that over-expression of NMNAT1 in skeletal muscle from middle-aged 10-month-old to 12-month-old mice strongly increased the expression of mitochondrial-encoded OXPHOS genes. Over-expression of NMNAT1 in primary myoblasts produced a similar effect. However, SIRT1 iKO myoblasts do not respond to increased NAD+, consistent with the idea that nuclear SIRT1 activity diminishes with age due to gradual reduction of NAD+ [17].

SIRT1 appears to play a central role in the detrimental effects of reduced nuclear NAD+ levels on OXPHOS and that role is surprisingly independent of PGC-1α/β. Through what downstream regulators does SIRT1 exert its OXPHOS- altering effects on the mitochondria? A critical clue is that SIRT1 iKO animals exhibit increased glycolysis, similar to that seen in solid tumors (the "Warburg" effect), as suggested by increased lactate levels and a switch from slow- twitch oxidative muscle fibers to fast-twitch glycolytic muscle fibers. Because increased glycolysis seen in solid tumors is associated with an increase in stability of the hypoxia-associated transcription factor HIF-1α, Gomes *et al.* hypothesized that HIF-1α would be elevated in SIRT iKO animals. Indeed, not only is HIF-1α protein expression elevated in SIRT1 iKO mice, but also in wild-type myoblasts that have reduced NAD+ resulting from shRNA knockdown of NMNAT1. It is possible to artificially stabilize HIF-a by reducing activity of HIF prolyl-hydroxylase 2 (encoded by EglN1). After knocking out EglN1, mitochondrial-encoded OXPHOS gene expression and mitochondrial DNA content were reduced to a similar extent to that seen in normal aging and SIRT1 iKO [17]. Most importantly, primary myoblasts that lack HIF-1α maintain mtDNA content and OXPHOS gene expression levels, even in the absence of SIRT1, suggesting that HIF-1α is downstream of SIRT1 and necessary for first-phase OXPHOS dysregulation. But then the question arises how is HIF-1α being stabilized?

Gomes *et al.* explore three possible known mechanisms of HIF-1α stabilization. First, they rule out that ROS originating at complex III is the source, because HIF-1α levels increase 6 hour after SIRT1 deletion, but ROS levels do not increase until 24 hour after deletion, and myoblasts engineered to lack mtDNA are thus unable to produce ROS and still exhibit stabilized HIF-1α. SIRT1 deacetylation of the key HIF-1α amino acid lysine 709 was ruled out by mutation to a form that either mimicked activation or that was unable to be acetylated. Von Hippel–Lindau (VHL) E3 ubiquitin ligase targets HIF-1α for degradation by recognizing hydroxylated prolines. No change in the hydroxylation of prolines in HIF-1α was observed in SIRT1 KO animals, but there was a direct correlation between levels of SIRT1 and VHL. SIRT1 deletion did not affect expression from the VHL promoter, which suggests that SIRT1 is regulating VHL levels post-translationally [19]. However, the exact mechanism remains unknown.

How do nuclear NAD+ levels, or nuclear localized HIF-1α affect mitochondrial-localized gene expression?

A survey of altered gene expression in SIRT1 iKO mice suggested that nuclear-encoded mitochondrial transcription factor A (TFAM) was a good candidate. Testing this hypothesis revealed that TFAM levels decrease 6 hour after SIRT1 KO, consistent with the decline of VHL and increased stabilization of HIF-1α. More importantly, forced expression of TFAM restores mitochondrial OXPHOS gene expression and ATP levels in SIRT1 iKO cells.

How is TFAM expression linked to SIRT1 and/or HIF-1α?

It is known that c-Myc, an important cell growth regulator and proto-oncogene co-operates with HIF-1α in cancer cells to reprogram metabolism. Consistent with a possible role for c-Myc, shRNA knockdown of c-Myc completely blocked the ability of ectopic SIRT1 to induce mitochondrially encoded mRNAs (phase 1 OXPHOS dysfunction). Also, over-expression of c-Myc prevented decrease of mitochondrially expressed OXPHOS genes and ATP levels (stage 1 dysfunction) after pharmacological inhibition of SIRT1 by the drug EX-527 [17]. It is curious that a similar experiment with the SIRT1 KO cells was not also performed. But the reported data suggest that c-Myc acts downstream of SIRT1.

c-Myc DNA-binding sites are found upstream of many mitochondrial biogenesis genes, and bioinformatic analysis revealed a c-Myc consensus binding site upstream of the TFAM promoter. A chromatin immunoprecipitation study demonstrated that c-Myc binds this site in cells. Mutation of this sequence reduced promoter activity by about half.

TFAM was already known to be inducible by PGC-1α, which was not affected by deletion of the c-Myc binding site. SIRT1 over-expression also induces TFAM, but this induction is dependent on the presence of the c-Myc binding site.

What is the link to HIF-1α?

It turns out that HIF-1α interacts with c-Myc to modulate its activity. Gomes *et al.* found that deletion of SIRT1 increased binding of c-Myc to HIF-1α, which in turn decreased c-Myc–mediated transcription as assessed by a c-Myc-dependent reporter. So a preliminary model was constructed in which SIRT1 normally destabilizes HIF-1α in the nucleus, allowing c-Myc to maintain expression of mitochondrial regulator TFAM, which in turn promotes normal levels of mitochondrially encoded OXPHOS genes [19] (**Figure 13.1**). If HIF-1α is instead stabilized by reduced SIRT1 activity, say for example by reduced nuclear NAD+ levels associated with aging, c-Myc declines. Then TFAM decreases and mitochondrial-encoded OXPHOS decreases (**Figure 13.1**).

The preceding work was performed in animals fed standard diets or cells with normal levels of glucose and nutritional factors. An important question is how this proposed mechanism would work when animals or cells are faced with low energy conditions. Under low energy conditions, 5¢-adenosine monophosphate-activated protein kinase (AMPK) senses low levels of ATP and phosphorylates PGC-1α, which then allows subsequent activation of PGC1-α by SIRT1 via deacetylation. Under normal energy conditions, PGC1-a's acetylation and activation state is regulated by histone deacetylase GCN5.20 Gomes *et al.* suggest that AMPK acts as a switch between PCG1-α–dependent and independent pathways and is responsible for the biphasic decline in OXPHOS mRNAs. Gomes *et al.* provide evidence that after deletion of SIRT1, AMPK is only activated at 48 hour, which is quite a long time after the down-regulation of mitochondrial-encoded OXPHOS mRNA but simultaneous with the decline in nuclear OXPHOS mRNAs. Expression of a dominant negative AMPK prevents AMPK activation and blocks the decrease in nuclear OXPHOS mRNAs seen in SIRT1 iKOs (stage 2 dysfunction). On the other hand, forced expression of mitochondrial TFAM prevents AMPK activation.

It should be noted that although AMPK activation is often considered as a possible goal of anti-aging therapies, the data of Gomes and co-workers suggest that AMPK activation in well-fed animals with reduced SIRT1 activity, such as might be seen in moderate old age, may help trigger irreversible mitochondrial damage.

As might be expected, caloric restriction (CR), which is known to extend life span and delay diseases of aging in numerous organisms including mice when initiated in young mice (6-weeks-old), completely prevented decreases in VHL, NAD+, ATP, mtDNA integrity, and expression of nuclear- and mitochondrial-encoded OXPHOS genes in moderately old 22-month-old mice. CR also prevented the increased HIF-1α levels seen in mice fed a standard diet [17]. However, the molecular underpinnings of CR remain murky. One simple hypothesis is that because CR prevents decreased NAD+, the set of molecular changes that lead to dysfunctional OXPHOS are prevented.

Of greater interest, when the 22-month "moderately" old mice were injected with NMN, a precursor to NAD+ that raises NAD+ levels *in vivo*, the decrease in VHL restored normal HIF-1α levels, reduced lactate, and increased ATP, and mitochondrially encoded OXPHOS genes were all reversed within 1 week. NMN treatment also reversed impaired insulin signaling and glucose uptake in muscle as well as switched the muscle to a more oxidative, slow-twitch phenotype. However, no improvement in muscle strength was observed. As expected, the reversal of mitochondrial dysfunction was not seen in EglN1 or SIRT iKO mice, because SIRT1 and EglN1 are downstream of NAD+ (**Figure 13.1**).

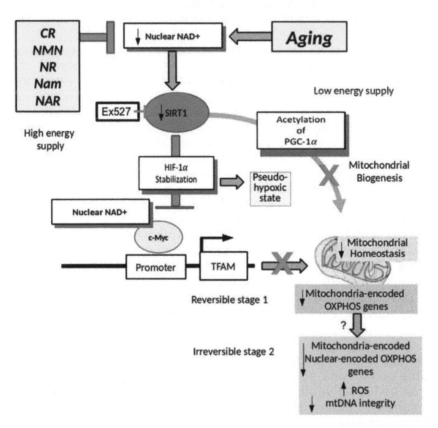

Figure 13.1 Two-stage model of mitochondrial dysfunction in aging. Decreased nuclear nicotinamide adenine dinucleotide (NAD+) levels lower SIRT1 activity. In a normal high-energy supply state, reduced SIRT1 levels stabilize the hypoxia master regulator HIF-1α leading to a pseudo-hypoxic cell state and reduced levels of free c-Myc. Decreased c-Myc reduces transcription of key mitochondrial homeostasis regulator mitochondrial transcription factor A (TFAM), which in turn causes decreased transcription of mitochondrial oxidative phosphorylation (OXPHOS) genes and lower OXPHOS, stage 1 dysfunction, which is reversible by restoring NAD+. After some time, a transition to stage-2 dysfunction occurs, in which nuclear and mitochondrial OXPHOS gene expression is reduced, reactive oxygen species (ROS) increase, and mitochondrial DNA (mtDNA) integrity decreases. Under low-energy conditions, low SIRT1 leads to reduced deacetylation and activity of mitochondria master regulator proliferator-activated receptor c co-activator (PCG-1α), reducing

mitochondrial biogenesis and homeostasis. CR, calorie restriction; NMN, nicotinamide mononucleotide; NR, nicotinamide riboside; Nam, nicotinamide; NAR, nicotinic acid riboside, HIF-1α, hypoxia-associated transcription factor.

NAD, a New Health Span Regulator?

These results have significant implications and provide a roadmap to begin to address aging-associated dysfunction. As Gomes *et al.* point out, induction of a tumor-like Warburg state may predispose cells to mutagenesis and cancer resulting from increased ROS. However, care must be taken with regard to tissue specificity of this pathway. SIRT1 iKO mice only show OXPHOS dysregulation in skeletal and cardiac muscle, and not in the liver, brain, or white adipose tissue. It is possible that other sirtuins may be important in non-muscle tissue or that this pathway is altered or even not present. Although it has been frequently reported that oxidative phosphorylation in other tissues such as the liver and brain is reduced, careful studies that pinpoint changes in expression of nuclear versus mitochondrial expressed genes are necessary to generalize this mechanism and/or to un- cover specific relevant mechanisms.

That type 2 diabetes can also be rescued in mice by injection of NAD+ precursor NMN suggests that NAD+ dysregulation may play a significant role in age-associated pathologies [21]. Perhaps the most significant aspect of this bi- phasic aging mechanism is that it represents another example of a reversal in an age-associated phenotype. However, caution is warranted: It was disappointing that muscle strength was not restored after NMN treatment. Perhaps this was due to the limited treatment period of only 1 week? It is most curious that longer periods of treatment have not been reported, given that the experiments were performed months ago.

A fundamental question remains regarding the cause of the decline in NAD+ levels or reduced NAD/NADH ratio. NAD+ is synthesized by several routes. Although NAD+ can be synthesized de novo from tryptophan, most NAD+ is made from nicotinic acid (NA) or nicotinamide (NAM), a.k.a the vitamin B3 using the salvage pathway. Synthesis of NAD+ from NA or NAM involves successive transfer of a phosphoribosyl followed by an adenylyl moiety. When starting from NA, a final ATP-dependent amidation step by NAD synthase is required to complete the synthesis. One key rate limiting enzyme is nicotinamide phosphoribosyl-transferase (NAMPT), which has been reported to be down-regulated in old age in rats [22] and mice [21] and may be responsible for the reported age-associated NAD+ deficits. Other possible ways that NAD+ may be dysregulated include increased expression of enzymes that consume large quantities of NAD+, such as PARP and CD38.

Moreover, because NAD+ appears to oppose HIF-1α and downstream ROS induction, it is reasonable to hypothesize that NAD+ may have anti-cancer or cancer preventive effects. A recent report suggests that NM or NA inhibits growth of aggressive human breast cancer xenografts in mice [23] through enhancement of mitochondrial complex I, which dovetails nicely with data that shows that reducing NAD+ levels increased metastasis in these cells. It should be noted that another group found that inhibiting NAMPT to reduce NAD+ levels killed human prostate cancer cells that over-expressed NAMPT [24]. Santidrian *et al.* speculate that FK866, a NAMPT inhibitor, may possess other anti-cancer activities beyond NAMPT inhibition, because they found that this inhibitor killed their breast cancer cells, but that RNA interference (RNAi) knockdown of NAMPT did not. Given the huge potential of highly tumorigenic cancer cells to evolve new phenotypes, it would not be surprising that NAD+ could be pro-oncogenic in some cases and anti-oncogenic in others. However, normal cells are more likely to respond in a predictable manner. If NAD+ is shown to consistently block HIF-1α, then it may consistently inhibit the earliest stages of cancer progression. Such a possibility is worth testing.

In addition to replication in mice and other model systems, these remarkable findings need to be confirmed by appropriate human studies as well.

Medical Implications

If the biphasic decline in OXPHOS observed in mice holds for humans, then preventing the initial decline in OXPHOS, or reversing the first phase of OXPHOS dysfunction, in which only mitochondrial gene expression is affected, should result in significant anti-aging benefit. An outstanding question is how much of the increased ROS generation that is observed in aging mammals is a consequence of the pathways described by Gomes *et al.* [17] It has long been hypothesized that blocking excessive ROS production would slow aging, and there is at least one example in which blocking ROS production restored aberrant stem cell function in old mice [1, 2].

That increasing NAD+ levels can rescue mitochondrial function in skeletal muscle and diabetes type 2 in old mice, [21] as well as potentially inhibit early stages of tumor progression, raises the possibility that simple manipulation of NAD+ by supplementation and exercise has great potential for maintaining human health. For example, mitochondrially localized SIRT3 is also dependent on NAD+. SIRT3 down-regulation with aging is tied to ROS production and can be reversed, rescuing stem cell function [1]. It will interesting to explore whether increasing NAD+ will increase mitochondrially localized SIRT3 to correct defects in hematopoietic stem cells. The most effective means may very well be the simplest.

Six weeks of moderate aerobic exercise has been reported to restore diminished NAD+ levels in the skeletal muscle of old (26 month) rats to levels near that seen in young animals [22]. Interestingly, SIRT1 levels actually were observed to increase with age and were reduced by exercise. Exercise has also been reported to increase NAD+ in mice [25]. However, SIRT1 activity decreased with age and was restored by exercise, as would be expected from its putative role in maintaining mitochondrial function. It would of great interest to know how well NAD+ levels were restored in tissues other than skeletal muscle. Given the involvement of skeletal and cardiac muscle in aging, it is tempting to hypothesize that the beneficial effects of exercise on NAD+ levels and mitochondrial function may be restricted to the few tissue types directly involved. On the other hand, given the well-known, but modest, benefits of exercise to life span and health span, it is tempting to hypothesize that modulation of NAD+ levels is one key mechanism by which exercise achieves its benefits. Finally, although moderate exercise is known to extend health span in humans, and has been correlated with lower mortality in old age, it is well understood that exercise does not actually prevent aging, or even prevent aging-associated decline in muscle strength and agility, as can be observed most simply in humans by the need of professional athletes to retire in their 30s or 40s. Restoration of youthful NAD+ levels by exercise may be insufficient to reverse aging-associated loss of muscle function.

Although Gomes and other workers injected NAD+ precursor NMN to attain biological benefit, there is a reasonable possibility that oral supplementation may be effective as well. NAD+ can apparently be metabolized after oral introduction in humans, [26] although its ability to alter intracellular NAD+ levels in different cell types and compartments is unknown. It's also promising that pM concentrations of NAD+ have been reported to be absorbed by numerous cell types [27]. Unfortunately, Nikiforov *et al.* [28] using some of the same cell lines reported by Billington *et al.*, report that NAD+ is not absorbed. Clearly, greater characterization of NAD+ uptake and pharmacokinetics is warranted.

NADH, the reduced form of NAD+, is commercially available as a nutriceutical. Given that it may very well be the NAD+/NADH ratio itself rather than absolute NAD+ levels that may be most important, NADH supplementation may not be wise. Fortunately, a study on the pharmacokinetics of NADH suggest that NADH is broken down before adsorption [26].

NA and NAM, both forms of vitamin B3, are commercially available. Although there are no studies that show people who regularly take vitamin B3 are biologically younger than negative controls, it is not unreasonable to believe that both NA and NAM will raise NAD+ levels, at least in younger people. The beneficial anti-breast cancer effects of NA and NAM on human xenografts in mice used a 1% solution delivered orally [23]. The apparent lack of any anti-aging effect of NAM may be due to the observed decline in key enzyme NAMPT with age [29]. A caveat of NAM is that it potentially can inhibit sirtuins, such as SIRT1 and SIRT1-consuming enzyme PARP1, by end product inhibition. Excess NAM over that which can be processed by NAMPT may therefore be counterproductive. NAMPT is rate limiting in the conversion of NAM into NAD+ (**Figure 13.2**).

Figure. 13.2 Pathways by which nicotinamide adenine dinucleotide (NAD+) precursors are converted into NAD+. (Top) Pathways. (Bottom) Structures of NAD+ and its precursors. QA, quinolinic acid; NA, nicotinic acid; QAPRT, quinolinic acid phosphoribosyl transferase; NAPRT, nicotinic acid phosphor- ibosyltransferase; NAMPT, nicotinamide phosphoribosyl transferase; Nam, nicotinamide; NAR, nicotinic acid riboside; NR, nicotinamide riboside; NRK, nicotinamide riboside kinase; NAMN, nicotinic acid

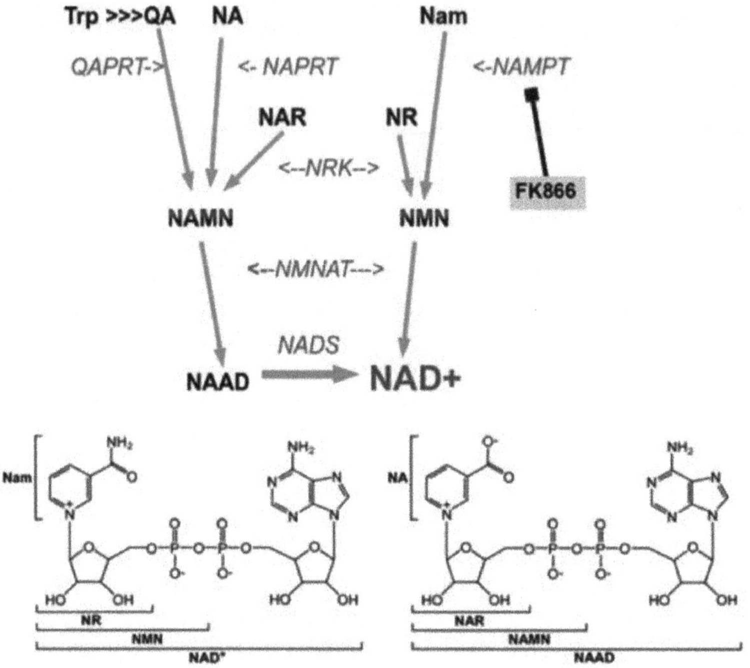

mononucleoside; NMN, nicotinamide mononucleotide; NMNAT, nicotinamide mononucleotide adenyltransferase; NADS, nicotinamide adenine dinucleotide synthetase; NAAD, nicotinic acid adenine dinucleotide.

The mechanisms that underlie the age-associated decrease in NAMPT remain unknown, but pose a significant problem for NAM supplementation as an anti-aging therapeutic. On the other hand, NA is converted by a different enzyme, NA phosphoribosyl transferase (NAPRT), into NAMN, which in turn is converted by sequential action of NNMAT and NADS into NAD+. The status of these enzymes during mammalian aging needs to be investigated, especially that of NAPRT, given that it is rate limiting for conversion of NA [30]. It would not be surprising to learn that NAPRT decreases with age.

Can the problems associated with age-associated reduction of NAMP be avoided? NMN, nicotinamide riboside (NR), and nicotinic acid riboside (NAR) avoid the requirement for NAMPT or NAPRT (**Figure 13.2**). NMN, the metabolite used in the Gomes *et al.* study, appears to be absent from dietary sources. There is evidence to suggest that NMN must first be metabolized to

NR to enter cells, and then after entering cells be retransformed into NMN [31].

Furthermore, oral NMN only increases NAD+ levels in the liver, not in muscle, which contrasts with oral NR present in dietary sources such as milk and yeast [31]. NR increases NAD+ in liver, skeletal muscle, and brown adipose tissue [31]. NR is probably a better candidate for oral supplementation. Recently, the ability of oral NR to promote increased NAD+ levels and health benefits in mice has been investigated (Canto, 2012). NR stimulated both nuclear-localized SIRT1 and mitochondrial-localized SIRT3 as well as their downstream effectors in a variety of cell types and tissues, including liver, skeletal muscle, and brown adipose tissue [31]. NR treatment increased energy expenditure and limited the weight gain associated with animals fed a high-fat diet (HFD), probably by enhancing the oxidative performance of skeletal muscle and brown adipose tissue. In mice fed a HFD, NR enhanced insulin sensitivity. However, NR did not induce NAD+ in brain or white adipose tissue. Differential expression of nicotinamide riboside kinase (NRK) activity (**Figure 13.2**), which converts NR into NMN, is likely responsible for the differential effects of NR supplementation.

Although NRK1 is ubiquitously expressed, NRK2 is expressed primarily in skeletal and cardiac muscle [31]. Thus, NR is a good candidate to enhance NAD+ levels in at least two important tissue types, but it is incapable of increasing NAD+ in normal brains. On the other hand, NR has been reported to partially restore cognition in an Alzheimer disease (AD) mouse model, [32] which suggests it probably enters the brain. It is possible that AD alters NRK expression or in some other way augments brain metabolism of NR into NAD+.

Because there appears to be no universal precursor to boost NAD+ throughout the body, are there any other ways to boost NAD+? Yes, it has been proposed that inhibiting enzymes that consume large amounts of NAD+, such as poly(ADP-ribose) polymerase (PARP) and CD38/CD157, might be an effective approach [33]. In animal models, potential anti-cancer drugs that inhibit PARP increase NAD+. Knockout of CD36 also raises NAD+ levels significantly. However, there are problems with each approach. PARP inhibition only affects nuclear NAD+ levels, and PARP inhibition is likely to damage the pancreas, given the pathology observed inPARP2-/- animals. Negative global effects may be anticipated given the central role of PARPs in maintaining the integrity of the genome. CD38 and CD157 are also potential therapeutic targets [33]. However, critical biochemical details remain unknown. For example, what fraction of CD38 is localized intracellularly? In any case, potential drugs to inhibit CD38 and CD157 to increase NAD+ are yet to be developed.

Resveratrol, with its "controversial" mechanism of action has been reported to raise NAD+ levels (for review see Mouchiroud *et al.* [33]. Resveratrol activates AMPK and SIRT1 indirectly and may activate SIRT1 directly as well by an allosteric mechanism. Resveratrol stimulates NAD+ in at least some cell types, and the most appealing recent evidence suggests that increased NAD+ results from stimulation of NADH dehydrogenases associated with mitochondrial complex I that increase the NAD+/NADH ratio by oxidation of NADH [34]. The actions of resveratrol may be too pleiotropic with negative effects, like prevention of the insulin-sensitizing benefits conferred by exercise.

CR confers all of the reported benefits of increased NAD+. Furthermore, CR raises NAD+ levels [17]. Although, CR may not extend life span in primates, it will be very interesting to re-explore the effects CR has on compartmentalized NAD+ levels and OXPHOS in various mammalian tissue types.

The working hypothesis of Gomes *et al*. implies that some aging-associated mechanism down-regulates NAMPT, resulting in reduced NAD+, which then initiates a chain of events leading to dysfunction of OXPHOS. One strategy to circumvent NAD+ decline is to prevent down-regulation of NAMPT or to boost its expression. Currently, there are no known drugs that up-regulate NAMPT. Identification of such therapeutics would likely be of significant benefit. A recent report implicates mir34a as a possible regulator of NAMPT [35] making mir34a a possible drug target to augment NAMPT. Development of an inducer of NAMPT may be complicated by the observation that although intracellular NAMPT decreases with age extracellular serum NAMPT increases with age. Unfortunately, extracellular NAMPT is a pro-inflammatory cytokine that may increase risk of stroke [36]. New drugs would be required to exclusively stimulate the expression of intracellular NAMPT.

Is global maintenance or restoration of NAD+ levelsdesirable? Probably, given that levels associated with younganimals or humans are presumably optimal. One caveatmight be noted that mice over-expressing SIRT1 arehealthier than control wild-type mice, but have similar lifespans to wild-type animals. Extended life span and someother health benefits only result if SIRT1 expression islimited to the brain, and then only if neurons in the dorsomedial and lateral hypothalamic nuclei are hyperactive [16].The problem with this argument is that SIRT1 expression isonly correlated with NAD+ expression, and NAD+ expression is expected to have far more pleiotropic and balanced effects than those triggered by SIRT1.

However, it is 391. apparent that NAD+ levels in the brain may significantly impact aging rate. NAD+ levels in a nearby region of the hypothalamus, the suprachiasmatic nucleus, may be important for maintaining a robust circadian rhythm, which declines with aging. SIRT1, acting as part of a signal-amplifying loop with NAMPT and PGC-1α, transcription- ally activates two key circadian regulators, BMAL1 and CLOCK. Aging-associated decreased SIRT1 levels cause disturbances in circadian rhythm, which probably have significant downstream effects throughout the organism. Forced expression of SIRT1 protects mice from circadian dysfunction [37]. It is quite possible that increasing NAD+ levels would also be beneficial.

Conclusion

Identification of reduced NAD+ levels as an initiator of biphasic mitochondrial OXPHOS dysfunction is significant for understanding the decline of mitochondrial function during aging. The reversibility of first-stage OXPHOS dysfunction by increasing NAD+ levels points the way to the development of new anti-aging therapeutics as well as suggesting the potential of NAD+ precursors such as NR to enhance health span. Together with previous reports of reversibility of aging-associated phenotypes, these data encourage a dedicated effort to develop a comprehensive roadmap of potentially reversible aging-associated pathways.

References

1. Brown K, Xie S, Qiu X, Mohrin M, Shin J, Liu Y, Zhang D, Scadden DT, Chen D. SIRT3 Reverses aging-associated degeneration. Cell Rep 2013;3:319–327.

2. Mendelsohn AR, Larrick JW. Rejuvenation of adult stem cells: Is age-associated dysfunction epigenetic? Rejuvenation Res 2013;16:152–157.

3. Mendelsohn AR, Larrick JW. Rejuvenation of Aging Hearts. Rejuvenation Res 2013;16:330–332.

4. Loffredo FS, Steinhauser ML, Jay SM, Gannon J, Pancoast JR, Yalamanchi P, Sinha M, Dall'Osso C, Khong D, Sha- drach JL, Miller CM, Singer BS, Stewart A, Psychogios N, Gerszten RE, Hartigan AJ, Kim MJ, Serwold T, Wagers AJ, Lee RT. Growth differentiation factor 11 is a circulating factor that reverses age-related cardiac hypertrophy. Cell 2013;153:828–839.

5. Mendelsohn AR, Larrick JW. The DNA methylome as a biomarker for epigenetic instability and human aging. Rejuvenation Res 2013;16:74–77.

6. DeCamp E, Clark K, Schneider JS. Effects of the alpha-2 adrenoceptor agonist guanfacine on attention and working memory in aged non-human primates. Eur J Neurosci 2011;34:1018–1022.

7. Carlson ME, Suetta C, Conboy MJ, Aagaard P, Mackey A, Kjaer M, Conboy I. Molecular aging and rejuvenation of human muscle stem cells. EMBO Mol Med 2009;1:381.

8. Villeda SA, Luo J, Mosher KI, Zou B, Britschgi M, Bieri G, Stan TM, Fainberg N, Ding Z, Eggel A, Lucin KM, Czirr E, Park J-S, Couillard-Despre's S, Aigner L, Li G, Peskind ER, Kaye JA, Quinn JF, Galasko DR, Xie XS, Rando TA, Wyss-Coray T. The ageing systemic milieu negatively regulates neurogenesis and cognitive function. Nature 2011;477:90–94.

9. Mendelsohn AR. Medical Implications of Basic Research in Aging, 1st ed. Eosynth, Palo Alto, CA, 2013.

10. Bratic A, Larsson N-G. The role of mitochondria in aging. J Clin Invest 2013;123:951–957.

11. Xu P, Sauve AA. Vitamin B3, the nicotinamide adenine dinucleotides and aging. Mech Ageing Dev 2010;131: 287–298.

12. Lin H. Nicotinamide adenine dinucleotide: Beyond a redox coenzyme. Org Biomol Chem 2007;5:2541–2554.

13. Bordone L, Cohen D, Robinson A, Motta MC, van Veen E, Czopik A, Steele AD, Crowe H, Marmor S, Luo J, Gu W, Guarente L. SIRT1 transgenic mice show phenotypes re- sembling calorie restriction. Aging Cell 2007;6:759–767.

14. Herranz D, Canamero M, Mulero F, Martinez-Pastor B, Fernandez-Capetillo O, Serrano M. Sirt1 improves healthy ageing and protects from metabolic syndrome-associated cancer syndrome. Nat Commun 2010;1:3.

15. Satoh A, Brace CS, Rensing N, Cliften P, Wozniak DF, Herzog ED, Yamada KA, Imai S. Sirt1 extends life span and delays aging in mice through the regulation of Nk2 homeobox 1 in the DMH and LH. Cell Metab 2013;18:416–430.

16. Gomes AP, Price NL, Ling AJY, Moslehi JJ, Montgomery MK, Rajman L, White JP, Teodoro JS, Wrann CD, Hub- bard BP, Mercken EM, Palmeira CM, de Cabo R, Rolo AP, Turner N, Bell EL, Sinclair DA. Declining NAD + induces

17. Decamp E, Clark K, Schneider JS. Effects of the alpha-2 adrenoceptor agonist guanfacine on attention and working memory in aged non-human primates. Eur J Neurosci 2011;34:1018–1022.

18. Wang M, Gamo NJ, Yang Y, Jin LE, Wang X-J, Laubach M, Mazer JA, Lee D, Arnsten AFT. Neuronal basis of age- related working memory decline. Nature 2011;476: 210–213.

19. Kwong LK, Sohal RS. Age-related changes in activities of mitochondrial electron transport complexes in various tis- sues of the mouse. Arch Biochem Biophys 2000;373: 16–22.

20. Gerhart-Hines Z, Rodgers JT, Bare O, Lerin C, Kim S-H, Mostoslavsky R, *et al.* Metabolic control of muscle mito- chondrial function and fatty acid oxidation through SIRT1/ PGC-1? EMBO J 2007;26:1913–1923.

21. Fernandez-Marcos PJ, Auwerx J. Regulation of PGC-1a, a nodal regulator of mitochondrial biogenesis. Am J Clin Nutr 2011;93:884S–890S.

22. Yoshino J, Mills KF, Yoon MJ, Imai S. Nicotinamide mononucleotide, a key NAD+ intermediate, treats the pathophysiology of diet and age-induced diabetes in mice. Cell Metab 2011;14:528–536.

23. Koltai E, Szabo Z, Atalay M, Boldogh I, Naito H, Goto S, Nyakas C, Radak Z. Exercise alters SIRT1, SIRT6, NAD and NAMPT levels in skeletal muscle of aged rats. Mech Ageing Dev 2010;131:21–28.

24. Santidrian AF, Matsuno-Yagi A, Ritland M, Seo BB, LeBoeuf SE, Gay LJ, Yagi T, Felding-Habermann B. Mitochondrial complex I activity and NAD + /NADH balance regulate breast cancer progression. J Clin Invest 2013;123:1068–1081.

25. Wang B, Hasan MK, Alvarado E, Yuan H, Wu H, Chen WY. NAMPT overexpression in prostate cancer and its contribution to tumor cell survival and stress response. Oncogene 2011;30:907–921.

26. Canto C, Jiang LQ, Deshmukh AS, Mataki C, Coste A, Lagouge M, Zierath JR, Auwerx J. Interdependence of AMPK and SIRT1 for metabolic adaptation to fasting and exercise in skeletal muscle. Cell Metab 2010;11:213–219.

27. Kimura N, Fukuwatari T, Sasaki R, Shibata K. Comparison of metabolic fates of nicotinamide, NAD+ and NADH administered orally and intraperitoneally; characterization of oral NADH. J Nutr Sci Vitaminol (Tokyo) 2006;52:142– 148.

28. Billington RA, Travelli C, Ercolano E, Galli U, Roman CB, Grolla AA, Canonico PL, Condorelli F, Genazzani AA. Characterization of NAD uptake in mammalian cells. J Biol Chem 2008;283:6367–6374.

29. Nikiforov A, Dolle C, Niere M, Ziegler M. Pathways and subcellular compartmentation of NAD biosynthesis in human cells from entry of extracellular precursors to mitochondrial NAD generation. J Biol Chem 2011;286: 21767–21778.

30. Choi SC, Yoon J, Shim WJ, Ro YM, Lim D-S. 5-azacytidine induces cardiac differentiation of P19 embryonic stem cells. Exp Mol Med 2004;36:515–523.

31. Hara N, Yamada K, Shibata T, Osago H, Hashimoto T, Tsuchiya M. Elevation of cellular NAD levels by nicotinic acid and involvement of nicotinic acid phosphoribosyl- transferase in human cells. J Biol Chem 2007;282:24574–24582.

32. Canto C, Houtkooper RH, Pirinen E, Youn DY, Oosterveer MH, Cen Y, Fernandez- Marcos PJ, Yamamoto H, Andreux PA, Cettour-Rose P, Gademann K, Rinsch C, Schoonjans K, Sauve AA, Auwerx J. The NAD+ precursor nicotinamide riboside enhances oxidative metabolism and protects against high-fat diet induced obesity. Cell Metab 2012;15: 838–847.

34. Gong B, Pan Y, Vempati P, Zhao W, Knable L, Ho L, Wang J, Sastre M, Ono K, Sauve AA, Pasinetti GM. Ni- cotinamide riboside restores cognition through an

upregulation of proliferator-activated receptor-c coactivator 1a regulated b-secretase 1 degradation and mitochondrial gene expression in Alzheimer's mouse models. Neurobiol Aging 2013;34:1581–1588.

35. Mouchiroud L, Houtkooper RH, Moullan N, Katsyuba E, Ryu D, Canto´ C, Mottis A, Jo YS, Viswanathan M, Schoonjans K, Guarente L, Auwerx J. The NAD + /sirtuin pathway modulates longevity through activation of mitochondrial UPR and FOXO signaling. Cell 2013;154:430–441.

36. Desquiret-Dumas V, Gueguen N, Leman G, Baron S, Nivet-Antoine V, Chupin S, Chevrollier A, Vessieres E, Ayer A, Ferre M, Bonneau D, Henrion D, Reynier P, Procaccio V. Resveratrol induces a mitochondrial complex I-dependent increase in NADH oxidation responsible for sirtuin activation in liver cells. J Biol Chem 2013:288: 36662–36675.

37. Choi S-E, Fu T, Seok S, Kim D-H, Yu E, Lee K-W, Kang Y, Li X, Kemper B, Kemper JK. Elevated microRNA-34a in obesity reduces NAD + levels and SIRT1 activity by directly targeting NAMPT. Aging Cell 2013;12:1062–1072.

38. Liu L-Y, Wang F, Zhang X-Y, Huang P, Lu Y-B, Wei E-Q, Zhang W-P. Nicotinamide phosphoribosyltransferase may be involved in age-related brain diseases. PLoS One 2012;7.

39. Chang H-C, Guarente L. SIRT1 mediates central circadian control in the SCN by a mechanism that decays with aging. Cell 2013;153:1448–1460.

Section III

Altering Epigenetics, Differentiation, And Engineering Rejuvenation

Chapter 14

Mesenchymal Stem Cells for Frailty?

Frailty is a medical syndrome associated with advancing age characterized by reduced functional reserve, strength, endurance and susceptibility to infection associated with high morbidity, hospitalization and death. Non-specific interventions to improve the health-span of affected patients include physical therapy, exercise, improved nutrition, etc. Among the hallmarks of aging, depletion of stem cells with resultant compromise of regeneration and repair of tissues informs a rational stem cell-based replacement strategy. This hypothesis has been evaluated in a randomized, double-blind, placebo-controlled clinical trial utilizing human allogeneic mesenchymal stem cells (allo-hMSCs), a facile, scalable stem cell replacement therapy [1]. Intravenous infusion of 100 or 200 million allo-hMSCs was deemed safe in aged frail individuals. However, modest improvement outcomes were limited to the lower dose, a finding that remains difficult to explain. Future studies are definitely warranted given the magnitude of this increasingly important medical syndrome.

Introduction

1. The problem: Frailty

The functional reserve of organs, tissues and cells decreases with advancing age. Limited functional reserve contributes to frailty, a syndrome that increases with aging. Unexplained weight loss, with weakness, slowness, easy exhaustion with reduced appetite and physical activity characterizes frailty [3]. A "Frailty Index" combines accumulated deficits of aging, including social, physical and cognitive impairments [4]. The health burden of frailty is significant and increasing with a prevalence over 10% in the elderly population [5].

2. Standard of Care

While no specific therapies alleviate or reverse frailty [6], afflicted patients are currently managed with physical therapy (e.g. aerobic/resistance training), nutritional support (e.g. calories, vitamin D) and optimized geriatric-specific medical and surgical care (e.g. attention to drug-drug interaction, dose attenuation). Clearly improved interventions are needed.

3. Hallmarks of Aging

The "hallmarks of aging" described by López-Otín et al. [7] can be grouped into three main categories. Group 1: Damage to cellular functions including genomic instability, telomere attrition, epigenetic alterations and loss of proteostasis. Group 2: antagonistic responses to such damage including deregulated nutrient sensing, altered mitochondrial function and cellular senescence. Group 3: integrative hallmarks that contribute to clinical phenotypes including stem cell exhaustion and altered intercellular communication. Group 3 ultimately contributes to the clinical manifestations of aging and frailty with physiological loss of reserve, organ decline and reduced function. [8, 9] Accordingly, a cell-based, regenerative treatment strategy is projected to ameliorate signs and symptoms of frailty [10-13]. Why Mesenchymal Stem Cells?

4. Mesenchymal Stem Cells

Almost 60 years ago Friedenstein *et al.* [14] described fibroblast-like plastic-adherent stromal cells comprising ~0.01% of the nucleated bone marrow population. In 2006, after many decades of confusion, the International Society for Cellular Therapy proposed minimal criteria for defining mesenchymal stem cells as a) plastic adherent; b) expression of CD105, CD73, and CD90 but NOT CD14/CD11b (monocyte, dendritic cell lineage), CD45 (common lymphocyte), CD79a/CD19/HLA-DR (B lymphocyte lineage), CD34 (hematopoietic lineage); c) capacity for multi-lineage differentiation [15].

MSC retain the capacity for post-natal self-renewal and differentiation into multiple lineages, ectoderm (epithelial and neural cells), mesoderm (connective stromal cells, cartilage cells, fat cells, bone cells) and endoderm (muscle, gut and lung). MSCs can be identified and expanded from multiple tissues among them peripheral blood, heart, adipose tissue, umbilical cord, placenta and bone marrow, the most common source [16].

For human therapeutic purposes, 10-20 mL of bone marrow is aspirated from the anterior iliac crest of healthy young (<45 year old) donors. Mononuclear cells are separated by density gradient centrifugation over Ficoll with subsequent adherence to plastic tissue culture flasks for two days in the presence of 20% fetal bovine substitute. Nonadherent cells are removed, and adherent cells are expanded for 2-3 weeks. A week or so after primary culture, fibroblast-like cells and small round-shaped cells (monocytes) form the heterogenous cell layer and colonies. Following trypsinization and subculture a more spindle-shaped appearance characterizes the greatly expanded cultures of therapeutic MSCs that can be cryopreserved for storage or shipment. Generally >99% of the administered cells are CD105+ by fluorescence-activated cell sorting (FACS) analysis. One can expect a yield of 50-400 million cells from a successful 10 mL bone marrow aspirate.

5. Mechanisms

MSCs target various tissues throughout the body to mediate remarkable repair and regenerative effects. These pro-regenerative effects result from a number of novel trophic activities (i.e. paracrine signaling, mitochondrial transfer, exosomes, etc.).

5.1. Immunomodulation Facilitates Use of Allogeneic MSC

MSCs interact with cells of both the innate and adaptive immune systems to mediate immunomodulatory and immunosuppressive activities [17,18]. Constitutive expression of major histocompatibility complex (MHC) class I, but not class II, and lack of T-cell co- stimulatory molecules e.g. CD40, CD80, CD86, or B7, contributes to the failure of MSCs to be destroyed by cytotoxic lymphocytes or natural killer cells [19]. Perhaps most importantly for the therapeutic use of allogeneic MSCs, host lymphocytes are not activated by allogeneic MSCs, which can be partially attributed to MSC elaboration of various immunomodulatory factors such as interleukins 2 and 10, interferon-gamma, TGF-beta1, hepatocyte growth factor, nitric oxide (NO), indoleamine 2,3-dioxygenase (IDO) and prostaglandin E2 (PGE2) [20-22].

5.2. Exosomes and Extracellular Vesicles

MSC-derived extracellular vesicles (EVs), including exosomes and microvesicles (MV), are involved in cell-to-cell communication, cell signaling, and altering cell or tissue metabolism at short or long distances in the body. MSC-derived exosomes contain cytokines and growth factors, signaling lipids, mRNAs, and regulatory miRNAs [23]. Lai *et al.* [24] reported that purified MSC-derived exosomes reduced infarct size in a murine ischemia/reperfusion model [23]. Apparently, MSCs release increased EVs under hypoxic conditions [25] providing a rationale for study of MSC-based therapy in chronic myocardial ischemia.

5.3. Transfer of Mitochondria

MSCs can connect to target cells via tunneling nanotubes (TNT) for transfer of mitochondria and other organelles. Tunneling nanotubes (TNTs) were initially reported in rat pheochromocytoma cells and immune cells Nanotubular highways for intercellular organelle transport [26,27]. Although MSCs were initially reported to transfer functional mitochondria to tumor cells via this mechanism [28], subsequent work reported delivery of mitochondria from MSC to endothelial cells, renal tubular cells, alveolar epithelial cells and cardiomyocytes [29-33]. TNTs are 50 to 1500 nm diameter, tubular structures spanning up to several hundred microns between two connected cells. TNTs facilitate transfer of various cellular components such as mitochondria, vesicles, endosomes, beta amyloid, viral particles, microRNA, prions, lysosomes, etc. via the TNT continuity of the plasma membrane and cytoplasm joining the cells (Vignais, 2017; [34]. TNT-mediated transfer of mitochondria from MSC: a) increased basal and maximal oxygen consumption in target HUVEC cells with reduction in glycolysis and lactate production [32], b) augmented ATP concentrations in alveolar cells [31], and c) induced cardiomyocyte reprogramming to a progenitor state [30]. Conversely, TNT mediated-acquisition of mitochondria from vascular smooth muscle cells increased the proliferation of the MSC. Unfortunately, this apparent beneficial trophic effect of MSC has a dark side: numerous studies indicate the MSCs can augment survival of leukemia-initiating cells [35], facilitate cancer cell metabolic reprogramming [36,37] and resistance to chemotherapy [38,39]. What role, if any this "metabolic transfusion" might play in the rejuvenation of older individuals by allo-huMSC remains to be determined.

5.4 Paracrine Effects, Anti-fibrosis, Anti-apoptosis

MSC augment cardiomyocyte survival and reduce apoptosis *in vivo* in acute MI models [40,41]. MSCs contribute to regulation of the extracellular matrix and thereby mediate antifibrotic effects [42] and tissue remodeling [43].

6. Demonstrated Benefits of MSC in Animal Models

Numerous studies have found benefit of MSC in various animal models. A summary of these can be found in Bianco [44] and more recently [45].

7. Most Human MSC Translational Studies are Negative

A recent review summarizes progress with clinical translation [46]: over 350 trials of MSC are documented in clinicaltrials.gov. Perhaps the most successful MSC trials have addressed the problem of graft-versus host-disease where the immunomodulatory function provides benefit. Therapy of osteoarthritis and low back pain appears promising and might support expanded use in frailty. Many human stem cell trials have focused on heart disease (acute/subacute MI, chronic myocardial ischemia, etc.) with adult bone marrow providing the most frequent source of stem cells. To reduce costs, standardize cell preparation and "industrialize" cell therapy, several groups have turned to allogeneic MSCs. Administration of allogeneic MSC has been shown to be safe in both animal models and multiple clinical trials. Unfortunately, to date overall outcomes of stem cell therapy to repair damaged hearts has been quite mixed.

For example, the ACCRUE database (meta-Analysis of Cell-based CaRdiac stUdy; NCT01098591) has collected individual patient data (IPD) from randomized, multinational and cohort studies of cell-based therapy in ischemic heart disease [47]. IPD-based meta-analysis of 12 randomized clinical trials (767 patients receiving intracoronary BM-derived or cardiosphere-derived cells after acute MI) demonstrated no clinical benefit versus 485 controls. Perhaps there are better applications of the allogeneic MSC technology?

8. Frailty: The Killer App for MSC?

Based on numerous studies supporting a potential benefit of MSC therapy for age-related frailty, the Interdisciplinary Stem Cell Institute located at the University of Miami Miller School of Medicine (Joshua M. Hare MD, Director) working with commercial partners, Longeveron LLC (Miami, FL) and EMMES Corporation (Rockville, MD) have been developing allogeneic MSCs. They now report the outcome of The AllogeneiC Human Mesenchymal Stem Cells in Patients with Aging FRAilTy via IntravenoUS Delivery (CRATUS) study (#NCT02065245). This was a Phase II randomized, double blind, placebo-controlled clinical trial of allogeneic human mesenchymal cells (allo-hMSC) for frailty associated with aging [1]. A total of 30 patients (mean age 75.5 +/-7.3) were enrolled, with ten patients receiving 100M allo-huMSC, ten patients receiving 200M allo-hMSC compared to 10 patients receiving "placebo".

Overall, the CRATUS trial demonstrated the feasibility and safety of administering allo-hMSCs at doses up to 200M. However, the outcomes were quite confusing because statistical significance was only found for a subset for the 100M group. For example the distance of six-minute walk improved from baseline to 6 month (346 to 411ft., $p = 0.011$) and the SPPB (short physical performance battery) score improved with a $p = 0.031$ significance. Hand grip strength did not improve, ejection fraction remained stable and FEV1 improved from 2.5 to 2.6 L/min ($p = 0.25$). Why would a therapy with purported global effects only move the bar on a subset of measures? Why would doubling the dose of a single injection eliminate any observable benefit?

DOSE: One hundred million cells infused into a textbook 5L human blood volume would immediately be diluted to ~50 cells/uL or an increase in the leukocyte count by about 1% (rough WBC count is ~5000/uL).

PHARMACODYNAMIC EFFECT: Prior work suggest that cell therapy is characterized by a non-linear dose response [45]. Some studies suggest a lower dose of cells is better [48,49], while others support a 'more is better" scenario.

MODEST EFFECT: Because the lifespan and survival of MSCs *in vivo* is limited one may question whether possible long term effects can be expected.

SMALL SAMPLE SIZE: While CRATUS was billed as a phase 2 clinical trial, in reality demonstration of safety of modest doses of allo-hMSC the stated primary outcome has been achieved, however any benefit or outcome above and beyond this would be considered gravy based on the small number enrolled. And in fact, this is what has been reported.

Medical Implications

MSC transplantation for frailty and aging is a potentially promising approach based on the data of the reported clinical trial. However, the data needs to be reproduced with more patients to strengthen the statistics. The large error bars in the data are likely due to significant patient to patient variation, and only study of larger numbers of patients can hope to overcome the problem in this study. It would be reassuring to see stronger correlations between each measure of frailty after treatment. The unusual dose response suggests that more doses be examined to determine the optimum dose and timing of repeat doses. It should be noted that many MSC studies report contradictory results, and such studies are clearly bedeviled by problems in experimental design. Perhaps the best hope for such experiments is a variation of the idea of "science by triangulation", where a series of experiments and trials by different investigators marginates the territory of true results.

The source of MSC may not be optimal as well. MSC are known to change during expansion, losing multi potent differentiation potential and even undergoing senescence. A promising new technology is to use MSC derived from induced pluripotent stem cells [50], which allows expansion of large numbers of "unaged cells" before differentiation into MSC.

Conventionally, MSC are thought to home in on and potentially engraft in areas of tissue damage. Although this has been observed in animal models, there is little evidence that this is a natural process in humans. In fact, neither in healthy individuals, nor in patients with end-stage liver disease, kidney disease or heart transplants are any MSC detected in human blood [51]. Presumably, the frailty studies and others that observe medical benefit after injection of MSC, are taking advantage of some innate potential of MSC that is not normally exploited by homeostasis. It would be useful to examine patient biopsies, e.g. from muscle, to look for long-term engraftment and markers of improved tissue homeostasis. One particularly interesting biomarker to examine would be the presence of senescent cells in the tissue of the elderly. There is preliminary evidence that senescent fibroblasts in the dermis can stimulate stem cell migration [52]. Do exogenously administered allo-huMSC home to senescent cells and modify their phenotype?

Given that the efficiency of engraftment may be low [45], it may also be useful to regionally transplant the MSC using a gel or other material to ensure that the MSC remain locally to facilitate persistence of MSC and long-term benefits.

Conclusion

Preliminary results from a human phase 2 trial on frailty show very modest benefit from injection of human allo-MSC at a 100 million cell dose. This trial needs to be expanded and repeated to establish its relevance to human health. The mechanisms that underlie any potential benefits remain to be elucidated.

References

1. Tompkins BA, DiFede DL, Khan A, Landin AM, Schulman IH, Pujol MV, *et al.* Allogeneic Mesenchymal Stem Cells Ameliorate Aging Frailty: A Phase II Randomized, Double- Blind, Placebo-Controlled Clinical Trial. J Gerontol A Biol Sci Med Sci 2017;72:1513–22. doi:10.1093/gerona/glx137.

2. Fried LP, Ferrucci L, Darer J, Williamson JD, Anderson G. Untangling the concepts of disability, frailty, and comorbidity: implications for improved targeting and care. J Gerontol A Biol Sci Med Sci 2004;59:255–63.

3. Fried LP, Tangen CM, Walston J, Newman AB, Hirsch C, Gottdiener J, *et al.* Frailty in older adults: evidence for a phenotype. J Gerontol A Biol Sci Med Sci 2001;56:M146-156.

4. Rockwood K, Mitnitski A. Frailty defined by deficit accumulation and geriatric medicine defined by frailty. Clin Geriatr Med 2011;27:17–26. doi:10.1016/j.cger.2010.08.008.

5. Collard RM, Boter H, Schoevers RA, Oude Voshaar RC. Prevalence of frailty in community-dwelling older persons: a systematic review. J Am Geriatr Soc 2012;60:1487–92. doi:10.1111/j.1532-5415.2012.04054.x.

6. Xue Q-L. The Frailty Syndrome: Definition and Natural History. Clin Geriatr Med 2011;27:1–15. doi:10.1016/j.cger.2010.08.009.

7. López-Otín C, Blasco MA, Partridge L, Serrano M, Kroemer G. The Hallmarks of Aging. Cell 2013;153:1194–217. doi:10.1016/j.cell.2013.05.039.

8. Sousa-Victor P, Muñoz-Cánoves P. Regenerative decline of stem cells in sarcopenia. Mol Aspects Med 2016;50:109–17. doi:10.1016/j.mam.2016.02.002.

9. Gonen O, Toledano H. Why Adult Stem Cell Functionality Declines with Age? Studies from the Fruit Fly Drosophila Melanogaster Model Organism. Curr Genomics 2014;15:231–6. doi:10.2174/1389202915666140421213243.

10. Raggi C, Berardi AC. Mesenchymal stem cells, aging and regenerative medicine. Muscles Ligaments Tendons J 2012;2:239–42.

11. Kanapuru B, Ershler WB. Inflammation, coagulation, and the pathway to frailty. Am J Med 2009;122:605–13. doi:10.1016/j.amjmed.2009.01.030.

12. Laschober GT, Brunauer R, Jamnig A, Singh S, Hafen U, Fehrer C, *et al.* Age-specific changes of mesenchymal stem cells are paralleled by upregulation of CD106 expression as a response to an inflammatory environment. Rejuvenation Res 2011;14:119–31. doi:10.1089/rej.2010.1077.

13. Rando TA, Wyss-Coray T. Stem Cells as Vehicles for Youthful Regeneration of Aged Tissues. J Gerontol A Biol Sci Med Sci 2014;69:S39–42. doi:10.1093/gerona/glu043.

14. Friedenstein AJ, Chailakhjan RK, Lalykina KS. The development of fibroblast colonies in monolayer cultures of guinea-pig bone marrow and spleen cells. Cell Tissue Kinet 1970;3:393–403.

15. Dominici M, Le Blanc K, Mueller I, Slaper-Cortenbach I, Marini F, Krause D, *et al.* Minimal criteria for defining multipotent mesenchymal stromal cells. The International Society for Cellular Therapy position statement. Cytotherapy 2006;8:315–7. doi:10.1080/14653240600855905.

16. Pittenger MF, Mackay AM, Beck SC, Jaiswal RK, Douglas R, Mosca JD, *et al.* Multilineage potential of adult human mesenchymal stem cells. Science 1999;284:143– 7.

17. Uccelli A, Moretta L, Pistoia V. Mesenchymal stem cells in health and disease. Nat Rev Immunol 2008;8:726–36. doi:10.1038/nri2395.

18. Ghannam S, Bouffi C, Djouad F, Jorgensen C, Noël D. Immunosuppression by mesenchymal stem cells: mechanisms and clinical applications. Stem Cell Res Ther 2010;1:2. doi:10.1186/scrt2.

19. Majumdar MK, Keane-Moore M, Buyaner D, Hardy WB, Moorman MA, McIntosh KR, *et al.* Characterization and functionality of cell surface molecules on human mesenchymal stem cells. J Biomed Sci 2003;10:228–41. doi:68710.

20. Nicola MD, Carlo-Stella C, Magni M, Milanesi M, Longoni PD, Matteucci P, *et al.* Human bone marrow stromal cells suppress T-lymphocyte proliferation induced by cellular or nonspecific mitogenic stimuli. Blood 2002;99:3838–43. doi:10.1182/blood.V99.10.3838.

21. Tse WT, Pendleton JD, Beyer WM, Egalka MC, Guinan EC. Suppression of allogeneic T-cell proliferation by human marrow stromal cells: implications in transplantation. Transplantation 2003;75:389–97. doi:10.1097/01.TP.0000045055.63901.A9.

22. Prockop DJ, Oh JY. Mesenchymal Stem/Stromal Cells (MSCs): Role as Guardians of Inflammation. Mol Ther 2012;20:14–20. doi:10.1038/mt.2011.211.

23. Phinney DG, Pittenger MF. Concise Review: MSC-Derived Exosomes for Cell-Free Therapy. Stem Cells Dayt Ohio 2017;35:851–8.doi:10.1002/stem.2575.

24. Lai RC, Arslan F, Lee MM, Sze NSK, Choo A, Chen TS, *et al.* Exosome secreted by MSC reduces myocardial ischemia/reperfusion injury. Stem Cell Res 2010;4:214–22. doi:10.1016/j.scr.2009.12.003.

25. Bian S, Zhang L, Duan L, Wang X, Min Y, Yu H. Extracellular vesicles derived from human bone marrow mesenchymal stem cells promote angiogenesis in a rat myocardial infarction model. J Mol Med Berl Ger 2014;92:387–97. doi:10.1007/s00109- 013-1110-5.

26. Rustom A, Saffrich R, Markovic I, Walther P, Gerdes H-H. Nanotubular highways for intercellular organelle transport. Science 2004;303:1007–10. doi:10.1126/science.1093133.

27. Önfelt B, Nedvetzki S, Yanagi K, Davis DM. Cutting Edge: Membrane Nanotubes Connect Immune Cells. J Immunol 2004;173:1511–3. doi:10.4049/jimmunol.173.3.1511.

28. Spees JL, Olson SD, Whitney MJ, Prockop DJ. Mitochondrial transfer between cells can rescue aerobic respiration. Proc Natl Acad Sci 2006;103:1283–8. doi:10.1073/pnas.0510511103.

29. Plotnikov EY, Khryapenkova TG, Galkina SI, Sukhikh GT, Zorov DB. Cytoplasm and organelle transfer between mesenchymal multipotent stromal cells and renal tubular cells in co-culture. Exp Cell Res 2010;316:2447–55. doi:10.1016/j.yexcr.2010.06.009.

30. Acquistapace A, Bru T, Lesault P-F, Figeac F, Coudert AE, Le Coz O, *et al.* Human mesenchymal stem cells reprogram adult cardiomyocytes toward a progenitor-like state through partial cell fusion and mitochondria transfer. Stem Cells Dayt Ohio 2011;29:812–24. doi: 10.1002/stem.632.

31. Islam MN, Das SR, Emin MT, Wei M, Sun L, Westphalen K, *et al.* Mitochondrial transfer from bone marrow-derived stromal cells to pulmonary alveoli protects against acute lung injury. Nat Med 2012;18:759–65. doi:10.1038/nm.2736.

32. Liu K, Ji K, Guo L, Wu W, Lu H, Shan P, *et al.* Mesenchymal stem cells rescue injured endothelial cells in an *in vitro* ischemia-reperfusion model via tunneling nanotube like structure-mediated mitochondrial transfer. Microvasc Res 2014;92:10–8. doi:10.1016/j.mvr.2014.01.008.

33. Pasquier J, Guerrouahen BS, Al Thawadi H, Ghiabi P, Maleki M, Abu-Kaoud N, *et al.* Preferential transfer of mitochondria from endothelial to cancer cells through tunneling nanotubes modulates chemoresistance. J Transl Med 2013;11:94. doi:10.1186/1479-5876-11-94.

34. Austefjord MW, Gerdes H-H, Wang X. Tunneling nanotubes. Commun Integr Biol 2014;7. doi:10.4161/cib.27934.

35. Moschoi R, Imbert V, Nebout M, Chiche J, Mary D, Prebet T, *et al.* Protective mitochondrial transfer from bone marrow stromal cells to acute myeloid leukemic cells during chemotherapy. Blood 2016;128:253–64. doi:10.1182/blood-2015-07-655860.

36. Morandi A, Indraccolo S. Linking metabolic reprogramming to therapy resistance in cancer. Biochim Biophys Acta 2017;1868:1–6. doi:10.1016/j.bbcan.2016.12.004.

37. Corbet C, Feron O. Cancer cell metabolism and mitochondria: Nutrient plasticity for TCA cycle fueling. Biochim Biophys Acta 2017;1868:7–15. doi:10.1016/j.bbcan.2017.01.002.

38. Scherzed A, Hackenberg S, Froelich K, Kessler M, Koehler C, Hagen R, *et al.* BMSC enhance the survival of paclitaxel treated squamous cell carcinoma cells *in vitro*. Cancer Biol Ther 2011;11:349–57.

39. Roodhart JML, Daenen LGM, Stigter ECA, Prins H-J, Gerrits J, Houthuijzen JM, *et al.* Mesenchymal Stem Cells Induce Resistance to Chemotherapy through the Release of Platinum-Induced Fatty Acids. Cancer Cell 2011;20:370–83. doi:10.1016/j.ccr.2011.08.010.

40. Gnecchi M, He H, Liang OD, Melo LG, Morello F, Mu H, *et al.* Paracrine action accounts for marked protection of ischemic heart by Akt-modified mesenchymal stem cells. Nat Med 2005;11:367–8. doi:10.1038/nm0405-367.

41. Nguyen B-K, Maltais S, Perrault LP, Tanguay J-F, Tardif J-C, Stevens L-M, *et al.* Improved function and myocardial repair of infarcted heart by intracoronary injection of mesenchymal stem cell-derived growth factors. J Cardiovasc Transl Res 2010;3:547– 58. doi:10.1007/s12265-010-9171-0.

42. Mias C, Lairez O, Trouche E, Roncalli J, Calise D, Seguelas M-H, *et al.* Mesenchymal stem cells promote matrix metalloproteinase secretion by cardiac fibroblasts and reduce cardiac ventricular fibrosis after myocardial infarction. Stem Cells Dayt Ohio 2009;27:2734–43. doi:10.1002/stem.169.

43. Serrano AL, Mann CJ, Vidal B, Ardite E, Perdiguero E, Muñoz-Cánoves P. Cellular and molecular mechanisms regulating fibrosis in skeletal muscle repair and disease. Curr Top Dev Biol 2011;96:167–201. doi:10.1016/B978-0-12-385940-2.00007-3.

44. Bianco P. "Mesenchymal" stem cells. Annu Rev Cell Dev Biol 2014;30:677–704. doi:10.1146/annurev-cellbio-100913-013132.

45. Golpanian S, Schulman IH, Ebert RF, Heldman AW, DiFede DL, Yang PC, *et al.* Concise Review: Review and Perspective of Cell Dosage and Routes of Administration From Preclinical and Clinical Studies of Stem Cell Therapy for Heart Disease. Stem Cells Transl Med 2016;5:186–91. doi:10.5966/sctm.2015-0101.

46. Trounson A, McDonald C. Stem Cell Therapies in Clinical Trials: Progress and Challenges. Cell Stem Cell 2015;17:11–22. doi:10.1016/j.stem.2015.06.007.

47. Gyöngyösi M, Wojakowski W, Lemarchand P, Lunde K, Tendera M, Bartunek J, *et al.* Meta-Analysis of Cell-based CaRdiac stUdiEs (ACCRUE) in patients with acute myocardial infarction based on individual patient data. Circ Res 2015;116:1346–60. doi:10.1161/CIRCRESAHA.116.304346.

48. Hare JM, Fishman JE, Gerstenblith G, DiFede Velazquez DL, Zambrano JP, Suncion VY, *et al.* Comparison of Allogeneic vs Autologous Bone Marrow–Derived Mesenchymal Stem Cells Delivered by Transendocardial Injection in Patients With Ischemic Cardiomyopathy. JAMA 2012;308:2369–79. doi:10.1001/jama.2012.25321.

49. Hamamoto H, Gorman JH, Ryan LP, Hinmon R, Martens TP, Schuster MD, *et al.* Allogeneic Mesenchymal Precursor Cell Therapy to Limit Remodeling After Myocardial Infarction: The Effect of Cell Dosage. Ann Thorac Surg 2009;87:794–801. doi:10.1016/j.athoracsur.2008.11.057.

50. Luzzani CD, Miriuka SG. Pluripotent Stem Cells as a Robust Source of Mesenchymal Stem Cells. Stem Cell Rev 2017;13:68–78. doi:10.1007/s12015-016-9695-z.

51. Hoogduijn MJ, Verstegen MMA, Engela AU, Korevaar SS, Roemeling-van Rhijn M, Merino A, *et al.* No evidence for circulating mesenchymal stem cells in patients with organ injury. Stem Cells Dev 2014;23:2328–35. doi:10.1089/scd.2014.0269.

52. Ohgo S, Hasegawa S, Hasebe Y, Mizutani H, Nakata S, Akamatsu H. Senescent dermal fibroblasts enhance stem cell migration through CCL2/CCR2 axis. Exp Dermatol 2015;24:552–4. doi:10.1111/exd.12701.

Chapter 15

Epigenetic Drift Is a Determinant of Mammalian Lifespan

The epigenome, which controls cell identity and function, is not maintained with 100 percent fidelity in somatic animal cells. Errors in the maintenance of the epigenome lead to epigenetic drift, an important hallmark of aging. Numerous studies have described DNA methylation clocks that correlate epigenetic drift with increasing age. The question of how significant a role epigenetic drift plays in creating the phenotypes associated with aging remains open. A recent study describes a new DNA methylation clock that can be slowed by caloric restriction (CR) in a way that correlates with the degree of lifespan and health-span extension conferred by CR, suggesting that epigenetic drift itself is a determinant of mammalian lifespan. Genetic transplantation using genomic editing of DNA methylation homeostatic genes from long-lived to short-lived species is one way to potentially demonstrate a causative role for DNA methylation. Whether the DNA methylation clock be reset to youthful state, eliminating the effects of epigenetic drift without requiring a pluripotent cell intermediate is a critical question with profound implications for the development of aging therapeutics. Methods that transiently erase the DNA methylation pattern of somatic cells may be developed that reset this aging hallmark with potentially profound effects on lifespan, if DNA methylation-based epigenetic drift really plays a primary role in aging.

Introduction

The epigenome, which controls cell identity and function, is not maintained with 100 percent fidelity in somatic animal cells. Errors in the maintenance of the epigenome lead to epigenetic drift [1,2], an important hallmark of aging [3]. Because changes in the epigenome can result in changes in gene expression [4], and such changes in turn can alter which and how many proteins are made by a cell, it is evident that epigenetic drift could significantly impact homeostasis over time resulting in phenotypes characteristic of aging.

Determining the relative contribution of each hallmark of aging is of great importance to understanding the mechanisms that underlie aging with the potential to increase healthspan and eventually lifespan. Maintenance of homeostasis, growth control and stress response at the cellular level are key mechanisms that are conserved in animals. Numerous key genes, such as Daf-2/insulin receptors, and related pathways when modified or mutated can extend lifespan in organisms ranging from invertebrates, such as worms (*C. Elegans*) and fruit flies (*Drosophila*), to mammals such as mice, rats and monkeys [5]. But characterizing the nature and contribution of the specific underlying molecular and cellular processes beyond the general idea that damage or entropy drives increasing dysfunction with age are critical to understanding aging. Unlike simple machines, biological systems possess varying degrees of regenerative/rejuvenative capacity that counteracts myriad forms of damage. The extent to which an animal's somatic cells can counter intrinsic or extrinsic entropic forces largely determines its lifespan. In the extreme, some organisms such as hydra appear immortal, in that they maintain a constant mortality with age [6]. The mechanism involves non-aging stem cells capable of replacing all cells in the organism. The differentiated cells in the hydra themselves likely age, but specialized mechanisms to maintain stem cells indefinitely must exist at least in hydra. Hydra have solved the problems of **extrinsic damage**, due in part to DNA and other biomolecule damage via radiation and the environment, and **intrinsic** damage due in part to problematic cell divisions and maintenance of cell state via the epigenome.

In animals with a finite lifespan (the vast majority of known species!), epigenetic drift occurs [4], however its relative importance compared to other hallmarks of aging such as cell senescence is a matter of debate. A simple prediction is that the most important hallmarks of aging will most closely correlate with chronological age in any specific organism and that differences between lifespans of organisms will also correlate quantitatively with the specific hallmark.

Patterns of DNA methylation at deoxycytosines in CpGs, a critical epigenetic modification at least in vertebrates, have been observed to change with age in relatively characteristic ways. These changes are especially significant in CpG islands (CGIs), clusters of CpGs that localize to promoter regions in mammals. CGIs tend to be unmethylated, while overall most CpGs which are localized to non-CGIs are methylated [7]. Various aging "clocks" based on sequencing of cells and tissues from young and old mice, rats, monkeys, humans and other mammals have been reported [8-12]. These clocks identify sets of specific DNA methylation changes that when statistically analyzed as a set, can be used to predict the chronological and perhaps even the biological age of an organism with accuracy in humans of the order of +/- 3.6 years for the Horvath clock [9] and 3.3 weeks in the mouse [13]. In addition, there are numerous reports that patterns of methylation of DNA can predict all-cause mortality in humans [14-18]. Correlations of increased epigenetic drift in DNA methylation patterns have been reported for cognitive and physical functioning [14], obesity [19], menopause [20], osteoarthritis [21], neurodegenerative diseases including Alzheimer's disease [22], Huntington's disease [23], and Parkinson's disease [24] and Down syndrome [25], lung cancer [26], HIV infection [27], while centenarians [18, 28] exhibit a more youthful less altered pattern.

Interestingly, these DNA methylation clocks in general did not correlate with transcriptional changes in the set of genes comprising the clock, which is surprising because DNA hypermethylation at promoters tends to repress transcription, while DNA hypomethylation tends to activate RNA transcription in mammals and probably all vertebrates. Transcriptional changes over time have been associated with aging [6,7]. Moreover, the changes in the clock genes are statistical, there is mosaicism at the individual cell level [30], which would suggest that adult organisms may carry a mixture of young, middle-aged and old cells at any point in their lifetime, with the mixture tending toward more old cells with increasing age. Not surprisingly, at least one of the more well- studied DNA methylation clocks is closely linked to cell proliferation, the greater number of cell divisions, the older the cell appears [9]. Moreover, a DNA methylation based mitotic clock for stem cells has been established that connects extent of cell proliferation with cancer [31]. Thus, diseases characterized by physical damage to tissues that provokes a repair response involving cell division exhibit an aged methylation phenotype. The processes of DNA methylation based epigenetic drift appears independent of replicative and cellular senescence in that a correlation of altered DNA methylation with cell passage persists in cell culture, but not with senescence status [32]. However, it seems likely that the role of pro-inflammatory signals from senescent cells on bystanders are likely to accelerate epigenetic drift in the bystanders.

Clearly, changes in methylation of DNA are potentially good biomarkers for aging in mammals, but are they actually one of the fundamental mechanisms that cause loss of homeostasis that is observed with aging? One complicating problem is that methylation of DNA at CpG plays a less critical role in invertebrate gene expression versus mammals. For example, in well-studied *Drosophila*, levels of CpG are very low and the regulatory role is unclear, and in *C. elegans*, CpG is essentially not present at all. However, epigenetic drift has been reported for *C. elegans* at the level of histone modifications H3K27me3 [33] [34], and *Drosophila* [35] and associated with "transcriptional drift"[36], increasing number of errors in the pattern of transcribed genes. There is speculation from work describing extensive methylation of DNA in pacific oysters that CpG DNA methylation may in fact, date to the common ancestor of eukaryotes [37], although its differential role in influencing gene expression versus stabilizing the genome and suppressing transposable elements may vary greatly through evolutionary time[38]. In vertebrates and mammals methylation of DNA at CpG modulates gene expression and plays a significant role in maintaining cell identity, as is clear from experiments in which treatment with 5-azacytidine, a DNMT inhibitor that hypomethylates DNA, can transform fibroblasts into myocytes, chondrocytes and adipocytes [39]. Clearly, alteration of methylation of DNA with aging could have profound effects on cell state and function.

Epigenetic Drift is a Determinant of Mammalian Lifespan

In work that extends our understanding of the possible role that DNA methylation-based epigenetic drift plays in determining lifespan, Maegawa *et al.* [40] show that the rate of epigenetic drift correlates with lifespan among mice, rhesus monkeys and humans. Furthermore, caloric restriction (CR), which extends lifespan in a large number of organisms, in monkeys and mice resulted patterns of methylation of DNA in blood cells significantly younger than *ad libitum* (AL) controls. The authors suggest in a somewhat circular fashion that CR slows aging in part through slowing epigenetic drift and that epigenetic drift may be a key determinant of mammalian lifespan [40]. Actually, more sophisticated experiments in which maintenance of methylation of DNA was altered directly by genetic means or drugs in the context of CR, would be needed to actually prove these hypotheses. A potentially transformative experiment would be to use CRISPR gene editing to substitute key DNA methylation metabolism genes DNMT1, DNMT2, DNMT3A, DNMT3B, TET1, TET2 and TET3 from a long-lived species, such as humans into short-lived mice, and examine the effect on genetic drift and lifespan.

In Maegawa et al.'s experiments, unlike much of the previous work that generated DNA methylation clocks the Digital Restriction Enzyme Analysis of Methylation (DREAM) sequencing method was used [40]. In this method DNA is digested by two restriction enzymes. One only cuts CCCGGG without a methylated CpG, leaving a blunt ended fragment cut in the middle of the recognition sequence, then another enzyme is used that will cut CCCGGG regardless of C(m)pG leaving a 5' overhand creating a methylation signature for next generation sequencing (NGS)[41]. This method is very sensitive, but will miss many methylated CpGs not in the recognition sequence. Analyzing 19 mice from 0.3- 2.8 years, 16 monkeys from 0.8 to 30 years and 16 humans from 0 (cord blood) to 86 years, using unsupervised hierarchical clustering, a standard statistical technique, found that for the subset of genes in unmethylated CGI sites (5%<) methylation went from $2 \pm 0.1\%$ in the young to $18 \pm 5\%$ in the old mice (p = 0.03), $2 \pm 0.3\%$ to $22 \pm 3\%$ in young vs. old monkeys (p = 0.002) and $3 \pm 0.5\%$ to $20 \pm 4\%$ in newborn vs. old humans (p = 0.009). The reverse pattern was seen for non-CGI sites with the most methylation (>90%): DNA methylation went from $94 \pm 0.4\%$ (young mice) to $78 \pm 4\%$ (old mice) (p = 0.003) and similarly from $94 \pm 0.3\%$ to $73 \pm 4\%$ in young vs. old monkeys (p = 0.007) and from $93 \pm 1\%$ in newborns to $74 \pm 2\%$ in newborns to old humans (p < 0.001). So which genes were involved? Ingenuity pathway analysis of hypermethylated genes showed enrichment for genes involved in development, signaling, growth, cell maintenance and in cancer and cardiovascular disease. Pathways tended to be conserved across species. They then repeated this analysis for granulocytes, T-cells and CD34+ cells to determine which of the analyzed genes might have cell-type specific methylation patterns, and were able to show that variation in cell numbers of these cells could not explain the variability, although they should have done a more comprehensive study looking at neutrophils, monocytes, eosinophils, and B-cells as well. Then focusing on promoter regions, Maegawa et al. find that the genes involved in "methylation drift" are conserved across all three species[40]. But keep in mind the potential artifacts from requiring the CCCGGG sequence to be present in order to be detected in any particular gene, which would occur 1 out of 4096 random DNA sequences.

How did the DREAM DNA methylation analysis compare to other studies using different techniques? There was overlap, but the DREAM method detected a much higher number of drifted genes. What about correlation with gene expression, which was generally not observed in previous reports? Using DREAM, Maegawa et al. found substantial correlation with gene expression. Genes with increased expression with age were significantly demethylated, and the smaller number of genes with reduced expression with age had increased DNA methylation. In order to confirm the data, another method of detecting DNA methylation was used: bisulfite pyrosequencing, in which treatment with bisulfite converts methylated cytosine to uracil, which sequences as a thymidine for 34 candidate mouse genes, 36 candidate monkey genes, and 16 human genes. Clear age-related patterns emerged, but with the caveat that some genes showed significant DNA methylation changes by bisulfite pyrosequencing that were undetected by DREAM, which is consistent with the more thorough capability of the former. The authors suggest that their DREAM analysis may underestimate the extent of conservation and alterations among species [40].

To determine a rate of age-related hypermethylation, Maegawa *et al.* considered 10 conserved hypermethylated genes and plotted the data against age to calculate drift rates of 4.1 ± 1.2% per year in mice, 0.34 ± 0.14% per year in monkeys, and 0.10 ± 0.02% per year in humans. The numbers were similar considering all tested hypermethylated genes regardless of conservation: 5.1 ± 0.4% per year in mice, 0.47 ± 0.02% per year in monkeys, 0.09 ± 0.01% per year in humans. This data is consistent with the idea that epigenetic drift is a determinant of maximum lifespan, but is only correlative. There was an inverse correlation in a log-log plot of methylation rate with maximum lifespan (**Figure 15.1**) [40]. In effect, Maegawa *et al.* have built a new DNA methylation aging clock. Interestingly some monkeys appear to have a methylation rate significantly lower than some humans, and there is a four fold difference in rates methylation rate for humans which may be due to noise, or to the possibility that the model needs refinement.

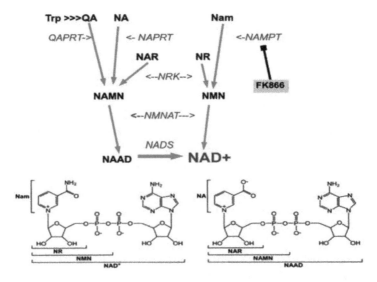

Figure 15.1 Maximum lifespan is correlated with methylation rate of change per year (adapted from Maegawa *et al. 2017*).

Because CR is known to extend lifespan in mice, and monkeys, the effect of CR on DNA methylation drift was examined using DREAM and pyrosequencing on blood cells in old mice (2.7 to 3.2 years) subjected to 40% CR from 0.3 years and on old monkeys (22-30 years) subjected to 30% CR from 7-14 years old. Caloric restriction slowed DNA methylation drift for both the mice and monkeys. The average methylation of all 24 genes was 26 ± 2% in AL old mice and 17 ± 0.7% in CR old mice and average methylation was 27 ± 0.7% in AL monkeys compared to 24 ± 0.9% in CR monkeys. The 12 CR mice had an average chronological age of 2.8 years and a "methylation age" of 0.8 years (3.5 fold improvement in epigenetic drift rate), and the 18 CR monkeys had an average chronologic age of 27 years with the predicted methylation age of 20 years[40]. The clock may need calibration, as 2.8 year old mice are reporting 0.8 years, are unlikely to live another 2 years or more as would be predicted from the clock. The decidedly smaller effect for monkeys may be due to a combination of less CR, starting CR later, or primates having less potential to improve epigenetic drift given inherently lower drift.

To determine tissue specificity of epigenetic drift, 12 hypermethylated and 3 hypomethylated genes were studied. Most of these genes showed age-associated DNA methylation drift in most tissues. Interestingly, as might be predicted from cell proliferation rates, kidney and liver showed less age-related hypermethylation, while the large intestine showed even larger drift than blood. On the other hand, blood, spleen, and kidney showed similar hypomethylation drift, while liver, small, and large intestine and bone marrow had reduced drift. [40] Since hypomethylation tends to be occurring at non- CGI locations it suggests that mechanisms other than proliferation rate may actually underlie this kind of epigenetic drift.

Given the hypothesis that telomere shortening is a potential biomarker for aging, as well as promoter of aging, quantitative PCR was used to examine telomere shortening in mice, monkeys and humans. Interestingly, only a small amount of telomere shortening was found with age, on which CR treatment had no measurable effect, in agreement with a previous report in monkeys [42], suggesting that telomere length is a poor biomarker for biological age.

As the authors point out, their data was cross-sectional, a longitudinal study would likely provide even more accurate data and better models [40]. Larger data sets and greater use of pyrosequencing across the whole genome on pure populations of cells will eventually yield far better data and models.

Maegawa *et al.* hypothesize that the most reproducible changes they observe are in stem or progenitor cells, given that differentiated cells might be lost upon cell death, which may be an oversimplification as some differentiated cells in the immune system, liver, kidneys etc. can be quiescent for long periods, and that differentiation does not automatically imply a post-mitotic state [40]. However, their hypothesis is strongly supported by emerging data. Epigenetic drift may cause loss of stem cell plasticity by aging and a key regulator of lifespan [30] Stem cell dysfunction and exhaustion have been linked to aging- associated dysfunction [43-45]. Given that epigenetic programs may be established and reset during the DNA replication to some extent, it is plausible that DNA methylation drift derives from accumulated random epigenetic errors during stem cell proliferation. They suggest that species-specific differences in rates of methylation drift relate to differing rates of stem cell turnover. This is plausible, although in need of supporting data.

We suggest that there are other intriguing possibilities. The fidelity of epigenetic maintenance in cell proliferation may be different between species. For example, the error rate of methylation maintenance has not been exhaustively studied. A rate of 10e-4 to 10e-5 loss/gains per division was observed for CpGs of the APRT gene in cultured mice kidney cells. [46] Small differences in the epigenetic maintenance rate per cell division could translate into large differences in the epigenetic drift rate per year. Another possibility is that there is a close link between DNA damage and repair capability and epigenetic drift. Cells from species with enhanced DNA repair capacity, which is associated with longevity [47], are likely to better maintain chromatin structure and patterns of DNA methylation after constant damage from environmental radiation. Consistent with such a hypothesis, CR or fasting enhances DNA repair in mammals and protects from DNA damage from chemotherapy and radiation damage in mice and humans [48], and CR helps to delay accelerated aging in a DNA repair deficient mouse model [49]. Perhaps the same mechanisms that protect from DNA damage, help maintain the methylome.

Because previous studies have shown that chronic inflammation, which is known to shorten lifespan, also accelerates methylation drift [50], and because so many diseases with an inflammatory component accelerate DNA methylation clocks it is tempting to speculate that increased numbers of senescent cells promoting inflammation may very well accelerate epigenetic drift, and that epigenetic drift may lead to cell stress that promotes cell senescence, a vicious cycle. For example, inhibition of DNA methyltransferases by 5-azacytidine or siRNA induces senescence in mesenchymal stem cells (MSCs) by altering DNA methylation and histones associated with promoters [51]. Could increased DNA methylation also trigger senescence? In support of the latter idea a stochastically acquired DNA methylation signature for senescence is acquired in subpopulations of MSCs over time [52].

Post-mitotic differentiated cells such as neurons may be subject to epigenetic drift with aging as well. For example, the epigenome in post-mitotic Purkinje cells is reported to be dynamic during development [53] and neuronal activity has been reported to modify patterns of DNA methylation [54]. Moreover, it has been suggested that at least some of the aging-associated DNA methylation changes observed with aging in the brain derives from neurons [55] and DNA methylation changes in synaptic genes in the prefrontal cortex associate with aging [56]. DNA damage from radiation and other external insults would be predicted to play a key role in post-mitotic cells. In a recent report, epigenetic drift associated with aging was hypothesized to play a role in altering autophagy in adult neurons in *C. elegans* [57]. Autophagy, typically a beneficial homeostatic process that extends lifespan and counters dysfunctions of aging, was transformed in older worms into a destabilizing process that *shortens* lifespan because autophagosomes lose their ability to resolve correctly with age. Worm lifespan could actually be extended 30% by inhibiting autophagy initiating factors such as bec-1 in adult worms, preventing the build up of toxic autophagosomes [57]. That potentially restricted and as yet uncharacterized changes in gene expression that occur during aging could so profoundly alter a homeostasis maintaining process, suggests that there are many ways even modestly altered gene expression can be amplified into pathological phenotypes. One caveat is that CpG DNA methylation plays no role in epigenetic drift in C. *elegans*, which lacks methylated CpG. However, epigenetics is far more complex than just DNA methylation. For example, it is known that a global decrease in histone modification H3K27me3 occurs in aging worms [33], although this aging-associated epigenetic change does not appear conserved in mouse satellite cells [58] or killifish [59].

Medical Implications

Although the existence of epigenetic drift and DNA methylation clocks is established, more work is needed using single cells and complete genome coverage to fully assess how DNA methylation comprehensively changes with aging. Furthermore, such studies need to assess the relative amounts of hydroxymethylcytosine as well as methylcytosine [60]. There is evidence that hydroxymethylcytosine plays a role in nucleosome positioning with distinctive roles in neurons and primordial germ cells [61]. To date, clocks of aging based on methylation of DNA have been derived from studies that ignore this potential complicating distinction, because the most frequently used techniques to detect DNA methylation report hydroxymethylcytosine as cytosine.

Clocks of epigenetic drift based on patterns of DNA methylation provide a powerful molecular biomarker for testing the effects of therapeutics on aging. When performed on cells from the same individual animal or human being, it should be possible to obtain an accurate assessment of at least one molecular hallmark of aging that corresponds well to biological age.

CR has been known for a long time as a means to slow aging in mammals, so it is gratifying to observe that alterations in methylation of DNA reflect a magnitude of change consistent with known effects on lifespan for mice and monkeys [62]. That the effect was reduced for monkeys, suggests that longitudinal studies in humans may be very beneficial in determining just how much potential CR has to extend the lifespan of humans. The recent CALERIE trial showed CR slowed measures of physiological aging in humans [63]. It is quite possible that there will be a large variation for individuals in potential benefits from CR, and from CR mimetics, such as rapamycin [64] caveat that CR sometimes activates mTOR (in opposition to the action of rapamycin, to achieve benefit, for example on the expansion of adult gut stem cells [65]. As for health-span, the effects of CR on cell physiology in humans and animal systems are under intense study. There are points of potential divergence between potential increased lifespan, health-span and negative tradeoffs due to metabolic alterations. For example, CR will, by necessity, reduce muscle mass. An interesting report suggests that CR can improve hematopoietic stem cell (HSC) function by increasing cell numbers and preventing a skewing toward myeloid lineages, but at the same time inhibits differentiation of HSC into lymphoid lineages and blocks proliferation of lymphoid progenitors, effectively impairing immune function [66]. So, it does a person little good if she is biologically younger than her untreated peers, but more prone to mortality. However, other reports suggest that lifelong CR had no effect on immune function [47, 48].

Can the epigenetic clock be reset?

Reprogramming a differentiated cell to a pluripotent state and then re-differentiating cells to the original cell type is the only known way to reverse epigenetic drift and reset the epigenome [69]. An outstanding question is does partial reprogramming via transient induction of IPS inducing factors actually reset the epigenetic state of a cell [70]. The answer to this question should be forthcoming with profound implications for the development of anti-aging therapeutics. A more modest approach, trans-differentiating one cell type (fibroblasts) into another cell type (neurons) appears to retain an epigenetic aging signature of the parental cell [71]. An interesting possibility is that DNA methylation inhibitors such as 5-azacytidine could be used during the transdifferentiation process to erase the aging-associated hypermethylation, and rejuvenate the cells. Potentially, cells may be cis-differentiated into their original phenotype or trans-differentiated into a key stem cell type to rejuvenate their epigenome and/or perhaps reconstitute a stem cell compartment. Determining which drugs or genetic manipulations can erase DNA methylation to change cell state [72], and then whether the correct DNA methylation pattern can be recovered subsequently will have profound impact on this strategy.

References

1. Martin GM. Epigenetic drift in aging identical twins. Proc Natl Acad Sci U S A 2005;102:10413–4. doi:10.1073/pnas.0504743102.
2. Fraga MF, Ballestar E, Paz MF, Ropero S, Setien F, Ballestar ML, *et al.* Epigenetic differences arise during the lifetime of monozygotic twins. Proc Natl Acad Sci U S A 2005;102:10604–9. doi:10.1073/pnas.0500398102.
3. López-Otín C, Blasco MA, Partridge L, Serrano M, Kroemer G. The Hallmarks of Aging. Cell 2013;153:1194–217. doi:10.1016/j.cell.2013.05.039.
4. Booth LN, Brunet A. The Aging Epigenome. Mol Cell 2016;62:728–44. doi:10.1016/j.molcel.2016.05.013.
5. Kenyon CJ. The genetics of ageing. Nature 2010;464:504–12. doi:10.1038/nature08980.

6. Schaible R, Scheuerlein A, Dańko MJ, Gampe J, Martínez DE, Vaupel JW. Constant mortality and fertility over age in Hydra. Proc Natl Acad Sci 2015;112:15701–6. doi:10.1073/pnas.1521002112.

7. Bird A. DNA methylation patterns and epigenetic memory. Genes Dev 2002;16:6–21. doi:10.1101/gad.947102.

8. Hannum G, Guinney J, Zhao L, Zhang L, Hughes G, Sadda S, et al. Genome-wide methylation profiles reveal quantitative views of human aging rates. Mol Cell 2013;49:359–67. doi:10.1016/j.molcel.2012.10.016.

9. Horvath S. DNA methylation age of human tissues and cell types. Genome Biol 2013;14:3156. doi:10.1186/gb-2013-14-10-r115.

10. De Paoli-Iseppi R, Deagle BE, McMahon CR, Hindell MA, Dickinson JL, Jarman SN. Measuring Animal Age with DNA Methylation: From Humans to Wild Animals. Front Genet 2017;8. doi:10.3389/fgene.2017.00106.

11. Bocklandt S, Lin W, Sehl ME, Sánchez FJ, Sinsheimer JS, Horvath S, et al. Epigenetic Predictor of Age. PLoS ONE 2011;6:e14821. doi:10.1371/journal.pone.0014821.

12. Garagnani P, Bacalini MG, Pirazzini C, Gori D, Giuliani C, Mari D, et al. Methylation of ELOVL2 gene as a new epigenetic marker of age. Aging Cell 2012;11:1132–4. doi:10.1111/acel.12005.

13. Stubbs TM, Bonder MJ, Stark A-K, Krueger F, von Meyenn F, Stegle O, et al. Multi-tissue DNA methylation age predictor in mouse. Genome Biol 2017;18. doi:10.1186/s13059-017-1203-5.

14. Marioni RE, Shah S, McRae AF, Chen BH, Colicino E, Harris SE, et al. DNA methylation age of blood predicts all-cause mortality in later life. Genome Biol 2015;16:25. doi:10.1186/s13059-015-0584-6.

15. Christiansen L, Lenart A, Tan Q, Vaupel JW, Aviv A, McGue M, et al. DNA methylation age is associated with mortality in a longitudinal Danish twin study. Aging Cell 2016;15:149–54. doi:10.1111/acel.12421.

16. Perna L, Zhang Y, Mons U, Holleczek B, Saum K-U, Brenner H. Epigenetic age acceleration predicts cancer, cardiovascular, and all-cause mortality in a German case cohort. Clin Epigenetics 2016;8. doi:10.1186/s13148-016-0228-z.

17. Chen BH, Marioni RE, Colicino E, Peters MJ, Ward-Caviness CK, Tsai P-C, et al. DNA methylation-based measures of biological age: meta-analysis predicting time to death. Aging 2016;8:1844–59. doi:10.18632/aging.101020.

18. Horvath S, Pirazzini C, Bacalini MG, Gentilini D, Di Blasio AM, Delledonne M, et al. Decreased epigenetic age of PBMCs from Italian semi-supercentenarians and their offspring. Aging 2015;7:1159–70.

19. Horvath S, Erhart W, Brosch M, Ammerpohl O, von Schönfels W, Ahrens M, et al. Obesity accelerates epigenetic aging of human liver. Proc Natl Acad Sci U S A 2014;111:15538–43. doi:10.1073/pnas.1412759111.

20. Levine ME, Lu AT, Chen BH, Hernandez DG, Singleton AB, Ferrucci L, et al. Menopause accelerates biological aging. Proc Natl Acad Sci U S A 2016;113:9327–32. doi:10.1073/ pnas.1604558113.

21. Vidal L, Lopez-Golan Y, Rego-Perez I, Horvath S, Blanco FJ, Riancho JA, et al. Specific increase of methylation age in osteoarthritis cartilage. Osteoarthritis Cartilage 2016;24:S63. doi:10.1016/j.joca.2016.01.140.

22. Levine ME, Lu AT, Bennett DA, Horvath S. Epigenetic age of the pre-frontal cortex is associated with neuritic plaques, amyloid load, and Alzheimer's disease related cognitive functioning. Aging 2015;7:1198–211.

23. Horvath S, Langfelder P, Kwak S, Aaronson J, Rosinski J, Vogt TF, et al. Huntington's disease accelerates epigenetic aging of human brain and disrupts DNA methylation levels. Aging 2016;8:1485–504. doi:10.18632/aging.101005.

24. Horvath S, Ritz BR. Increased epigenetic age and granulocyte counts in the blood of Parkinson's disease patients. Aging 2015;7:1130–42.

25. Horvath S, Garagnani P, Bacalini MG, Pirazzini C, Salvioli S, Gentilini D, et al. Accelerated epigenetic aging in Down syndrome. Aging Cell 2015;14:491–5. doi:10.1111/acel.12325.

26. Levine ME, Hosgood HD, Chen B, Absher D, Assimes T, Horvath S. DNA methylation age of blood predicts future onset of lung cancer in the women's health initiative. Aging 2015;7:690–700.

27. Horvath S, Levine AJ. HIV-1 Infection Accelerates Age According to the Epigenetic Clock. J Infect Dis 2015;212:1563–73. doi:10.1093/infdis/jiv277.

28. Horvath S, Mah V, Lu AT, Woo JS, Choi O-W, Jasinska AJ, et al. The cerebellum ages slowly according to the epigenetic clock. Aging 2015;7:294–306.

29. Bahar R, Hartmann CH, Rodriguez KA, Denny AD, Busuttil RA, Dolle MET, et al. Increased cell-to-cell variation in gene expression in ageing mouse heart. Nature 2006;441:1011–4. doi:10.1038/nature04844.

30. Issa J-P. Aging and epigenetic drift: a vicious cycle. J Clin Invest 2014;124:24–9. doi:10.1172/JCI69735.

31. Yang Z, Wong A, Kuh D, Paul DS, Rakyan VK, Leslie RD, et al. Correlation of an epigenetic mitotic clock with cancer risk. Genome Biol 2016;17:205. doi:10.1186/s13059-016-1064-3.

32. Lowe D, Horvath S, Raj K. Epigenetic clock analyses of cellular senescence and ageing. Oncotarget 2016;7:8524–31. doi:10.18632/oncotarget.7383.

33. Maures TJ, Greer EL, Hauswirth AG, Brunet A. H3K27 Demethylase UTX-1 Regulates C. elegans Lifespan in a Germline-Independent, Insulin-Dependent, Manner. Aging Cell 2011;10:980–90. doi:10.1111/j.1474-9726.2011.00738.x.

34. Ni Z, Ebata A, Alipanahiramandi E, Lee SS. Two SET domain containing genes link epigenetic changes and aging in Caenorhabditis elegans. Aging Cell 2012;11:315–25. doi:10.1111/j.1474-9726.2011.00785.x.

35. Wood JG, Hillenmeyer S, Lawrence C, Chang C, Hosier S, Lightfoot W, et al. Chromatin remodeling in the aging genome of Drosophila. Aging Cell 2010;9:971–8. doi:10.1111/j.1474-9726.2010.00624.x.

36. Rangaraju S, Solis GM, Thompson RC, Gomez-Amaro RL, Kurian L, Encalada SE, et al. Suppression of transcriptional drift extends C. elegans lifespan by postponing the onset of mortality. ELife n.d.;4. doi:10.7554/eLife.08833.

37. Wang X, Li Q, Lian J, Li L, Jin L, Cai H, et al. Genome-wide and single-base resolution DNA methylomes of the Pacific oyster Crassostrea gigas provide insight into the evolution of invertebrate CpG methylation. BMC Genomics 2014;15:1119. doi:10.1186/1471-2164-15-1119.

38. Benayoun BA, Pollina EA, Brunet A. Epigenetic regulation of ageing: linking environmental inputs to genomic stability. Nat Rev Mol Cell Biol 2015;16:593–610. doi:10.1038/nrm4048.

39. Taylor SM, Jones PA. Multiple new phenotypes induced in 10T1/2 and 3T3 cells treated with 5-azacytidine. Cell 1979;17:771–9.

40. Maegawa S, Lu Y, Tahara T, Lee JT, Madzo J, Liang S, et al. Caloric restriction delays age-related methylation drift. Nat Commun 2017;8. doi:10.1038/s41467-017-00607-3.

41. Jelinek J, Madzo J. DREAM: A Simple Method for DNA Methylation Profiling by High- throughput Sequencing. Methods Mol Biol Clifton NJ 2016;1465:111–27. doi:10.1007/978-1-4939-4011-0_10.

42. Smith DL, Mattison JA, Desmond RA, Gardner JP, Kimura M, Roth GS, et al. Telomere Dynamics in Rhesus Monkeys: No Apparent Effect of Caloric Restriction. J Gerontol A Biol Sci Med Sci 2011;66A:1163–8. doi:10.1093/gerona/glr136.

43. Beerman I, Bock C, Garrison BS, Smith ZD, Gu H, Meissner A, et al. Proliferation- Dependent Alterations of the DNA Methylation Landscape Underlie Hematopoietic Stem Cell Aging. Cell Stem Cell 2013;12:413–25. doi:10.1016/j.stem.2013.01.017.

44. Schultz MB, Sinclair DA. When stem cells grow old: phenotypes and mechanisms of stem cell aging. Development 2016;143:3–14. doi:10.1242/dev.130633.

45. Oh J, Lee YD, Wagers AJ. Stem cell aging: mechanisms, regulators and therapeutic opportunities. Nat Med 2014;20:870–80. doi:10.1038/nm.3651.

46. Rose JA, Yates PA, Simpson J, Tischfield JA, Stambrook PJ, Turker MS. Biallelic Methylation and Silencing of Mouse Aprt in Normal Kidney Cells. Cancer Res 2000;60:3404–8.

47. MacRae SL, Croken MM, Calder RB, Aliper A, Milholland B, White RR, et al. DNA repair in species with extreme lifespan differences. Aging 2015;7:1171–82.

48. Dorff TB, Groshen S, Garcia A, Shah M, Tsao-Wei D, Pham H, et al. Safety and feasibility of fasting in combination with platinum-based chemotherapy. BMC Cancer 2016;16:360. doi:10.1186/s12885-016-2370-6.

49. Vermeij WP, Dollé MET, Reiling E, Jaarsma D, Payan-Gomez C, Bombardieri CR, et al. Diet restriction delays accelerated aging and genomic stress in DNA repair deficient mice. Nature 2016;537:427–31. doi:10.1038/nature19329.

50. Issa J-PJ, Ahuja N, Toyota M, Bronner MP, Brentnall TA. Accelerated Age-related CpG Island Methylation in Ulcerative Colitis. Cancer Res 2001;61:3573–7.

51. So A-Y, Jung J-W, Lee S, Kim H-S, Kang K-S. DNA Methyltransferase Controls Stem Cell Aging by Regulating BMI1 and EZH2 through MicroRNAs. PLOS ONE 2011;6:e19503. doi:10.1371/journal.pone.0019503.

52. Franzen J, Zirkel A, Blake J, Rath B, Benes V, Papantonis A, et al. Senescence- associated DNA methylation is stochastically acquired in subpopulations of mesenchymal stem cells. Aging Cell 2017;16:183–91. doi:10.1111/acel.12544.

53. Zhou FC, Resendiz M, Lo C-L, Chen Y. Cell-Wide DNA De-Methylation and Re- Methylation of Purkinje Neurons in the Developing Cerebellum. PLOS ONE 016;11:e0162063. doi:10.1371/journal.pone.0162063.

54. Guo JU, Ma DK, Mo H, Ball MP, Jang M-H, Bonaguidi MA, *et al.* Neuronal activity modifies DNA methylation landscape in the adult brain. Nat Neurosci 2011;14:1345– 51. doi:10.1038/nn.2900.

55. Oh G, Ebrahimi S, Wang S-C, Cortese R, Kaminsky ZA, Gottesman II, *et al.* Epigenetic assimilation in the aging human brain. Genome Biol 2016;17:76. doi:10.1186/s13059- 016-0946-8.

56. Ianov L, Riva A, Kumar A, Foster TC. DNA Methylation of Synaptic Genes in the Prefrontal Cortex Is Associated with Aging and Age-Related Cognitive Impairment. Front Aging Neurosci 2017;9. doi:10.3389/fnagi.2017.00249.

57. Wilhelm T, Byrne J, Medina R, Kolundžić E, Geisinger J, Hajduskova M, Neuronal inhibition of the autophagy nucleation complex extends life span in post- reproductive C. elegans. Genes Dev 2017;31:1561–72. doi:10.1101/gad.301648.117.

58. Liu L, Cheung TH, Charville GW, Hurgo BMC, Leavitt T, Shih J, *et al.* Chromatin Modifications as Determinants of Muscle Stem Cell Quiescence and Chronological Aging. Cell Rep 2013;4:189–204. doi:10.1016/j.celrep.2013.05.043.

59. Baumgart M, Groth M, Priebe S, Savino A, Testa G, Dix A, *et al.* RNA-seq of the aging brain in the short-lived fish N. furzeri-conserved pathways and novel genes associated with neurogenesis. Aging Cell 2014;13:965–74. doi:10.1111/acel.12257.

60. Song C-X, Szulwach KE, Fu Y, Dai Q, Yi C, Li X, *et al.* Selective chemical labeling reveals the genome-wide distribution of 5-hydroxymethylcytosine. Nat Biotechnol 2011;29:68–72. doi:10.1038/nbt.1732.

61. Teif VB, Beshnova DA, Vainshtein Y, Marth C, Mallm J-P, Höfer T, *et al.* Nucleosome repositioning links DNA (de)methylation and differential CTCF binding during stem cell development. Genome Res 2014;24:1285–95. doi:10.1101/gr.164418.113.

62. Mattison JA, Colman RJ, Beasley TM, Allison DB, Kemnitz JW, Roth GS, *et al.* Caloric restriction improves health and survival of rhesus monkeys. Nat Commun 2017;8. doi:10.1038/ncomms14063.

63. Belsky DW, Huffman KM, Pieper CF, Shalev I, Kraus WE. Change in the Rate of Biological Aging in Response to Caloric Restriction: CALERIE Biobank Analysis. J Gerontol A Biol Sci Med Sci 2017. doi:10.1093/gerona/glx096.

64. Gillespie ZE, Pickering J, Eskiw CH. Better Living through Chemistry: Caloric Restriction (CR) and CR Mimetics Alter Genome Function to Promote Increased Health and Lifespan. Front Genet 2016;7. doi:10.3389/fgene.2016.00142.

65. Igarashi M, Guarente L. mTORC1 and SIRT1 Cooperate to Foster Expansion of Gut Adult Stem Cells during Calorie Restriction. Cell 2016;166:436–50. doi:10.1016/ j.cell.2016.05.044.

66. Tang D, Tao S, Chen Z, Koliesnik IO, Calmes PG, Hoerr V, *et al.* Dietary restriction improves repopulation but impairs lymphoid differentiation capacity of hematopoietic stem cells in early aging. J Exp Med 2016;213:535–53. doi:10.1084/jem.20151100.

67. Tomiyama AJ, Milush JM, Lin J, Flynn JM, Kapahi P, Verdin E, *et al.* Long-term calorie restriction in humans is not associated with indices of delayed immunologic aging: A descriptive study. Nutr Healthy Aging n.d.;4:147–56. doi:10.3233/NHA-160017.

68. Rando TA, Chang HY. Aging, Rejuvenation, and Epigenetic Reprogramming: Resetting the Aging Clock. Cell 2012;148:46–57. doi:10.1016/j.cell.2012.01.003.

69. Okita K, Ichisaka T, Yamanaka S. Generation of germline-competent induced pluripotent stem cells. Nature 2007;advanced online publication. doi:10.1038/nature05934

70. Ocampo A, Reddy P, Martinez-Redondo P, Platero-Luengo A, Hatanaka F, Hishida T, *et al. in vivo* Amelioration of Age-Associated Hallmarks by Partial Reprogramming. Cell 2016;167:1719–1733.e12. doi:10.1016/j.cell.2016.11.052.

71. Mertens J, Paquola ACM, Ku M, Hatch E, Böhnke L, Ladjevardi S, *et al.* Directly Reprogrammed Human Neurons Retain Aging-Associated Transcriptomic Signatures and Reveal Age-Related Nucleocytoplasmic Defects. Cell Stem Cell 2015;17:705–18. doi:10.1016/j.stem.2015.09.001.

72. Lewis C, Brewster B, Tian E, Shi Y. Direct Reprogramming Facilitated by Small Molecules. J Stem Cell Transplant Biol 2015;01.

Chapter 16

Rejuvenation by Partial Reprogramming of the Epigenome

Epigenetic variation with age is one of the most important hallmarks of aging. Resetting or repairing the epigenome of aging cells in intact animals may rejuvenate the cells and perhaps the entire organism. In fact, differentiated adult cells, which by definition have undergone some epigenetic changes, are capable of being rejuvenated and reprogrammed to create pluripotent stem cells and viable cloned animals. Apparently, such reprogramming is capable of completely resetting the epigenome. However, attempts to fully reprogram differentiated cells in adult animals have failed in part because reprogramming leads to formation of teratomas. A preliminary method to partially reprogram adult cells in mature Hutchinson-Guilford progeria (HGPS) mice by transient induction of the Yamanaka factors OSKM (Oct4/Sox2/Klf4/c-Myc) appears to ameliorate aging-like phenotypes in HGPS mice, and promote youthful regenerative capability in middle-aged wild type individuals exposed to beta cell and muscle cell specific toxins. However, whatever epigenetic repair is induced by transient reprogramming does not endure and may be due to the induction of key homeostatic regulators instead. Some of the effect of transient reprogramming may result from increased proliferation and enhanced function of adult stem cells. Partial reprogramming may point the way to new anti-aging and pro-regenerative therapeutics. Re-differentiation of cells into their pre-existing phenotype with simultaneous epigenomic rejuvenation is an interesting variation that also should be pursued. However, discovery of methods to more precisely repair the epigenome is the most likely avenue to the development of powerful new anti-aging agents.

Introduction

Alterations of the epigenetic state/epigenome constitute an important hallmark of aging [1]. Indeed, epigenetic variation with age may be the most important hallmark of aging, because it has been shown in many organisms, including mammals, that adult cells, which by definition have undergone some aging, are capable of being rejuvenated and reprogrammed2 [3]. For example, viable cloned animals have been created by somatic nuclear transfer or incorporation of derived embryonic-stem cell-like induced pluripotent stem cells (iPS). Such iPS cells were prepared by ectopic expression of a defined set of reprogramming factors [Oct4/Sox2/Klf4/c-Myc (OSKM)], first shown by Yamanaka in 20064, and expanded to diverse sets of biochemical agents [5]. iPS cells can be used to create animals possessing the DNA and mitochondria of the originating cell by for example, tetraploid complementation where the iPS cells are injected into a blastocyst formed by fusion of two blastomeres. Because at least some iPS cells can form entire normal animals, a full erasure of a cell's previous epigenetic state and complete amelioration of aging-induced damage is possible.

Can all mammalian cell types carrying a diploid genome be reprogrammed? Possibly. Adult cells that can be reprogrammed to pluripotency are completely rejuvenated suggesting that any damage or loss of critical information with time that is associated with aging can be reversed in these cells. At least some post-mitotic terminally differentiated cells such as neurons [6] can be reprogrammed. Moreover, even senescent, post-mitotic stressed/injured, cells can be successfully rejuvenated by reprogramming [7].

Perhaps the most reductionist view of these results support epigenetic theories of aging [8-10] whereby instability of the epigenome over time results in diminished cellular function and eventually cellular, tissue and organ dysfunction that drives aging. The cause of such instability may be as simple as the consequences of accumulated molecular insults or just an inherent lack of fidelity in maintenance of the epigenome by key regulatory enzymes. Although a hot topic of current research, the fidelity of epigenetic maintenance is not well characterized in mammalian cells. Insights into cell heterogeneity and aging will be a consequence of better understood and quantified molecular mechanisms. If epigenetic theories of aging are valid, then resetting or repairing the epigenome of aging cells in intact animals may rejuvenate the cells and perhaps the entire organism.

Given that pluripotent reprogramming can rejuvenate single cells, several teams of scientists investigated the unlikely but appealing hypothesis that reprogramming a subset of cells in mice by induction of the Yamanaka factors could rejuvenate cell and organismal function. If reprogramming rejuvenates single cells, why not an entire animal? Of course, researchers performing these experiments likely expected and encountered a major problem. Although global induction of OSKM, the Yamanaka factors, indeed resulted in the formation of pluripotent cells *in vivo*, potentially fatal teratomas were also formed [11,12]. There is also a question how induction of OSKM affects different cell types, especially stem cells and post- mitotic cells. These results have thus limited enthusiasm for using reprogramming as a pro-regenerative, anti-aging manipulation. However, the question remains: Is there another way to use reprogramming technology to repair the aging epigenome?

in vivo Amelioration of Age-Associated Hallmarks by Partial Reprogramming

Ocampo and colleagues at the Salk Institute (San Diego, CA) now report a preliminary answer of "yes." Ocampo *et al.* have discovered a "partial reprogramming" technique that can apparently overcome the effects of "aging", at least in cell culture of near senescent fibroblasts, in mice carrying a mutation that confers the premature aging Hutchinson-Guilford progeria (HGP) phenotype, and promotes modest regenerative-based recovery from streptozotocin-induced pancreatic damage, and from cardiotoxin-induced muscle damage [13].

But there is a very large caveat. These are preliminary experiments not directly performed on old animals. HGP mice and enhanced regeneration in middle-aged mice are not truly representative of biological aging: care must be taken in concluding that the results actually apply beyond their specialized domain.

Ocampo *et al* used LAKI-4F and 4F mice. LAKI mice carry the HGP G609G mutation in the lmna gene, which leads to a truncated form of lamin A, aka progerin, responsible for the premature aging symptoms of HGPS. Many of "symptoms" of aging are also observed in LAKI mice including weight loss and dysfunction in several organs including skin, kidney, spleen and tissues including endothelial and smooth muscle cells. Unlike most human patients who are heterozygous for progerin, LAKI mice are homozygous for HGP G609G, which presumably worsens the pathology. LAKI 4F and 4F (wt) mice also carry a doxycycline inducible OSKM polycistronic cassette (4F) [13].

Ocampo and colleagues hypothesized that since reprogramming is a multistage process and early stages retain the initial cell differentiation state, that partial reprogramming may have a beneficial effect on regeneration and the epigenome without causing pathological changes to intact animals. Initial experiments in cultured LAKI 4F tail tip fibroblasts, showed that transient induction of OSKM for two to four days did not extinguish expression of thy1, a fibroblast specific marker, nor induce intermediate stage markers of reprogramming such as SSEA1 or later stage markers of reprogramming such as Nanog. However, transient expression did reduce histone gamma-H2AX expression, a marker of DNA damage, as well as reduce regulators associated with senescence and the p53 pathway such as p16ink4a, p21cip, MMP13 and IL-6. As expected for an early stage of cellular reprogramming, two epigenetic markers of heterochromatin, down regulated H3K9me3 and up regulated H4K20me3 were restored to normal levels. The abnormal nuclear architecture induced by Lmna G609G that is thought to play a significant role in its premature aging effects was restored to near normal morphology by transient OSKM induction. These effects were dependent on the continued expression of OSKM and were quickly lost when OSKM expression was extinguished. Progerin expression was unaffected by OSKM induction and individual expression of Oct4, Sox2, Klf4, or c-Myc did not improve nuclear morphology. Short term restoration of H3K9me3 expression levels is observed as early as 12 hours, and treatment with a h3K9 methyltransferase inhibitor prevented the restoration of near normal nuclear architecture suggesting transient epigenetic remodeling may drive the beneficial effects of transient OSKM expression. The authors conclude that several molecular hallmarks of physiological aging that are observed in HGP fibroblasts were ameliorated by transient induction of OSKM including accumulation of DNA damage, senescence, epigenetic dysregulation and nuclear envelope morphological changes [13].

Similar experiments were performed in 4F mice, which are wild type for Imna, and in late passage cells from 4F mice (which are essentially pre-senescent). Some of the results observed for LAKI 4F derived cells were replicated: reduced amount of DNA damage marker gamma-H2AX, normalized expression of H3K9me, and down-regulated expression of the p53 pathway and senescence-associated gens expression such as p16ink4a, MMP13 and IL-6 as compared to non-OSKM induced cells [13]. However, given that complete reprogramming has an even more beneficial effect on the hallmarks of aging at least for individual cells, these results were not particularly remarkable. The more important question is what happens in animals?

The key difference between Ocampo's and previous work is the empirical discovery that transient, cyclic induction of the OSKM Yamanaka factors for two days ("on the weekend!") by doxycycline, followed by 5 days without the inducer appears to be well tolerated in LAKI F4 mice. This regimen prevented the appearance of teratomas in mice carrying a single copy of the OSKM cassette, even after 35 cycles (weeks). These mice appear healthy and do not lose weight, suggesting that transient cyclic induction of the Yamanaka factors is not toxic. No iPS cells were detected, which suggests that some semblance of normal cell differentiation was maintained under these conditions [13]. This is not surprising as reprogramming has been observed to be a multistage process, and the earliest stages involve changes that do not effect cell differentiation directly [14]. One anomaly that the authors reported as expected is that levels of reactive oxygen species (ROS) are reduced after transient OSKM induction. Decreased ROS levels do occur in IPS cells, but it has been reported that ROS levels actually increase in the earliest stage of reprogramming, and that this increase is necessary for later efficient IPS cell formation [15].

Cyclic treatment of LAKI 4F mice with repeated transient cycles of OSKM induction resulted in an increase of median lifespan from 18 to 24 weeks, and of maximum lifespan from 21 to 29 weeks in the LAKI F4 mice. Doxycycline-stimulated LAKI 4F mice showed improvement in the appearance of skin, kidney, spleen, stomach and other areas of the GI tract, increased epidermal and dermal thickness, reduced skin keratinization, partially restored vascular smooth muscle cells, and decreased bradycardia compared to un-induced control animals. However, there were no apparent histological differences in liver, heart and skeletal muscle between treated and untreated animals [13]. Brain is not normally affected by progerin expression.

At the cellular level, cyclic transient induction of OSKM increased proliferation to more normal levels in the stomach, kidneys and skin. The liver of treated animals contained fewer cells staining positive for senescence marker beta galactosidase, suggesting reduced cell stress and senescence. It would be interesting to know if transient OSKM can reverse the senescent state as has been reported for constitutive OSKM. With regards to stem cells, treatment resulted in increased numbers of pax7 satellite muscle cells, and cytokeratin [15] positive hair follicle stem cells which probably indicates increased regenerative capacity [13]. Other adult stem cell populations such as MSCs, ADSCs or progenitor cell populations were not examined.

The authors hypothesize that taken together these results suggest that transient OSKM induction may prevent several critical hallmarks of aging including dysfunctional epigenetic changes, depletion of stem cell populations, decline of regenerative capacity, and accumulation of senescent cells. However, such sweeping conclusions await experiments in normally aging animals as care must be taken in generalizing about aging phenomena from HGPS mice [16,17].

In order to indirectly address whether cyclic transient OSKM induction has anti-aging effects in wild type mice, 4F (wt) mice were subjected to injurious agents that affect metabolism or muscle function in both young (2-month-old) and middle aged (12-month-old) mice. Specifically, first Ocampo *et al.* showed that young mice are more resistant to the effects of streptozotocin (STZ) than middle aged mice by 1) inducing a diabetes type I like state in young and middle- aged mice by treatment with low dose STZ, a glucose analog that kills pancreatic beta cells, and 2) performing a glucose tolerance test to assess function two weeks after injury to allow tissue repair to occur. Young STZ-treated mice had better glucose tolerance than older mice, Next they pretreated middle-age mice with the hope of either rejuvenating them or conferring STZ resistance similar to young cells. Thus, these mice were given transient, cyclic OSKM treatments for 3 weeks, then given STZ to damage the beta cells, followed by glucose tolerance testing at 2 weeks. Induction of OSKM in STZ-treated mice resulted in better glucose tolerance than in non-induced STZ mice, suggesting that pretreatment with transient OSKM expression confers a degree of protection from STZ toxicity on pancreatic beta cells. An increase in beta cell numbers in OSKM induced STZ treated mice supported this contention. Ocampo et al propose that OSKM-induced mice have better beta cell regenerative capacity than control middle-aged mice [13]. A more thorough molecular analysis of the treated beta cells may shed light on the precise mechanism of protection from STX.

To model sarcopenia, the loss of skeletal muscle with age that is at least partially due to the loss of numbers and function of satellite cells, Ocampo et al used cardiotoxin (CTX)-induced muscle injury of the antero-tibialis muscle of young and middle-aged mice. Skeletal muscle from young mice recovered more quickly from CTX injury than middle-aged mice. OSKM induction was not performed similarly to the other animal experiments because they wanted to ensure that muscle was exposed to doxycycline. Instead, doxycycline, the inducer of OSKM expression was injected directly into the muscle of middle aged mice weekly for three weeks. It is quite possible that muscle localized doxycycline persists far longer than systemic doxycycline, given that strong OSKM expression was observed at 3 days, suggesting that longer OSKM exposure may be important for different cell types, especially those known to be recalcitrant to standard OSKM reprogramming. The mice were then treated with CTX and muscle fiber area was assessed after 10 days. OSKM pre-treatment resulted in increased total muscle fiber as well as increased numbers of pax7 satellite cells, consistent with a pro- regenerative effect [13].

Future studies need to be performed on normal aging animals and include data on known biomarkers of aging. Even in the young or middle age animals used in the current study more details about epigenetic changes including DNA methylation, histone modifications, and the transcriptome of differentiated cells are essential to understand the effects of inducible OSKM on the epigenome and regeneration. It has been observed that more prolonged induction of OSKM induces telomerase [18]., but typically telomerase induction is not characteristic of the preliminary stage of OSKM reprogramming. Thus it will be interesting to investigate the status of telomeres and telomerase, a critical epigenetic phenotye, which associates with some aging phenotypes.

Medical Implications

It is highly unlikely that any direct use of Yamanaka factors would be developed therapeutically and potential future development depends on the nature of the beneficial mechanisms by which transient induction of OSKM alters cell physiology to confer an aging benefit. Can reprogramming be the key to repairing the epigenome and would reprogramming the epigenome indeed have significant pro-regenerative and rejuvenative effects?

To answer these questions requires first answering the question: did transient induction of OSKM actually repair the epigenome? In one sense, yes, clearly DNA gammaH2AX damage- associated loci were reduced, as were the number of senescent cells, and H3K9me3 and H4K20me3 levels were normalized, as was nuclear staining of lamin A/C and morphology in cells from LAKI mice. However, in another sense, the results are disappointing, as the epigenetic effects were transient, they did not endure – a "reset" of the epigenome did not occur, since a new two-day induction of OSKM was necessary every 7 days to maintain the partially normalized phenotypes. If the ultimate goal of an epigenetic repair strategy is to actually repair and/or reset the epigenome of differentiated cells, it is possible that even induction of powerful sets of reprogramming factors for short amounts of time is insufficient and that other approaches will need to be developed.

However, if the epigenome is not being repaired then what is happening? There are several possibilities. Transient epigenome repair that does not change the underlying age-associated alternations in the epigenome may occur or perhaps, the transient induction of OSKM is inducing other pro-homeostatic factors that counter the HG progeria phenotype and are capable of temporarily altering the epigenome. It is well known that multiple interventions can beneficially affect HGP 19., such as blocking farnesylation or reducing mTOR activity. Two such alterations are decrease of growth master regulator mTOR activity and increase of oxidation protective master gene NRF2 activity [2]. Interestingly, expression of SOX2 can inhibit mTOR activity in at least some cell types such as fibroblasts. Also of interest is the induction of NRF2 by OSKM in the earliest phase of reprogramming. In fact NRF2 is needed for efficient reprogramming, especially in the earlier stages [21]. So do these factors confer any benefit to HGP, to preventing senescence, or to reduce damage of STZ to the pancreas or cardiotoxin damage to muscle? The answer is probably yes to at least some of these phenotypes.

Of great interest is that reduction of mTOR activity by rapamycin and stimulation of NRF2 activity, are both known to suppress the HGP phenotype. NRF2 is sequestered by the mutant HG progeria lamin A/C, and increased expression of NRF2 is needed to overcome the toxic effects of this sequestration. The epigenome and nuclear morphology of HGP patient cells is restored to normal by NRF2 reactivation [20]. Although it is unknown whether HGP mice ectopically expressing activated NRF2 live longer than untreated mice, it would be surprising if this were not the case. Rapamycin whose primary effect is to lower mTOR activity, does extend lifespan of HGP as well as wild type mice. In fact, rapamycin has been reported to induce the expression of Oct4 and Sox2, two of the Yamanaka reprogramming factors, as well as Nanog, which can alternatively act as a reprogramming factor [22] suggesting that rapamycin may be one component of a viable drug-based method to transiently induce OSKM.

Can NRF2 recapitulate the pro-regenerative effects of OSKM? Interestingly, induction of NRF2 by pterostilbene can ameliorate STZ-induced diabetes in mice, and NRF2 activity is necessary for recovery from cardiotoxin-induced muscle damage [23] although the effects of enhanced NRF2 activity have not been investigated on muscle damage. NRF2 augments skeletal muscle regeneration after ischemic perfusion injury [24]. Moreover, increased NRF2 expression delays senescence in cultured fibroblasts [25]. In fact, induction of NRF2 alone could explain many of the results seen in Ocampo *et al.* For example, early induction of NRF2 via increased ROS, may quickly result in a rapid drop in ROS via induction of antioxidant enzymes such as superoxide dismutase, possibly explaining the seeming anomalous result of Ocampo *et al.* that transient OSKM induction results in reduced ROS. If induction of a specific regulator such as NRF2 does play a key role, then activating drugs or natural substances such as sulphorane or pterostilbene, known inducers of NRF2 activity, might be a useful therapeutic approach for HGPS, and possibly have anti-aging activity as well. It would also be of interest to see if elevation of NRF2 directly promotes resistance to STZ and CTX, perhaps by optimizing mitochondrial function in relevant stem cells, as observed for transient OSKM induction.

It would certainly be of interest to study the complete set of proteins with altered expression induced by two day OSKM treatment. NRF2 and mTOR would probably be good candidates to start with and could even provide an alternative hypothesis for the potential benefits of transient induction of OSKM on aging. Coincidentally inhibition of mTOR by rapamycin is associated with increased longevity in old mice. NRF2 activation is associated with long-lived animals [26]. and botanically derived Protandim, another NRF2 activator, extended median lifespan in male mice [27]. Both would provide ready mechanisms for enhancement of longevity, should that be observed in subsequent experiments on aging in normal mouse strains.

If reprogramming even partially and/or transiently effects epigenomic repair/arrest or rejuvenation, it will of utility to identify small molecular drugs that have similar effects. Already, combinations of chemical agents have been described that can at least transform fibroblasts into iPS cells. As already mentioned, rapamycin is an attractive agent with known anti-aging activity that had been reported to induce a subset of the Yamanaka factors. While any subsequent development would be contingent on a multitude of factors from toxicology/safety testing to actual tissue targeting and clinical evaluation, a long road ahead is waiting.

To determine the precise epigenetic/epigenomic repairs will require better characterization of changes to the epigenomic state during aging. Discovery of and repair of aging-related epigenetic changes may be accelerated by CRISPR/cas9 directed epigenomic regulators [28-31] to make specific changes at critical loci.

Given the increased numbers of satellite and hair follicle stem cells observed by Ocampo *et al.*, it's possible that the major effect of transient OSKM is not really to repair the epigenome, but to increase the number and enhance the function of progenitor and stem cells in the animal. This raises the question whether OSKM expression which ultimately can induce a primitive pluripotent stem cell state is enhancing the expression of other stem cell master regulators involved in maintenance of the stem cell state, or whether this effect results from enhanced activity of homeostatic regulators such as NRF2 or perhaps both.

Another related idea would be to attempt to reset the differentiation state of stem cells, progenitor cells and terminally differentiated cells by "re-differentiating" them to their preexisting phenotype, similar to transdifferentiation, with the caveat that the epigenome may need to be perturbed during the re-differentiation process to effect repair, given that epigenomic defects remain during transdifferentiation of fibroblasts from old individuals into neurons [32]. It is likely that post-mitotic differentiated cells will be more difficult to re-differentiate than progenitor or stem cells, but we believe that "re-differentiation" combined with appropriate epigenetic perturbation/engineering is a promising way to effect rejuvenation. This approach has been under active investigation by two of us (A.R.M. and J.L.L.).

Conclusion

Partial reprogramming may point the way to new anti-aging and pro-regenerative therapeutics. However, discovery of methods to more precisely repair the epigenome is the most likely avenue to the development of powerful new anti-aging agents.

References

1. López-Otín C, Blasco MA, Partridge L, Serrano M, Kroemer G. The Hallmarks of Aging. Cell 2013;153:1194–217. doi:10.1016/j.cell.2013.05.039.

2. Pal S, Tyler JK. Epigenetics and aging. Sci Adv 2016;2. doi:10.1126/sciadv.1600584.

3. Sen P, Shah PP, Nativio R, Berger SL. Epigenetic Mechanisms of Longevity and Aging. Cell 2016;166:822–39. doi:10.1016/j.cell.2016.07.050.

4. Takahashi K, Yamanaka S. Induction of Pluripotent Stem Cells from Mouse Embryonic and Adult Fibroblast Cultures by Defined Factors. Cell 2006;126:663–76.

5. Eguchi T, Kuboki T. Cellular Reprogramming Using Defined Factors and MicroRNAs. Stem Cells Int 2016;2016. doi:10.1155/2016/7530942.

6. Kim J, Lengner CJ, Kirak O, Hanna J, Cassady JP, Lodato MA, et al. Reprogramming of postnatal neurons into induced pluripotent stem cells by defined factors. Stem Cells Dayt Ohio 2011;29:992– 1000. doi:10.1002/stem. 641.

7. Lapasset L, Milhavet O, Prieur A, Besnard E, Babled A, Aït-Hamou N, et al. Rejuvenating senescent and centenarian human cells by reprogramming through the pluripotent state. Genes Dev 2011;25:2248–53. doi:10.1101/gad.173922.111.

8. Booth LN, Brunet A. The Aging Epigenome. Mol Cell 2016;62:728–44. doi:10.1016/j.molcel.2016.05.013.

9. Rando TA, Chang HY. Aging, Rejuvenation, and Epigenetic Reprogramming: Resetting the Aging Clock. Cell 2012;148:46–57. doi:10.1016/j.cell.2012.01.003.

10. Benayoun BA, Pollina EA, Brunet A. Epigenetic regulation of ageing: linking environmental inputs to genomic stability. Nat Rev Mol Cell Biol 2015;16:593–610. doi:10.1038/nrm4048.

11. Abad M, Mosteiro L, Pantoja C, Cañamero M, Rayon T, Ors I, et al. Reprogramming in vivo produces teratomas and iPS cells with totipotency features. Nature 2013. doi:10.1038/nature12586.

12. Ohnishi K, Semi K, Yamamoto T, Shimizu M, Tanaka A, Mitsunaga K, et al. Premature Termination of Reprogramming in vivo Leads to Cancer Development through Altered Epigenetic Regulation. Cell 2014;156:663–77. doi:10.1016/j.cell.2014.01.005.

13. Ocampo A, Reddy P, Martinez-Redondo P, Platero-Luengo A, Hatanaka F, Hishida T, et al. in vivo Amelioration of Age-Associated Hallmarks by Partial Reprogramming. Cell 2016;167:1719– 33.e12. doi:10.1016/j.cell.2016.11.052.

14. Wu J, Yamauchi T, Belmonte JCI. An overview of mammalian pluripotency. Development 2016;143:1644–8. doi:10.1242/dev.132928.

15. Zhou G, Meng S, Li Y, Ghebremariam YT, Cooke JP. Optimal ROS signaling is critical for nuclear reprogramming. Cell Rep 2016;15:919–25. doi:10.1016/j.celrep.2016.03.084.

16. Burtner CR, Kennedy BK. Progeria syndromes and ageing: what is the connection? Nat Rev Mol Cell Biol 2010;11:567–78. doi:10.1038/nrm2944.

17. Scaffidi P, Misteli T. Reversal of the cellular phenotype in the premature aging disease Hutchinson-Gilford Progeria Syndrome. Nat Med 2005;11:440–5. doi:10.1038/nm1204.

18. Marión RM, Silanes IL de, Mosteiro L, Gamache B, Abad M, Guerra C, et al. Common Telomere Changes during in vivo Reprogramming and Early Stages of Tumorigenesis. Stem Cell Rep 2017;8:460–75. doi:10.1016/j.stemcr.2017.01.001.

19. Blondel S, Jaskowiak A-L, Egesipe A-L, Le Corf A, Navarro C, Cordette V, et al. Induced Pluripotent Stem Cells Reveal Functional Differences Between Drugs Currently Investigated in Patients With Hutchinson-Gilford Progeria Syndrome. Stem Cells Transl Med 2014;3:510–9. doi:10.5966/sctm.2013-0168.

20. Kubben N, Zhang W, Wang L, Voss TC, Yang J, Qu J, et al. Repression of the Antioxidant NRF2 Pathway in Premature Aging. Cell 2016;165:1361–74. doi:10.1016/j.cell.2016.05.017.

21. Hawkins KE, Joy S, Delhove JMKM, Kotiadis VN, Fernandez E, Fitzpatrick LM, *et al.* NRF2 Orchestrates the Metabolic Shift during Induced Pluripotent Stem Cell Reprogramming. Cell Rep 2016;14:1883–91. doi:10.1016/j.celrep.2016.02.003.

22. Pospelova TV, Bykova TV, Zubova SG, Katolikova NV, Yartzeva NM, Pospelov VA. Rapamycin induces pluripotent genes associated with avoidance of replicative senescence. Cell Cycle Georget Tex 2013;12:3841–51. doi:10.4161/cc.27396.

23. Shelar SB, Narasimhan M, Shanmugam G, Litovsky SH, Gounder SS, Karan G, *et al.* Disruption of nuclear factor (erythroid-derived-2)-like 2 antioxidant signaling: a mechanism for impaired activation of stem cells and delayed regeneration of skeletal muscle. FASEB J Off Publ Fed Am Soc Exp Biol 2016;30:1865–79. doi:10.1096/fj.201500153.

24. Al-Sawaf O, Fragoulis A, Rosen C, Keimes N, Liehn EA, Hölzle F, *et al.* Nrf2 augments skeletal muscle regeneration after ischaemia-reperfusion injury. J Pathol 2014;234:538–47. doi:10.1002/path.4418.

25. Kapeta S, Chondrogianni N, Gonos ES. Nuclear Erythroid Factor 2-mediated Proteasome Activation Delays Senescence in Human Fibroblasts. J Biol Chem 2010;285:8171–84. doi:10.1074/jbc. M109.031575.

26. Bruns DR, Drake JC, Biela LM, Peelor FF, Miller BF, Hamilton KL. Nrf2 Signaling and the Slowed Aging Phenotype: Evidence from Long-Lived Models. Oxid Med Cell Longev 2015;2015. doi:10.1155/2015/732596.

27. Strong R, Miller RA, Antebi A, Astle CM, Bogue M, Denzel MS, *et al.* Longer lifespan in male mice treated with a weakly estrogenic agonist, an antioxidant, an α-glucosidase inhibitor or a Nrf2- inducer. Aging Cell 2016;15:872–84. doi:10.1111/acel.12496.

28. Liu XS, Wu H, Ji X, Stelzer Y, Wu X, Czauderna S, *et al.* Editing DNA Methylation in the Mammalian Genome. Cell 2016;167:233–47.e17. doi:10.1016/j.cell.2016.08.056.

29. Hilton IB, D'Ippolito AM, Vockley CM, Thakore PI, Crawford GE, Reddy TE, *et al.* Epigenome editing by a CRISPR/Cas9-based acetyltransferase activates genes from promoters and enhancers. Nat Biotechnol 2015;33:510–7. doi:10.1038/nbt.3199.

30. Enríquez P. CRISPR-Mediated Epigenome Editing. Yale J Biol Med 2016;89:471–86.

31. Thakore PI, Black JB, Hilton IB, Gersbach CA. Editing the Epigenome: Technologies for Programmable Transcriptional Modulation and Epigenetic Regulation. Nat Methods 2016;13:127– 37. doi:10.1038/nmeth.3733.

32. Mertens J, Paquola ACM, Ku M, Hatch E, Böhnke L, Ladjevardi S, *et al.* Directly Reprogrammed Human Neurons Retain Aging-Associated Transcriptomic Signatures and Reveal Age-Related Nucleocytoplasmic Defects. Cell Stem Cell 2015;17:705–18. doi:10.1016/j.stem.2015.09.001.

Chapter 17

Restoring Quiescence and Overcoming Senescence

Elderly humans gradually lose strength and the capacity to repair skeletal muscle. Skeletal muscle repair requires functional skeletal muscle stem (satellite) and progenitor cells (SMSCs). Diminished stem cell numbers and increased dysfunction correlate with the observed gradual loss of strength during aging. Recent reports attribute the loss of stem cell numbers and function to either increased entry into a pre-senescent state or the loss of self- renewal capacity due to an inability to maintain quiescence resulting in stem cell exhaustion. Earlier work has shown that exposure to factors from blood of young animals and other treatments could restore SMSC function. However, cells in the pre-senescent state are refractory to the beneficial effects of being transplanted into a young environment. Entry into the pre-senescent state results from loss of autophagy, leading to increased ROS and epigenetic modification at the CDKN2A locus due to decreased H2Aub, up-regulating cell senescence biomarker p16ink4a. However, the pre-senescent SMSCs can be rejuvenated by agents that stimulate autophagy, such as the mTOR inhibitor rapamycin. Autophagy plays a critical role in SMSC homeostasis. These results have implications for the development of senolytic therapies that attempt to destroy p16ink4a expressing cells, since such therapies would also destroy a reservoir of potentially rescuable regenerative stem cells. Other work suggests that in humans loss of SMSC self-renewal capacity is primarily due to decreased expression of sprouty [1]. DNA hypomethylation at the SPRY1 gene locus down regulates sprouty1, causing inability to maintain quiescence and eventual exhaustion of the stem cell population. A unifying hypothesis posits that in aging humans, first loss of quiescence occurs, depleting the stem cell population, but that remaining SMSCs are increasingly subject to pre- senescence in the very old.

Introduction

Aging reduces repair and regenerative capacity in all organs and tissues. Loss of regenerative capacity is attributable to decreased progenitor and stem cell function [1]. Maintenance of stem function requires self-renewal and capacity to differentiate in response to appropriate signals. Aging reduces stem cell function by multiple mechanisms including altered epigenetics and cell depletion due to cell death, differentiation, or cell senescence [1]. Loss of stem cell self-renewal is typically observed. For example, with increasing age in mammals, melanocyte stem cells in hair follicles tend to differentiate into melanocytes resulting in grey hair and the net loss of stem cells [2]. Stem cell populations may become exhausted by over-proliferation as has been observed with skeletal muscle satellite (or stem) cells (SMSCs), a.k.a., satellite cells, that lose the ability to remain quiescent [3-5].

Broadly, there are two classes of stem cells, those that undergo frequent renewal, exemplified by HSCs and those that undergo infrequent renewal, exemplified by SMSCs. These two classes may face different hurdles to maintain function. Infrequent renewal requires that stem cells have an efficient means of clearing metabolic waste and repairing DNA damage in the absence of cell divisions. Autophagy, whereby cells phagocytose organelles and proteins, is a major mechanism of maintaining homeostasis and may play a special role during quiescence when clearance of waste products by dilution associated with proliferation is not available.

Adult SMSCs play a key role in maintenance of skeletal muscle tissue. Satellite cells are normally quiescent, that is, they do not proliferate unless muscle is injured. SMSCs express the master transcription factor Pax7, which is required for their survival. SMSCs both self-renew and differentiate during repair of muscle.

Although old dysfunctional SMSCs can be rejuvenated by exposure to factors in blood from young animals [6], or by inhibiting TGF-beta [7] and other treatments, there is evidence that satellite cells eventually become unresponsive [4]. Such apparent irreversible loss of satellite stem cell function in old animals has been attributed to cell senescence, a term that encompasses multiple phenotypes in which vertebrate cells are irreversibly quiescent, and may express a variety of associated biomarkers such as elevated beta-galactosidase, p16ink4a, ROS levels, secretion of pro-inflammatory cytokines, increased amounts of heterochromatin etc. [8]

Pre-senescent muscle stem cells are rejuvenated by stimulation of autophagy.

In a potentially insightful study, Garcia-Prat and colleagues show that senescent SMSCs from old mice and people can be rejuvenated by treatment with drugs that stimulate autophagy, suggesting that autophagy plays a key role in the maintenance of stem cell function and prevention of cellular senescence [9] SMSCs from old animals enter a senescent or pre-senescent state in which they become non-functional and express p16ink4a [4], a cyclin dependent kinase inhibitor that targets CDK4 and CDK6, preventing cell cycle progression out of the G0 phase of the cell cycle. That senescent SMSCs can be induced to proliferate and are subsequently capable of producing new differentiated muscle cells, suggests that such cells are actually not senescent but rather "pre-senescent," since their post-mitotic state is reversible.

Garcia-Prat et al. were interested in determining how proteostasis contributed to the maintenance of quiescence in SMSCs. They determined by transcriptomic analysis that expression of autophagic genes were most closely associated with the quiescent state of SMSCs and that autophagic gene expression decreased with increasing age. Autophagy, the self-degradation process that targets organelles and proteins to autophagosomes for destruction in lysosomes has long been implicated in aging and longevity [10]. Using transgenic mice that express LC3, a protein associated with autophagosomes, tagged with GFP (GFP-LC3) as a reporter, Garcia-Prat observed that quiescent SMSCs isolated from old mice (20 to 24 months) stained somewhat more than young mice, suggesting that they had more autophagosomes.

However, when the SMSCs were incubated with bafilomycin, an inhibitor of lysosome degradation which increases GFP-LC3 staining when autophagy is active, only cells from young animals (3 months) accumulated more GFP-LC3. Garcia-Prat concluded that young SMSCs were undergoing constitutive autophagy, while old SMSCs had impaired autophagic activity. Markers of impaired autophagy were detected in old satellite cells, including the accumulation of autophagic vesicles, aggregated clearance regulator p62, and aggregated ubiquitin inclusions, consistent with a defect in autophagy [9].

Treatment of mice with autophagy stimulating drugs rapamycin, a mTOR inhibitor with reported anti-aging activity, or spermidine for two weeks restored levels of autophagy of SMSCs isolated from old mice to levels similar to that of young mice with concomitant reduction of markers of impaired autophagy. Although the satellite cells isolated from old (20-24 month) mice were more dysfunctional than those from young mice, these cells were not considered to be senescent [9].

To study the role of autophagy in mice with senescent satellite cells, satellite cells from 28-month-old geriatric mice were compared to 20-24 month old mice and 3-month-old young mice. To more carefully determine autophagy status, Garcia-Prat *et al.* transfected the isolated satellite cells with a mRFP–GFP–LC3 reporter, which distinguishes between unfused autophagosomes (red + green = yellow) and phagosomes fused to lysosomes (red only, because GFP is inactivated by low pH). Only young satellite cells stain red, consistent with lysosomal fusion and active autophagy. After bafilomycin treatment, only young satellite cells showed increased yellow staining consistent with the formation of new autophagosomes. On the other hand, geriatric satellite cells stained even more strongly for p62 and ubiquitin aggregates, consistent with a strong block in autophagic clearance. To investigate whether restoration of autophagy could restore function and reverse the irreversible senescent state of the geriatric satellite cells, animals were treated with rapamycin for two weeks, satellite cells were isolated by FACS and then engrafted into pre-injured muscle in young mice. Autophagy restored expansion of the geriatric SMSCs with increased numbers of cells expressing Pax7, Ki67, MyoD or myogenin after four days.

MyoD and myogenin expression indicated that cells were undergoing active muscle differentiation. Expression of senescent biomarkers p16ink4a and gammaH2AX, were reduced. Treatment with rapamycin or spermidine also reduced the number of cells staining for the presence of senescence-associated β-galactosidase (SA-β-gal+). To confirm that autophagy and not some other anti-aging property of rapamycin or spermidine was casual, experiments were performed using cells rescued by forced expression of autophagy master regulator Atg7. These cells behaved similarly to those treated with rapamycin, i.e., satellite cells from geriatric mice were rejuvenated with cell cycle re-entry, cell proliferation, new muscle fiber formation and concomitant reduction of senescence markers [9].

Taken together, these data demonstrate that normal stem cell function was restored, and markers of so-called irreversible senescence were reduced, suggesting that stimulation of autophagy rejuvenates senescent cells, perhaps requiring that these senescent cells be relabeled as pre-senescent to avoid problems with convention.

To prove that loss of autophagy could be causal, reciprocal experiments in which autophagy is blocked in young satellite cells were conducted in transgenic mice expressing Atg7 flanked by loxP sites to promote excision in the presence of Cre (Atg7ΔPax7 mice) or Cre fused to the estrogen receptor (Cre-ER) to confer inducibility driven by the muscle stem cell specific Pax7 promoter (Atg7ΔPax7ER mice). These transgenic mice either delete Atg7 in all satellite cells or can be made to delete Atg7 in satellite cells after administration of tamoxifen. Atg7ΔPax7 mice are severely deficient in satellite cells. When tamoxifen is used to delete Atg7 from Atg7ΔPax7ER young mice, the satellite cell population is again severely depleted within 30 days. Together these results suggest that basal autophagy is necessary for maintenance of satellite cell function. The remaining cells in both of these cases showed signs of senescence including increased p16ink4a, as well as cyclin dependent kinase inhibitors p21cip1 and p15ink4b and DNA damage gammaH2AX with no evidence of appropriate cell differentiation into muscle fibers. In response to injury, Pax7+ satellite cells in Atg7ΔPax7 mice showed little ability to expand and rapid conversion to cells expressing senescence biomarkers SA-β Xgal and gamma H2AX. When tagged with GFP, few GFP+ muscle fibers formed. As expected, rapamycin and spermidine had no effect on Atg7 null satellite cells incapable of autophagy confirming that these drugs exert their rejuvenative effect on SMSCs by stimulating autophagy [9].

Given the decreased autophagy observed in old and geriatric satellite cells, Garcia- Prat hypothesized that decreased mitophagy might be important. Mitophagy is essentially autophagy of mitochondria; so this makes sense. As expected, there was an accumulation of mitochondria seen in Atg7 null satellite cells, and a decrease in healthy mitochondria in both geriatric satellite cells and Atg7 null cells from young mice, as determined by the deceased ratio of TMRN, a dye that is sensitive to mitochondrial membrane potential, to Mitotracker green, a dye that stains mitochondria. In Atg7 null young cells and in wild type geriatric satellite cells, loss of mitophagy was observed to result in increased ROS, DNA damage markers like gamma H2AX and parkin, which marks old or damaged mitochondria for degradation. Consistent with this hypothesis, adding bafilomycin to young satellite cells not only blocked autophagy, but also mitophagy and simultaneously increased ROS levels [9].

Are increased levels of ROS required for the effects of impaired autophagy in old and geriatric satellite cells? To answer this question, old mice were treated with the antioxidant Trolox, a vitamin E derivative.

Satellite cells derived from Trolox-treated mice showed increased autophagy as evidenced by an increased number of GFP-LC3 staining and decreased amounts of p62 and ubiquitin conjugates. The mRFP–GFP–LC3 reporter showed increased autophagic flux. Treatment of geriatric satellite cells with Trolox and subsequent transplantation into young injured muscle restored satellite cell expansion, rescued the proliferative and regenerative capacity and reduced the expression of senescence markers. These data together support the authors' contention that impaired autophagy increases ROS driving progression toward senescence [9].

However, the data also support the idea that increased ROS contributes to inhibiting autophagy, which should be further investigated.

It has been previously observed that decreasing polycomb repressive complex-1 (PRC1)-mediated H2A monoubiquitination of lysine 119 (H2Aub) at the Cdkn2a gene locus, which encodes p16ink4a and ARF, drives p16 INK4a induction and senescence in geriatric mouse satellite cells. In Atg7 null and geriatric satellite cells, Trolox treatment reduced senescence and increased proliferation. These results are generally consistent with the notion that ROS production is necessary for induction and maintenance of cell senescence[8], Knockdown of p16ink4a by shRNA also reduced [4] the number of senescent SA-β-gal+ cells and increased regeneration in Atg7 null satellite cells. Since the authors postulate that epigenetic alteration of the CDKN2A locus is dependent on ROS, which in turn is dependent on decreased autophagy, it would be of great interest to know which epigenetic changes underlie the decreased autophagy in satellite cells.

What about human satellite cells?

The significance of Garcia-Prat's results depend upon whether similar autophagic driven phenotypes are observed and amenable to amelioration by treatments that stimulate autophagy or reduce ROS in human cells. A key concern is that human satellite cells appear to differ somewhat from murine satellite cells in subtle ways, including how Pax7 drives myogenic master regulators such as myf5 [11].

In earlier work from the same research group, Sousa-Victor *et al.* showed that senescence biomarkers p16ink4a and IGFbp5 were expressed only in CD56+ cells (a marker for both muscle stem and progenitor cells) in cryosections from muscle biopsies of geriatric humans (83 +/-7 years old) and not in biopsies from young adults (~30 year old) [4]. Furthermore proliferative potential in culture was reduced in satellite cells isolated from geriatric human subjects compared to adult controls. RNAi knockdown of p16ink4a restored geriatric cell proliferation by reducing senescence [4]. Garcia-Prat extend this result by showing that satellite cells isolated from geriatric humans show defective organelle and protein clearance similar to that seen for murine cells, which are strongly linked to increased ROS levels [9].

Similar to the effect on mouse satellite cells, treatment of human satellite cells in culture with rapamycin reduced the expression of biomarkers of Similar to the effect on mouse satellite cells, treatment of human satellite cells in culture with rapamycin reduced the expression of biomarkers of senescence, and restored the number of mitochondria and protein aggregates and ROS levels to near normal levels.

Taken together these results strongly support a role for autophagy in maintenance of human muscle stem cells and for the possibility of reversing old dysfunctional pre-senescent muscle stem cells by stimulating autophagy and/or ameliorating aging-associated elevated ROS levels.

Loss of Stem Cell Self-renewal: An Alternate Explanation for Loss of Human SMSC Function

Not too fast: there is evidence for an alternative hypothesis: loss of capability to maintain quiescence leads to stem cell exhaustion without senescence.

Critically, Bigot *et al.* find that the percentage of senescent cells as determined by staining for p16ink4a mRNA and percentage of cells that are SA-β-gal+ is the same for CD56+ SMSCs isolated from young (15-years-old to 20-years-old) and old humans (72-years-old to 80-years-old). Furthermore, proliferative capacity in culture and average telomere length did not differ between young and old isolates. Senescent phenotypes are only observed after extended serial passage in culture. These data are not consistent with the senescence hypothesis advanced by Garcia-Prat *et al.*, but instead led Bigot *et al.* to pursue loss of self-renewal capacity as the prime culprit for loss of muscle stem cells with age. Stem cells can either self- renew, or differentiate into muscle precursor cells or mature muscle cells. Differentiation involves asymmetric or symmetric divisions. In culture, the majority of CD56+ cells differentiate and fuse to form multinucleated myotubes, while a minority of cells remain mononucleated.

Most of the mononucleated cells from old humans express myosin heavy chain (MHC) and are unable to reattach and continue to proliferate after passaging with trypsin. Only a small number of a desmin-expressing myogenic cells remain after replating. By contrast, most mononucleated cells from young humans remain myogenic (express desmin) and can continue to proliferate after trypsinization and replating. Similar results are seen when human cells are transplanted into young immunocompromised mice that have been stimulated to regenerate muscle. Post-engraftment 8.1% of engrafted young cells express the Pax7 cell marker, compared to 3.5% of engrafted old human cells. These data are consistent with the hypothesis that old human CD56+ SMSCs have lost capacity for self-renewal [5].

Moreover, Bigot *et al.* show that CD56+ muscle progenitor cells actually are more capable of fusing to form myotubes than young CD56+ SMSCs cells, and concomitantly these myotubes differentiate more rapidly, expressing cell proteins associated with mature muscle, such as MHC 3 and myosin light chain 1, more rapidly then in myotubes from young subjects [5].

Bigot *et al.* tied the loss of muscle progenitor cell self-renewal to epigenetic changes. DNA methylome array analysis showed increased DNA methylation throughout the genome in old SMSCs. To test whether DNA methylation played a critical role, cells were treated with 5-aza-2'-deoxycytidine, a drug that reduces DNA methylation. Such treatment restored the number of Pax7+ cells derived form elderly subjects. The number of MHC+ mononucleated cells was decreased, consistent with the explanation that DNA methylation played a causal role in the loss of self-renewal seen in CD56+ cells from elderly subjects [5].

Expression of genes associated with stimulating myogenesis, such as Wnt3a were hypomethylated making them permissive for expression, while genes associated with satellite cell self-renewal such as Notch1 and SPRY1 (sprouty1) were hypermethylated and downregulated. Interestingly, 5-aza-2'-deoxycytidine treatment did not consistently alter expression of Notch1, or its co-regulator MAML1, but the expression of SPRY1 was restored to levels similar to that seen in young subjects. RNAi knockdown of SPRY1 in CD56+ cells from young subjects reduced the capacity for self-renewal similar levels seen in cells from old subjects, suggesting that SPRY1 down-regulation could be causal [5]. These results are consistent with earlier work showing that SPRY1 plays a critical role in the maintenance of quiescence in satellite cells [12] and that increased FGF2 expression in the stem cell niche down-regulates SPRY1 leading to loss of quiescence during aging[3]. Interestingly, Bigot *et al.* observed increased FGF2 expression in human muscle biopsies from old subjects, although not in culture, which suggests that extrinsic changes in the stem cell environment can not be ruled out as a mechanism for loss of the capacity for self-renewal [5].

Reconciliation?

On the surface, these reports present two compelling, though apparently contradictory descriptions of how skeletal muscle stem cell loss occurs. However, there are significant technical differences that may be explanatory. The work of Garcia-Prat *et al.*, is consistent with senescence playing a key role in loss of SMSCs, was mostly performed using mice. They isolated Pax7+ cells as SMSCs which are considered to be true satellite stem cells. However, Bigot *et al.* used only human cells in culture. They isolated CD56+ human muscle progenitor cells as SMSCs. Their CD56+ SMSCs include Pax7+ satellite stem cells as a small (5-10%) subpopulation. Bigot *et al.* were careful to ensure that cells underwent a minimum number of doublings in culture before analysis. Another key difference is that Sousa-Victor *et al.* and Garcia-Prat *et al.* used substantially older human subjects (83 +/- 7 years) for their studies than Bigot *et al.* Older subjects would be more likely to carry senescent cells, which may serve as a partial explanation for the differences between the results reported by the two research groups.

To reconcile these studies, one explanation may be that in humans, stem cell self- renewal capacity is indeed lost with age as observed by Bigot *et al.*, but that in extreme old age, the few remaining Pax7+ cells may become senescent as evidenced by the cryosection data of Garcia-Prat and Sousa-Victor.

Perhaps the statistical consequences of using the larger population of CD56+ cells and using "younger" subjects as the source for the elderly cells, prevented Bigot *et al.* from observing statistically significant cell senescence. If our explanation is true, then maintaining SPRY1 expression to prevent stem-cell exhaustion may be more important for old subjects, but reversal of senescence may become more medically relevant for very old, truly geriatric subjects.

Medical Implications

Loss of skeletal muscle stem cell function with age is likely due to a combination of loss of progenitor and stem cell self-renewal capacities and entry into a pre-senescent state wherein cells express p16ink4a, but can potentially still be rescued. Stimulation of autophagy by putative anti-aging drugs such as rapamycin and/or reduction of ROS by antioxidants may rescue cells in the pre-senescent state. However, these studies are preliminary pre-clinical studies which need confirmation and careful replication in humans.

There is evidence that stimulation of autophagy has some anti-aging benefit. Caloric restriction and rapamycin treatment in particular are known to stimulate autophagy and have been shown to increase life- and health-span in adult mice. However, in the specific context of preserving muscle function in the elderly, rapamycin or caloric restriction present a more complex picture. Rapamycin is reported to interfere with muscle mass increase induced by contraction, suggest that it may counteract exercise-based approaches to treating sarcopenia [13]. On the other hand, rapamycin has been reported to be beneficial in syndromes that involve loss of stem cells or induction of stem cell senescence, such as Duchenne muscular dystrophy [14,15] or lamin A/C progerias [16].

Rapamycin has been reported to induce miRNA-21 in some cell types [17] which in turn can inhibit SPRY1 in other cell types [18]: if these pathways are active in muscle tissue, then rapamycin may act to deplete SMSCs via decreasing spouty1 and quiescence maintenance. Although this outcome is consistent with the hypothesis of Bigot *et al.*, it will need to be confirmed by subsequent studies.

Of more general interest is that a pre-senescent state in which stem cells express senescence biomarker p16ink4a can be reversed. Expression of high levels of p16ink4a has been considered a hallmark of senescence [19], though its clear that over-expression of p16ink4a could sometimes be overcome [19].

Perhaps p16ink4a should be considered a biomarker of deep-quiescence or pre-senescence rather than senescence, which may have profound implications for basic and applied research.

The idea that destruction of senescent cells, i.e., "senolysis," will be of benefit to aging mammals, such as mice and humans, has become quite popular. There are studies that indicate that targeted destruction of p16ink4a expressing cells extends life- and health-span or confers other anti-aging benefits [20-24]. Lifespan extension by ablation of p16ink4a expressing cells remains controversial, as the reported 25% extended lifespan was relative to a vehicle control group of mice that had a significantly shortened lifespan to what is typically observed for the particular mouse strain studied [25]. However, if the results of Garcia-Prat *et al.* are confirmed and extended to other stem cells, then senolytic approaches that may provide some short-term health benefits, while unfortunately and simultaneously destroying reservoirs of potentially recoverable regenerative activity, thus capping potential health gains. To avoid such pitfalls, it may behoove anti-aging therapeutic drug designers to develop treatments to first rescue pre-senescent stem cells, before destroying p16ink4a- expressing "senescent" cells.

Conclusion

Aging results in epigenetic changes that alter muscle stem cell function, resulting in loss of self-renewal capacity or induction of senescence. The relative importance of each of these mechanisms in humans remains to be elucidated. Both may be subject to therapeutic intervention. The existence of potentially recoverable pre-senescent stem cells, should inform the development of senolytic drugs in order to prevent unintentional reduction of regenerative capacity.

References

1. Liu L, Rando TA. Manifestations and mechanisms of stem cell aging. J Cell Biol 2011;193:257–66. doi:10.1083/jcb.201010131. Inomata K, Aoto T, Binh NT, Okamoto N, Tanimura S, Wakayama T, *et al.* Genotoxic Stress Abrogates Renewal of Melanocyte Stem Cells by Triggering Their Differentiation. Cell 2009;137:1088–99. doi:10.1016/j.cell.2009.03.037.
2. Chakkalakal JV, Jones KM, Basson MA, Brack AS. The aged niche disrupts muscle stem cell quiescence. Nature 2012;490:355–60. doi:10.1038/nature11438.
3. Sousa-Victor P, Gutarra S, García-Prat L, Rodriguez-Ubreva J, Ortet L, Ruiz-Bonilla V, *et al.* Geriatric muscle stem cells switch reversible quiescence into senescence. Nature 2014;506:316–21. doi:10.1038/nature13013.
4. Bigot A, Duddy WJ, Ouandaogo ZG, Negroni E, Mariot V, Ghimbovschi S, *et al.* Age-Associated Methylation Suppresses SPRY1, Leading to a Failure of Re-quiescence and Loss of the Reserve Stem Cell Pool in Elderly Muscle. Cell Rep 2015;13:1172–82. doi:10.1016/j.celrep.2015.09.067.
5. Conboy IM, Conboy MJ, Wagers AJ, Girma ER, Weissman IL, Rando TA. Rejuvenation of aged progenitor cells by exposure to a young systemic environment. Nature 2005;433:760–4. doi:10.1038/nature03260.

6. Carlson ME, Conboy MJ, Hsu M, Barchas L, Jeong J, Agrawal A, *et al.* Relative roles of TGF-β1 and Wnt in the systemic regulation and aging of satellite cell responses. Aging Cell 2009;8:676–89. doi:10.1111/j.1474-9726.2009.00517.x.]

7. Childs BG, Durik M, Baker DJ, van Deursen JM. Cellular senescence in aging and age- related disease: from mechanisms to therapy. Nat Med 2015;21:1424–35. doi:10.1038/nm.4000.

8. García-Prat L, Martínez-Vicente M, Perdiguero E, Ortet L, Rodríguez-Ubreva J, Rebollo E, *et al.* Autophagy maintains stemness by preventing senescence. Nature 2016;529:37–42. doi:10.1038/nature16187.

9. Mizushima N. Autophagy: process and function. Genes Dev 2007;21:2861–73. doi:10.1101/gad.1599207.

10. Bareja A, Holt JA, Luo G, Chang C, Lin J, Hinken AC, *et al.* Human and Mouse Skeletal Muscle Stem Cells: Convergent and Divergent Mechanisms of Myogenesis. PLOS ONE 2014;9:e90398. doi:10.1371/journal.pone.0090398.

11. Shea KL, Xiang W, LaPorta VS, Licht JD, Keller C, Basson MA, *et al.* Sprouty1 Regulates Reversible Quiescence of a Self-Renewing Adult Muscle Stem Cell Pool during Regeneration. Cell Stem Cell 2010;6:117–29. doi:10.1016/j.stem.2009.12.015.

12. Drummond MJ, Fry CS, Glynn EL, Dreyer HC, Dhanani S, Timmerman KL, *et al.* Rapamycin administration in humans blocks the contraction-induced increase in skeletal muscle protein synthesis. J Physiol 2009;587:1535–46. doi:10.1113/jphysiol.2008.163816.

13. Eghtesad S, Jhunjhunwala S, Little SR, Clemens PR. Rapamycin Ameliorates Dystrophic Phenotype in mdx Mouse Skeletal Muscle. Mol Med 2011;17:917–24. doi:10.2119/molmed.2010.00256.

14. Sakuma K, Aoi W, Yamaguchi A. The Intriguing Regulators of Muscle Mass in Sarcopenia and Muscular Dystrophy. Front Aging Neurosci 2014;6. doi:10.3389/fnagi.2014.00230.

15. Ramos FJ, Chen SC, Garelick MG, Dai D-F, Liao C-Y, Schreiber KH, *et al.* Rapamycin reverses elevated mTORC1 signaling in lamin A/C-deficient mice, rescues cardiac and

16. Jin C, Zhao Y, Yu L, Xu S, Fu G. MicroRNA-21 mediates the rapamycin induced suppression of endothelial proliferation and migration. FEBS Lett 2013;587:378–85. doi:10.1016/j.febslet.2012.12.021.'

17. Jin X-L, Sun Q-S, Liu F, Yang H-W, Liu M, Liu H-X, *et al.* microRNA 21-mediated suppression of Sprouty1 by Pokemon affects liver cancer cell growth and proliferation. J Cell Biochem 2013;114:1625–33. doi:10.1002/jcb.24504.

18. Boquoi A, Arora S, Chen T, Litwin S, Koh J, Enders GH. Reversible cell cycle inhibition and premature aging features imposed by conditional expression of p16Ink4a. Aging Cell 2015;14:139–47. doi:10.1111/acel.12279.

19. Roos CM, Zhang B, Palmer AK, Ogrodnik MB, Pirtskhalava T, Thalji NM, *et al.* Chronic senolytic treatment alleviates established vasomotor dysfunction in aged or atherosclerotic mice. Aging Cell 2016. doi:10.1111/acel.12458.

20. Chang J, Wang Y, Shao L, Laberge R-M, Demaria M, Campisi J, *et al.* Clearance of senescent cells by ABT263 rejuvenates aged hematopoietic stem cells in mice. Nat Med 2016;22:78–83. doi:10.1038/nm.4010.

21. Zhu Y, Tchkonia T, Pirtskhalava T, Gower AC, Ding H, Giorgadze N, *et al.* The Achilles' heel of senescent cells: from transcriptome to senolytic drugs. Aging Cell 2015:n/a – n/a. doi:10.1111/acel.12344.

22. Xu M, Palmer AK, Ding H, Weivoda MM, Pirtskhalava T, White TA, *et al.* Targeting senescent cells enhances adipogenesis and metabolic function in old age. Elife 2015;4:e12997. doi:10.7554/eLife.12997.

23. Baker DJ, Wijshake T, Tchkonia T, LeBrasseur NK, Childs BG, van de Sluis B, *et al.* Clearance of p16Ink4a-positive senescent cells delays ageing-associated disorders. Nature 2011;advance online publication. doi:10.1038/nature10600.

24. Baker DJ, Childs BG, Durik M, Wijers ME, Sieben CJ, Zhong J, *et al.* Naturally occurring p16Ink4a-positive cells shorten healthy lifespan. Nature 2016;530:184–9. doi:10.1038 /nature16932.

Chapter 18

Thymus Maintenance and Regeneration by Specific Molecular Factors

Although the thymus plays a key role in T cell maturation in mammals, the thymus begins to atrophy and involute at sexual maturity. The diminished thymic micro-environment is thought to contribute to reduced adaptive immune function during aging, leading to the increased likelihood of infectious diseases and cancer. Caloric restriction or ectopic expression of prolongevity growth factor FGF21 have been reported to maintain the thymus in aging mice. Moreover forced expression of transcription factor FoxN1 has been shown to almost completely rejuvenate thymi from old mice, restoring their youthful state. These results open the way for development of potential drugs to restore immune function in the elderly.

Introduction

The thymus is a lymphoid organ where T-cells develop from hematopoietic progenitor cells into thymocytes and then mature T-cells. In the thymus, T-cells are also instructed to differentiate between self and non-self to create a tolerant T-cell repertoire. Once mature, T-cells emigrate to the peripheral immune system [1].

Involution of the thymus in mammals, including humans, is an early hallmark of aging that precedes most apparent age-related loss of function in other tissues. High levels of sex hormones at puberty are thought to direct thymic involution. It is thought that the resulting loss of the thymic microenvironment significantly contributes to degradation of immune function in old age, especially to the loss of acquired immune function. Decreased T-cell immune surveillance may be responsible for the increased susceptibility of the elderly to infectious diseases and cancer [2]. Treatments to prevent or reverse thymic involution could significantly impact healthspan.

Understanding the molecular mechanisms by which the thymus is maintained and whether repair or regenerative pathways continue to operate in the thymus could lead to new therapeutics. Although treatments as simple as short periods of fasting may be sufficient to rejuvenate stem cells (HSCs) [3], T cells derived from these HSCs presumably still require thymic function for efficient maturation.

FGF21 Protects Against Thymic Involution

Youm *et al.* report that ectopic expression of FGF21, a prolongevity growth factor that can extend murine lifespan up to 40% [4], maintained the thymus during aging in mice [5]. To understand which factors correlate with age-associated thymic involution, Youm *et al.* performed microarray analysis of gene expression in the thymus during aging in mice. FGF21 expression was observed to decline with age, a result that was confirmed by real-time quantitative PCR. Caloric restriction (CR) which is known to preserve the thymus structurally, increased FGF21 expression in the thymus. Consistent with a role for FGF21 in maintaining the thymus, the receptors for FGF21 are present in the thymus and either unaltered during aging (FGFR2, FGFR3, and FGFR4), or actually increased (beta-klotho and FGFR1).

Specifically, beta-klotho, which is the co-receptor required for FGF21 binding and function, is expressed in a subset of thymus epithelial cells (TEC): those expressing Keratin 8, which are presumed to be thymic nurse cells, those expressing FoxN1, which is the master transcription factor for thymopoeisis, and endothelial cells of double-walled post capillary venules, which allow import and export of CD4 and CD8 T lymphocytes [5].

To examine whether ectopic expression of FGF21 had a beneficial effect of the thymus, Youm *et al* studied thymus function in aging FGF-21-transgenic (FGF21tg) mice that have circulating levels of FGF21 50 to 100 times more than wt controls. FGF21tg mice, which have been reported to live 40% longer than wt controls[4], are smaller and weigh less than normal mice. The thymus and spleens of the FGF21tg mice are actually smaller than wt controls. However, if the mice are normalized by weight, then the FGF21tg mice have relatively bigger thymuses and spleens than wt mice. FGF21-tg mice possess increased numbers of T lymphocytes subtypes including CD4+, CD8+, CD4+CD8+ and CD4-CD8- cells.

14-month-old FGF21tg mice displayed preservation of cellularity in the medulla and cortex of the thymus unlike normal aged controls which showed the hallmark atrophy of these structures. Interestingly the increased number of white adipocytes that is associated with atrophy of the thymus in normal animals, is almost completely absent in the FGF21tg animals. Instead brown adipocytes are seen adjacent to the thymus, consistent with a role for FGF21 in promoting brown adipose tissue, which is actually more closely related to skeletal muscle than white adipose tissue and known to play a role in generation of body heat and weight maintenance. Consistent with observations, there were significantly less inflammation- associated macrophages with large spululite crystals and lipid drops in the Fgf21tg mice. Ectopic expression of FGF21 appears to decrease lipotoxicity in the thymus.

T-cell development and differentiation require thymus stem cells (TSCs) which include both medullary (mTECs) and cortical TECs (cTECs). Ectopic expression of FGF21 increases the number of cTECs and prevents the accumulation of thymic fibroblasts associated with atrophy. FGF21 expression activated ERK signaling in TSCs, and increased expression of TEC-specific genes including Eva, Il7, and Fgf7 suggesting that FGF21 maintains the micro- environment.

Thymic atrophy is associated with a reduced frequency of earliest thymocyte progenitors (ETPs) which mature into T cells under the influence of the stromal micro-environment. FGF21tg mice had significantly higher number of ETPs at 14 months than wt controls. Peripherally, Fgf23tg mice had increased numbers of naive CD4 and CD8 cells (CD62L-CD44hi) and a reduced number of effector memory cells (CD62L−CD44hi) unlike normal animals which showed an inverted numbers of naive and effector memory cells, associated with aging dysfunction. These data suggest that peripheral T-cell function may be maintained better in the FGF21g mice compared to wt.

Although thymic involution decreases T cell function, it is well known that pre-existing peripheral naive T-cells are able to compensate somewhat for the loss of naive T-cell export from the thymus. However, the compensatory mechanism still results in a reduced T-cell repertoire in aging mice. Sequence analysis of complementary determining region 3, which is edited during T cell maturation, showed that FGF21tg mice had a peripheral T cell repertoire that appeared more similar to young mice than to middle-aged controls as assayed by T cell receptor excision (TREC) DNA circles) [5]. The authors hypothesize that increased production and export of T cells from the thymus is responsible for the increased repertoire.

If FGF21 plays an essential role in the maintenance of the thymus then it is expected that mice lacking FGF21 would show more rapid decline in T-cell function and earlier thymal involution. FGF21 knockout mice (Fgf21-/-), by 1 year of age, possessed far fewer naive T cells and greater numbers of effector memory cells than wild type controls. Moreover, FGF21- /- mice had a greater reduction of thymic cellularity suggesting an increased rate of thymic involution. To further establish the role of FGF21 in the maintenance of the thymus and T-cell function, FGF21-/- animals were lethally irradiated and received a hematopoetic stem cell transplant (HSCT). This model parallels the diminished ability of the thymus to reconstitute T cells seen in elderly humans who are given radiation and HSCT. There was significantly greater mortality in irradiated FGF21-/- mice than in wt mice that received HSCT. In survivors, lack of FGF21 strongly reduced reconstitution of the thymus as well as reducing the number of peripheral CD4+CD8+ T lymphocytes [5].

The conclusion that FGF21 acts directly on the thymus and not T-cells is strengthened by the lack of expression of the obligate FGF21 co-receptor beta-klotho on thymocytes or mature T cells. Boosting FGF21 levels or stimulating the FGF21 signaling pathway downstream are potential paths to creating therapeutics that maintain the thymus in aging humans. However, there is much work to be done and potential complications that need to be addressed (see Medical Implications).

Ectopic expression of FoxN1 rejuvenates the thymus in old mice. The transcription regulator FoxN1 has been implicated in thymus maintenance and function. Mice engineered to have reduced postnatal levels of FoxN1 show rapid thymus degeneration [6] Zook et al observed that ectopic expression of FoxN1 in TECs using the keratin 14 promoter could ameliorate some of the aging-associated decline seen during aging in murine thymi [7]. However, eventually thymi ectopically expressing FoxN1 did degenerate to some extent.

In spite of the mixed results of Zook *et al.*, Bredenkamp *et al.* hypothesized that ectopic expression of FoxN1 in the same cells that normally express FoxN1 would regenerate atrophied thymi [8]. To test this hypothesis, Bredenkamp *et al.* engineered a trangenic mouse model that allows conditional over-expression of FoxN1 only in TEC cells by expressing FoxN1 from a construct that contains a "stop" cassette that prevents translation flanked by loxP sites, upstream of DNA that expresses a fusion of FoxN1 to the estrogen receptor. The site specific recombinase CRE is expressed from the TEC cell-specific FoxN1 promoter. In this way, the stop cassette is only removed in TEC cells, since only they express CRE. The ER-FoxN1 confers tamoxifen inducibility by using the ER domain to sequester FoxN1 in an inactive form until the addiction of tamoxifen, which then alters the confirmation of the estrogen receptor, allowing the fused FoxN1 to function. So these mice express both native FoxN1 from its own promoter and can be induced to over express FoxN1 in TEC cells using tamoxifen [8].

Middle-aged (12-months-old) and old mice (24-month-old) were treated with tamoxifen for one month. Etopic expression of FoxN1 regenerated old thymi so that they appear almost identical to young thymi in architecture, patterns of gene expression and function. These results are even more impressive results than those seen for ectopic expression of FGF21. Ectopic expression of FoxN1 increased thymocyte cell numbers approximately 2.6-2.7 fold with appropriate increases in CD4+, CD8+ and CD4+CD8+ T-cells. The ETP population increased to juvenile levels as well [8]. The results of forced expression of FoxN1 are remarkable. Although the restoration of thymic size was earlier shown to be induced also by castration or keratinocyte growth factor, unlike ectopic FoxN1, these treatments do not restore thymoyte numbers and function [9].

Structurally, tamoxifen induction of FoxN1 restores both the cortical and medullary regions of the thymus, including the medullary islets, and increases the numbers of cTECs and mTECs to levels seen in young animals. The (UEA-1)hi mTEC subpopulation, which has proposed to regulate medullary organization and is downregulated with age is also restored. Concomitant with the increases in TEC cell numbers was an increase in the proportion of proliferating TECs, especially among progenitor cTECs (MHC Class IIhi) and both progenitor and differentiated mTECs. Consistent with the observed increased cell division, TECS showed increased levels of ΔNp63, a marker for proliferative potential in epithelial cells [8].

The gene expression of multiple biomarkers of thymic function were restored to youthful levels including TEC development regulators dll4, Ccl25, Kitl, FgfR2IIIb, TRP63 and Cxcl12. Expression of AIRE, which plays a ket role in instructing T-ells to The gene expression of multiple biomarkers of thymic function were restored to youthful levels including TEC development regulators dll4, Ccl25, Kitl, FgfR2IIIb, TRP63 and Cxcl12. Expression of AIRE, which plays a ket role in instructing T-ells to distinguish self from non-self, was also restored to young levels in mTECs. Key components of Wnt signaling which play an important role in thymic function were also restored to levels observed in young mice [8].

As with ectopic expression of FGF21, ectopic expression of FoxN1 increased numbers of naive peripheral T-cells to levels seen in young animals as measured by increased numbers of CD45RBlo expressing "recent thymic emigrants" (RTEs) and about a 2 fold increase of TRECs. Together these data suggest that after FoxN1 ectopic expression, the number of T cells in the peripheral immune system of old mice has been restored [8], although T-cell function was not directly tested in these experiments.

Medical Implications

Preservation of the thymus may be an obvious goal for maintaining health-span, but just restoring a youthful thymic size or even simply maintaining apparent thymic structure do not necessarily result in better immune function. For example, in studies to evaluate the function of adaptive immunity after caloric restriction (CR), mice were challenged with West Nile Virus (WNV), which takes about 10 days to cause serious pathological changes. In these mice, CR maintains the thymus similarly to ectopic FGF21 expression. Survival of a WNV challenge requires acquired immunity. Surprisingly, both old and young CR mice were more susceptible to WNV, than young or old untreated mice, even when the old control mice possessed almost completely atrophied thymi [10] While maintaining the thymus may be an obvious goal for anti-aging therapies, potential therapeutic strategies must avoid subtle pitfalls that actually cause detrimental changes to T-cell mediated immunity, including some which seem to occur during CR. What's of great interest here is that CR is known to stimulate expression of FGF21. Youm et al. directly hypothesize that CR may maintain the thymus via FGF21 induction. So the question arises whether the detrimental effects of CR on acquired immune function, which are linked to impaired function of peripheral CD4+ and Cd8+ T lymphocytes, are avoided when thymi are maintained by FGF21 alone, or by an agent that can induce FGF21 such as metformin or AICAR [11]. Although increased numbers of CD4+ and CD8+ T lymphocytes are observed in mice ectopically expressing FGF21 or FoxN1, adaptive immune function was not directly examined. Without additional studies to clarify functional capability in FGF21-maintained thymi or FoxN1-rejuvenated thymi, caution is warranted.

Mere increases in FGF21 do not always correlate with health-span in humans, as obese subjects consistently express increased levels of FGF21. High levels of FGF21 are correlated with metabolic syndrome by increased glycemia, fasting insulin and triglycerides [12]. Of interest is that high FGF21 levels are actually predictive of Type 2 Diabetes [13, 14]. These data suggest that a FGF21 resistant state may be common in humans, especially those with metabolic syndrome [15]. Bearing these caveats in mind, agents such as the AMPK agonist metformin, which is used to treat type 2 diabetes is likely to increase FGF21 levels, while simultaneously opposing the FGF21 resistant scenarios seen in metabolic syndrome [11].

Most studies on the effects of small molecule inducers of FGF21 have focused on the liver, the major source of FGF21 in the blood. It will be of interest to know whether AMPK agonists such as metformin and AICAR or PPAR alpha agonist fenofibrate [16,17] can induce FGF21 in the thymus as well, or if merely increasing systemic plasma levels is sufficient to maintain the thymus similar to that seen with the FGF21 ectopic expression experiments.

Also, it will interesting to ascertain whether metformin, AICAR or fenofibrate can overcome the age-associated decline of FGF21 which appears to become resistant to re- induction by at least some experimental manipulations. This FGF21 resistance was due to epigenomic changes at the FGF21 gene, specifically increased DNA methylation [18].

FoxN1 seems to have the remarkable property of regenerating the thymus even in old mice. It represents an interesting exemplar of a single transcription factor that is capable of directing regeneration of an organ. Interestingly, although ectopic expression of FoxN1 may rejuvenate old atrophied thymi, over-expression of FoxN1 in late development in mice leads to neonatal lethality. In juvenile mice, FoxN1 actually leads to permeabilzed skin and reduced T and B lymphopoiesis [12], These results to not preclude development of drugs designed to increase FoxN1 expression in TEC cells to rejuvenate aging thymi, but, combined with the less spectacular ectopic FoxN1 expression results of Zook *et al*, optimization and timing of therapy (outside of old age) may present drug development problems.

Conclusion

Recent work suggests that decline of thymus structure and function with aging is not inevitable. CR and FGF21, which is associated with some of the pro-longevity and pro- healthspan benefits of CR [20] are capable of maintaining the aging thymus in mice when ectopically expressed [5]. Even more encouraging is that forced expression of FoxN1 in the thymus is able to restore thymus structure and apparent peripheral naive T-cell numbers to youthful levels even after the severe thymic atrophy associated with old age. Should these results be reinforced by subsequent studies, development of new therapeutics that target these factors may be on the horizon.

References

1. Boehmer H von. The Thymus in Immunity and in Malignancy. Cancer Immunol Res 2014;2:592-7. doi:10.1158/2326-6066.CIR-14-0070.
2. Palmer DB. The Effect of Age on Thymic Function. Front Immunol 2013;4. doi:10.3389/fimmu. 2013.00316.
3. Cheng C-W, Adams GB, Perin L, Wei M, Zhou X, Lam BS, *et al*. Prolonged fasting reduces IGF-1/PKA to promote hematopoietic-stem-cell-based regeneration and reverse immunosuppression. Cell Stem Cell 2014;14:810–23. doi:10.1016/j.stem.2014.04.014.
4. Zhang Y, Xie Y, Berglund ED, Coate KC, He TT, Katafuchi T, *et al*. The starvation hormone, fibroblast growth factor-21, extends lifespan in mice. ELife 2012;1
5. Youm Y-H, Horvath TL, Mangelsdorf DJ, Kliewer SA, Dixit VD. Prolongevity hormone FGF21 protects against immune senescence by delaying age-related thymic involution. Proc Natl Acad Sci 2016;113:1026–31. doi:10.1073/pnas.1514511113.

6. Chen L, Xiao S, Manley NR. Foxn1 is required to maintain the postnatal thymic microenvironment in a dosage-sensitive manner. Blood 2009;113:567–74. doi:10.1182/blood-2008-05-156265.

7. Zook EC, Krishack PA, Zhang S, Zeleznik-Le NJ, Firulli AB, Witte PL, et al. Overexpression of Foxn1 attenuates age-associated thymic involution and prevents the expansion of peripheral CD4 memory T cells. Blood 2011;118:5723–31. doi:10.1182/blood-2011-03-342097.

8. Bredenkamp N, Nowell CS, Blackburn CC. Regeneration of the aged thymus by a single transcription factor. Development 2014;141:1627–37. doi:10.1242/dev.103614.

9. Griffith AV, Fallahi M, Venables T, Petrie HT. Persistent degenerative changes in thymic organ function revealed by an inducible model of organ p regrowth. Aging Cell 2012;11:169–77. doi:10.1111/j.1474-9726.2011.00773.x.

10. Goldberg EL, Romero-Aleshire MJ, Renkema KR, Ventevogel MS, Chew WM, Uhrlaub JL, et al. Lifespan-extending caloric restriction or mTOR inhibition impair adaptive immunity of old mice by distinct mechanisms. Aging Cell 2015;14:130–8. doi:10.1111/acel.12280.

11. Nygaard EB, Vienberg SG, Ørskov C, Hansen HS, Andersen B. Metformin Stimulates FGF21 Expression in Primary Hepatocytes. Exp Diabetes Res 2012;2012:1–8. doi:10.1155/2012/465282.

12. Zhang X, Yeung DCY, Karpisek M, Stejskal D, Zhou Z-G, Liu F, et al. Serum FGF21 Levels Are Increased in Obesity and Are Independently Associated With the Metabolic Syndrome in Humans. Diabetes 2008;57:1246–53. doi:10.2337/db07-1476.

13. Chavez AO, Molina-Carrion M, Abdul-Ghani MA, Folli F, DeFronzo RA, Tripathy D. Circulating Fibroblast Growth Factor-21 Is Elevated in Impaired Glucose Tolerance and Type 2 Diabetes and Correlates With Muscle and Hepatic Insulin Resistance. Diabetes Care 2009;32:1542–6. doi:10.2337/dc09-0684.

14. Chen C, Cheung BMY, Tso AWK, Wang Y, Law LSC, Ong KL, et al. High Plasma Level of Fibroblast Growth Factor 21 Is an Independent Predictor of Type 2 Diabetes A 5.4-year population-based prospective study in Chinese subjects. Diabetes Care 2011;34:2113–5. doi:10.2337/dc11-0294.

15. Fisher ffolliott M, Chui PC, Antonellis PJ, Bina HA, Kharitonenkov A, Flier JS, et al. Obesity Is a Fibroblast Growth Factor 21 (FGF21)-Resistant State. Diabetes 2010;59:2781–9. doi:10.2337/db10-0193.

16. Badman MK, Pissios P, Kennedy AR, Koukos G, Flier JS, Maratos-Flier E. Hepatic fibroblast growth factor 21 is regulated by PPARalpha and is a key mediator of hepatic lipid metabolism in ketotic states. Cell Metab 2007;5:426–37. doi:10.1016/j.cmet.2007.05.002.

17. Gälman C, Lundåsen T, Kharitonenkov A, Bina HA, Eriksson M, Hafström I, et al. The circulating metabolic regulator FGF21 is induced by prolonged fasting and PPARalpha activation in man. Cell Metab 2008;8:169–74. doi:10.1016/j.cmet.2008.06.014.

18. Reis MD dos S, C somos K, Dias LPB, Prodan Z, Szerafin T, Savino W, et al. Decline of FOXN1 gene expression in human thymus correlates with age: possible epigenetic regulation. Immun Ageing 2015;12:18. doi:10.1186/s12979-015-0045-9.

19. Ruan L, Zhang Z, Mu L, Burnley P, Wang L, Coder B, et al. Biological significance of FoxN1 gain-of-function mutations during T and B lymphopoiesis in juvenile mice. Cell Death Dis 2014;5:e1457. doi:10.1038/cddis.2014.432.

20. Mendelsohn AR, Larrick JW. Fibroblast growth factor-21 is a promising dietary restriction mimetic. Rejuvenation Res 2012;15:624–8. doi:10.1089/rej.2012.1392.

Chapter 19

Aging Stem Cells Lose the Capability to Distribute Damaged Proteins Asymmetrically

Understanding the interplay between reversible epigenetic changes and potentially more difficult to reverse accumulation of damaged macromolecules is a central challenge in developing treatments for aging-associated dysfunction. One hypothesis is that epigenetic drift leads to subtle losses of homeostatic maintenance mechanisms, that in turn, lead to the accumulation of damaged macromolecules, which then further degrade homeostasis. A key mechanism of maintaining optimal cell function is asymmetrical division, whereby cellular damage is segregated away from cells that need to undergo further proliferation, such as stem cells. Such asymmetrical distribution of damaged macromolecules has been observed during cell division in many organisms, from yeast to human embryonic stem cells, and depends on diffusion barriers (DBs) in the membrane of the endoplasmic reticulum (ER). In a recent study, these results have been extended to neural stem cells (NSCs), in which the ability of the ER DB to promote asymmetrical distribution of damaged proteins deteriorates with age. NSC function declines with age as proliferative capacity is reduced. The loss of asymmetric protein distribution correlates with the loss of NSC proliferative capacity. Ectopic expression of progerin, an altered form of lamin A, is associated with the premature aging disorder, Hutchinson–Gilford progeria syndrome (HGPS). Progerin's expression also increases with normal aging due to mis-splicing, weakening the ER DB. Recent work suggests that many cell signaling pathway changes associated with HGPS are replicated during normal aging in cultured cells. Moreover, the detrimental changes associated with progerin expression in HGPS are partially reversible experimentally after treatment with statins, a farnesyltransferase inhibitor, a isoprenylcysteine carboxyl methyl- transferase inhibitor, or sulforaphane. It will be of great interest if these compounds can also reverse the aging-associated permeability of the ER DB and restore stem cell function.

Introduction

Some of the dysfunction associated with aging may occur through intracellular accumulation of damaged macromolecules. Because molecular errors, such as protein misfolding, are fundamental to living systems, evolution has had to develop mitigating strategies to ensure survival.

One strategy used by living systems to maximize cellular fitness is to distribute damaged macromolecules asymmetrically. For example, extrachromosomal DNA circles and protein aggregates are retained preferentially by mother yeast cells and excluded from daughter yeast cells [1, 2]. Similarly, damaged proteins segregate asymmetrically in Drosophila melanogaster somatic stem cells (especially age-associated [2-4] hydroxynonenal (HNE) modified proteins) [3] Assymetric distribution of and damaged proteins is found in cultured human cells such as HEK293 cells or human embryonic stem cells (ESCs) [4, 5]. The daughter cell receiving more of the damaged proteins is less fit and less capable of proliferation, whereas the cell receiving less of the damaged proteins is more fit and capable of proliferation. Not surprisingly, some have postulated that this mechanism may play a critical role in aging, for example, by generating cells with degraded function. This hypothesis is clearly an over-simplification, because this asymmetry does not for account for other kinds of damage or loss of regulatory information, such as errors in maintenance of the epigenome.

In mammals, these damaged macromolecules are sorted to two types of inclusion bodies —the juxta-nuclear quality control (JUNQ) compartment for ubiquitinylated proteins and the inclusion protein deposit (IPOD) compartment. These compartments can be inherited asymmetrically in mammalian cells through partitioning of vimentin, which associates with damaged proteins [5]. Because asymmetric diffusion though the endoplasmic reticulum (ER) is involved in the segregation of damaged macromolecules in yeast, it is reasonable to determine whether asymmetric diffusion plays a similar role in mammalian cells and how it may contribute to aging.

Asymmetric Diffusion Is a Mechanism for Segregating Age-Associated Damage in MammalianNeural Stem Cells

In a report extending our understanding of the role asymmetrical cell divisions plays in mammalian stem cell maintenance, Moore and colleagues [6] have found that neural stem cells (NSCs) generate a lateral diffusion barrier (DB) in the ER membrane that promotes asymmetric distribution of damaged proteins to daughter cells, which have a more restricted cell fate. However, the DB becomes gradually more inefficient with age, causing NSCs to become less fit and less capable of proliferation by accumulating damaged proteins.

To study asymmetrical distribution of proteins in NSCs, Moore *et al.* used fluorescence loss in photobleaching (FLIP) assays, whereby a green fluorescent protein (GFP) reporter was fused to sequences targeting it to the lumen of the ER (LumER–GFP) or the membrane of the ER (MemER–GFP). Cell cycle stage was identified by an engineered biosensor for the expression of histone H2B, which is normally expressed during S phase. Histone H2B is fused with a red fluorescent protein, mCherry. Photobleaching of LumER–GFP in electroporated NSCs from the dentate gyrus of young rats showed no difference of distribution of dark photo-bleached GFP in the daughter cells. By contrast, photobleaching of MemER– GFP showed loss of fluorescence up to the cleavage plane. Only one of the two daughter cells was affected, suggesting that NSCs generate a DB relative to the cleavage plane. These results show that the DB is associated with the membrane of the ER, not the lumen [6].

To investigate whether the DB was maintained with age, Moore *et al.* compared the proliferative rate of NSCs from middle-aged rats (9 months) to young (1.5 month) rats using an assay based on incorporation of 5-ethynyl-2'-deoxyuridine (EdU) and staining for its presence with fluorescently labeled antibodies. As expected, isolated NSCs from middle-aged rats proliferated more slowly than those from young rats. Gene expression profiling showed little difference between the NSCs from the middle-aged and young rats, although these kinds of experiments are subject to sensitivity concerns. However, unlike NSCs from young rats, photo-bleached MemER–GFP in NSCs from middle-aged rats distributed more symmetrically, demonstrating a loss of the DB in NSCs with age, even before overt transcriptional changes were observed. Appropriate controls for differential cellular diffusion rates using fluorescence recovery after photobleaching (FRAP) or for anaphase-telophase duration, ruled out the most likely experimental artifacts [6].

Moore *et al.* then exploited an important confluence be- tween the nuclear envelope (NE), the ER, and aging. The NE and lamin A, a NE-associated protein, are known to be incorporated into the ER during mitosis in mammalian cells [6]. Moreover, Hutchinson–Gilford progeroid syndrome (HGPS) results from mutations in the gene that encodes lamin through the introduction of a splice site (C1824T) that results in the deletion of 50 amino acids. Progerin lacks the ZmpSte24 cleavage site normally found in lamin A, causing progerin to be permanently anchored to the inner nuclear membrane due to constitutive farnesylation [7]. HGPS demonstrates many signs of premature aging, and importantly progerin also ac- cumulates during aging in wild-type individuals lacking HGPS mutations. Ectopic cellular expression of progerin acts in a dominant negative fashion to induce dysfunction associated with HGPS and aging. Using retroviral vectors to de- liver progerin to young mouse NSCs (the role of progerin in murine cells is more well studied than in rat cells) caused mouse NSCs to distribute MemER–GFP symmetrically in FLIP experiments, similar to the results seen in old NSCs. In control cells lacking ectopic progerin expression, MemER–GFP distributes asymmetrically in young mouse NSCs, similar to what is observed for rat NSCs. As might be expected, young mouse NSCs that ectopically express progerin proliferate more slowly than negative control young mouse NSCs [6]. These experiments suggest that progerin disrupts the DB and that lamin-dependent mechanisms may be necessary for normal DB function.

The NSC experiments described so far were performed in cell culture. To determine whether such effects are also observed for NSCs in their native niche, Moore *et al.* electroporated day 13 mouse embryos with LumER–GFP or MemER–GFP. Ex vivo slices were made at day 14, and single-trace FLIP experiments were performed on apical and basal progenitor cells. As for the adult NSCs, LumER– GFP showed symmetrical distribution. For MemER–GFP, a subset (25%) of apical and basal progenitors showed asymmetric distribution, although the majority of progenitors did not. The authors suggest that this may contribute to the heterogeneity typically seen in these cells types [6]. One obvious hypothesis is that creation of a DB may be required for a subset of cells, perhaps those that are destined to be- come adult NCSs, and thereby are required to maintain the stem cell lineage identity longer.

Does the establishment of a DB affect damaged proteins? It is known that a subset of proteins destined for destruction are tagged with ubiquitin. Although some of these ubiquiti-nylated proteins are tagged stochastically for turnover, others are tagged only after being recognized as damaged. Similar to results from stem cells in *Drosphila* melanogaster embryos and to mammalian stem cells in culture, [3-5] ubiquitinated proteins asymmetrically distribute between daughter cells in NSCs from young mice. On the other hand, ubiquitinated proteins distributes more symmetrically in NSCs from old mice or in NSCs from young mice that ectopically over-express progerin. Symmetric distribution of damaged proteins correlates with the weaker DB seen in older NSCs.

To better establish a connection with distribution of damaged proteins, a vimentin–GFP biosensor was used. Vimentin has been reported to segregate asymmetrically with mis- folded proteins in mammalian cells [5]. In these experiments, vimentin co-segregated with ubiqutin 96% of the time by co-staining analysis and 71% of the time using the vimentin-GFP biosensor. Interestingly, the daughter cells that received more vimentin-GFP divided more slowly than their sister cells that received less, similar to what was observed for human HEK293 cells and ESCs [4, 5]. In day 14 mouse embryos that had been electroporated with vimentin-GFP a day prior, vimentin-GFP associated with cells having longer cell cycles, which are known to be more differentiated. Differentiated cells such as neurons, which exit the cell cycle preferentially, receive more of the damaged proteins than do the NSCs.

Does this same pattern of excluding damaged proteins from NSCs hold in adult mice? In nestin-GFP transgenic mice, which express GFP from the NSC-specific nestin promoter, sections were stained with antibodies to ubiquitin to assess damaged proteins—doublecortin to identify new neurons and GFP to identify NSCs. In young mice, neurons contained more ubiquitin, and presumably more damaged protein than NSCs. By contrast, in 12-month-old mice, there was little difference in ubiquitinated protein levels between NSCs and neurons [6]. These data are consistent with the hypothesis that weakening of the DB with age contributes to a more symmetric distribution of damaged proteins and possibly with subtle degradation of NSC function with age. However, whether these increased amounts of damaged proteins actually degrade cell function beyond slowing proliferation remains to be elucidated.

Because progerin expression is known to increase with age, it would have been of interest to stain for progerin levels in the middle-aged/old mice and rats to see if the levels are consistent with the experiments reported by Moore *et al.* on asymmetric distribution of damaged proteins. Given the power of CRISPR technology, [8] it may be possible to engineer directly mice that only express wild-type (wt) lamin and cannot make progerin by deleting the wt lamin gene (LMNA) and replacing it with an engineered cDNA encoding lamin that can not mis-splice. It would be interesting to observe whether the DB of NSCs in such animals weakens with age.

Medical Implications

The medical implications of loss of a DB in stem cells with age are potentially profound. Restoration of the DB may rescue stem cell function in older adults. Much depends on the mechanism. If aberrant expression of lamin, a particularly increased expression of progerin, plays a role in loss of the DB, then reduction of progerin levels may rescue NSC and possibly other stem cell functions. Progerin expression is associated with other alterations in cells, including reduced proteasome activity and autophagy, double-stranded DNA breaks, global epigenomic changes to histones, such as loss of H3K9me3, H3K27me3 levels, down-regulation of HSP90, etc. [7] Progerin has been postulated to play an important role in normal aging as well [9]. Sixty-five major signaling pathways are activated similarly in HGPS and in old normal human fibroblasts in culture [10]. The specific epigenetic changes that activate the cryptic splicing site in the LMNA gene that allows progerin expression in aging mammals re- main to be elucidated. But the idea that it may be possible to manipulate the epigenome to prevent progerin expression is an attractive one.

What potential treatments could restore DB? If the progerin hypothesis is correct, the same drugs that partially block progerin in cell culture and mouse models might restore the DB, including statins, a farnesyltransferase inhibitor, or an isoprenylcysteine carboxyl methyltransferase (ICMT) inhibitor [11-14]. An interesting recent result is that sulforaphane, an anti-oxidant found in cruciferous vegetables that can stimulate autophagy and proteasome activity, clears progerin in fibroblasts derived from human patients in cell culture [15]. Sulforaphane and related compounds may be useful therapeutically for both HGPS and for aging-associated loss of stem cell function resulting from progerin expression.

Conclusion

Evolutionarily conserved asymmetrical distribution of damaged macromolecules to daughter cells that are destined to become quiescent may play a critical role in maintaining stem cell function. Evidence supports the establishment of a DB in the membrane of the ER as a key conserved mechanism to enforce asymmetrical distribution of damaged proteins in NSCs. Ultimately, the same molecular changes that lead to loss of the DB, for example, those that induce progerin expression with age, may be reversible.

References

1. Clay L, Caudron F, Denoth-Lippuner A, Boettcher B, Bu- velot Frei S, Snapp EL, Barral Y. A sphingolipid-dependent diffusion barrier confines ER stress to the yeast mother cell. eLife 2014;3. doi:10.7554/eLife.01883.
2. Shcheprova Z, Baldi S, Frei SB, Gonnet G, Barral Y. A mechanism for asymmetric segregation of age during yeast budding. Nature 2008;454:728–734.

3. Bufalino MR, DeVeale B, van der Kooy D. The asymmetric segregation of damaged proteins is stem cell–type dependent. J Cell Biol 2013;201:523–430.

4. Fuentealba LC, Eivers E, Geissert D, Taelman V, De Ro bertis EM. Asymmetric mitosis: Unequal segregation of proteins destined for degradation. Proc Natl Acad Sci USA 2008;105:7732–7737.

5. Ogrodnik M, Salmonowicz H, Brown R, Turkowska J, S´redniawa W, Pattabiraman S, Amen T, Abraham A-c, Eichler N, Lyakhovetsky R, Kaganovich D. Dynamic JUNQ inclusion bodies are asymmetrically inherited in mammalian cell lines through the asymmetric partitioning of vimentin. Proc Natl Acad Sci USA 2014;111:8049–8054.

6. Moore DL, Pilz GA, Arau´zo-Bravo MJ, Barral Y, Jessberger S. A mechanism for the segregation of age in mammalian neural stem cells. Science 2015;349:1334–1338.

7. Arancio W, Pizzolanti G, Genovese SI, Pitrone M, Giordano C. Epigenetic involvement in Hutchinson-Gilford progeria syndrome: A mini-review. Gerontology 2014;60: 197–203.

8. Cong L, Ran FA, Cox D, Lin S, Barretto R, Habib N, Hsu PD, Wu X, Jiang W, Marraffini LA, Zhang F. Multiplex genome engineering using CRISPR/Cas systems. Science 2013;339:819–823.

9. Olive M, Harten I, Mitchell R, Beers J, Djabali K, Cao K, Erdos MR, Cecilia Blair C, Funke B, Smoot L, Gerhard-Herman M, Machan JT, Kutys R, Virmani R, Collins FS, Wight TN, Elizabeth G. Nabel EF, Leslie B. Gordon LB. Cardiovascular pathology in Hutchinson- Gilford progeria: Correlation with the vascular pathology of aging. Arterioscler Thromb Vasc Biol 2010;30: 2301–2309.

10. Aliper AM, Csoka AB, Buzdin A, Jetka T, Roumiantsev S, Moskalev A, Zhavoronkov A. Signaling pathway activation drift during aging: Hutchinson-Gilford progeria syndrome fibroblasts are comparable to normal middle-age and old- age cells. Aging 2015;7:26–37.

11. Fong LG, Frost D, Meta M, Qiao X, Yang SH, Coffinier C, Young SG. A protein farnesyltransferase inhibitor ameliorates disease in a mouse model of progeria. Science 2006; 311:1621–1623.

12. Capell BC, Olive M, Erdos MR, Cao K, Faddah DA, Tavarez UL, Conneely KN, Qu X, San H, Ganesh SK, Chen X, Avallone H, Kolodgie FD, Virmani R, Nabel EG, Collins FS. A farnesyltransferase inhibitor prevents both the onset and late progression of cardiovascular disease in a progeria mouse model. Proc Natl Acad Sci USA 2008;105:15902–15907.

13. Yang SH, Qiao X, Fong LG, Young SG. Treatment with a farnesyltransferase inhibitor improves survival in mice with a Hutchinson-Gilford progeria syndrome mutation. Bio- chim Biophys Acta 2008;1781:36–39.

14. Ibrahim MX, Sayin VI, Akula MK, Liu M, Fong LG, Young SG, Bergo MO. Targeting isoprenylcysteine methylation ameliorates disease in a mouse model of progeria. Science 2013;340:1330–1333.

15. Gabriel D, Roedl D, Gordon LB, Djabali K. Sulforaphane enhances progerin clearance in Hutchinson–Gilford progeria fibroblasts. Aging Cell 2015;14:78–91.

Chapter 20

Stem Cell Depletion by Global Disorganization of the H3K9me3 Epigenetic Marker in Aging

Epigenomic change and stem cell exhaustion are two of the hallmarks of aging. Accumulation of molecular damage is thought to underlie aging, but the precise molecular composition of the damage remains controversial. That some aging phenotypes, especially those that result from impaired stem cell function, are reversible suggest that such "damage" is repairable. Evidence is accumulating that dysfunction in aging stem cells results from increasing, albeit, subtle disorganization of the epigenome over time. Zhang *et al.* (2015) report that decreasing levels of WRN, Werner's syndrome (WS) helicase, with increasing age results in loss of heterochromatin marks in mesenchymal stem cells (MSCs) and correlates with an increased rate of cellular senescence. Although WRN plays a role in DNA repair, WRN exerted its effects on aging via maintaining heterochromatin, evidenced by reduced levels of interacting chromatin regulators heterochromatin protein 1a (HP1α), suppressor of variegation 3- 9 homolog 1 (SUV39H1), and lamina-associated polypeptide 2β (LAP2β) as well as modified histone H3K9me3. Reducing expression of chromatin modeling co-factors SUV39H1 or HP1α in wild-type MSCs recapitulates the phenotype of WRN deficiency, resulting in reduced H3K9me3 levels and increased senescence without induction of markers of DNA damage, suggesting that chromatin disorganization and not DNA damage is responsible for the pathology of WS during aging in animals. Ectopic expression of HP1α restored H3K9me3 levels and repressed senescence in WRN-deficient MSCs. That HP1α can also suppress senescence in Hutchinson–Gilford progeria syndrome (HGPS) and extend life span in flies when over-expressed suggests that HP1α and H3K9me3 play conserved roles in maintenance of cell state. H3K9me3 levels are dynamic and expected to be potentially responsive to manipulation by extrinsic factors. Recent reports that migration inhibitory factor (MIF) or periodic fasting rejuvenate old MSCs provide the opportunity to link intrinsic and extrinsic mechanisms of aging in novel and potentially medically important ways and may lead to anti-aging treatments that reorganize the epigenome to rejuvenate cells and tissues.

Introduction

The story of the 12 blind men characterizing an elephant is a relevant analogy to the history of research into the mechanisms of aging. However, recently a consensus on the hallmarks of aging is being formed, and among these hallmarks are stem cell depletion and epigenomic alterations [1].

Stem cells can be eliminated by apoptosis (cell death), asymmetric division, differentiation, or cell senescence. Stem cell function also deteriorates before actual irreversible loss. In the latter case, various factors or treatments appear to re- store youthful stem cell function. For example, hematopoietic stem cells (HSCs) can be rejuvenated by fasting, reducing protein kinase A activity, [2] or increasing levels of Wnt5a [3]. Skeletal muscle satellite stem cells can be rejuvenated by inhibitors of transforming growth factor-β (TGF-β) [4].

The epigenome appears to undergo specific changes with aging, including characteristic patterns of deoxycytosine methylation that are strongly correlated with chronological age and can be used to weakly predict mortality when the difference between biological age and chronological age in blood cells is greater than 5 years [5]. Other changes in the epigenome include epigenetic drift in gene expression and various defined changes to chromatin, including loss of global heterochromatin, increased localized heterochromatin, acetylation of histone H4K16, trimethylation of H4K20 and H3K4, as well as reduced H3K9 methylation and H3K27 trimethylation. Changes in some of these signals have been associated with longevity. Heterochromatin protein 1a (HP1α) levels decrease with aging in animals from flies to mice. Loss-of-function mutations in HP1α decreased longevity in *Drosophila*, whereas limited over-expression modestly increased longevity [6].

Outstanding questions include: (1) How are the intrinsic epigenomic changes that occur during aging related to stem cell exhaustion and loss? and (2) Can extrinsic factors reverse stem cell aging?

Werner's Helicase and SUV39H1 Are Necessary for Maintenance of the Epigenome in Adult Stem Cells

A recent report uncovered evidence of a critical new and previously undetected function for Werner's helicase (WRN), a multi-functional helicase involved in DNA repair and telomere maintenance, whereby WRN was previously thought to exert its effects on accelerated aging. WRN associates with the heterochromatin maintenance proteins suppressor of variegation 3-9 homolog 1 (SUV39H1) and HP1α. Patients with Werner's syndrome (WS) have loss or reduction-of-function recessive WRN mutations resulting in many characteristics of aging, including alopecia, wrinkling, atrophied skin, scleroderma, lipodystrophy, cataracts, osteoporosis, atherosclerosis, type II diabetes, grey hair, and an increased frequency of certain cancers, especially sarcomas. Zhang et al. [7] hypothesized that some of the phenotypes of WS are due to defects in mesenchymal stem cell (MSC) function. MSCs are multi-potent mesoderm-derived cells that differentiate into osteoblasts, adipocytes, chondrocytes, and myocytes—cell types contributing to the pathology of WS.

To study the effects of WRN in isogenic cells, Zhang et al. used homologous recombination to knock out the two exons that encode the helicase domain of WRN in human embryonic stem cells (ESCs), resulting in cells producing no detectable WRN by western analysis (WRN-/-). Unlike WS patient- derived induced pluripotent cells (iPSCs), these ESCs maintained a normal karyotype and could differentiate into cells representative of each of the three germ layers. ESCs were cultured to direct their differentiation into CD83, CD90, CD105+ MSCs, capable of differentiating into osteoblasts, chondrocytes, and adipocytes. WRN-/- cells display pre- mature replicative senescence after just five to six passages in culture, as assessed by loss of proliferation and expression of senescence-associated (SA) β-galactosidase, p21ink4a, p21waf1, and SA secretory phenotype protein expression. WRN-/- MSCs were quickly lost when transplanted into muscle of immunocompromised severe combined immunodeficient/non-obese diabetic (SCID/NOD) mice compared to wild-type cells, suggesting loss of function. Expression of DNA damage markers increased 53BP1, gamma-H2AX, and ataxia telangiectasia mutated/ATM and Rad3-related kinase (ATM/ATR) substrate phosphorylation. Lentiviral vector transduction of wild-type WRN complemented the defects. Telomerase activity was reduced in the WRN-/- MSCs, although premature senescence could not be attributed solely to shortening of the telomeres [7].

WRN-/- MSCs show progressive disorganization of heterochromatin as assessed by the DNA stain Hoechst 33342, and by electron microscopy (EM) and immunostaining for inner nuclear membrane proteins lamina-associated poly- peptide 2β (LAP2b) and lamin B receptor (LBR). LAP2β anchors HP1α to heterochromatin. A key difference was reduced expression of H3K9me3, which marks heterochroma tin, whereas euchromatin histone modifications H3K27me3 and H3K4me2 were mostly unaffected. DNA methylation at 5-methylcytosine was unaffected globally, although subtle changes cannot be ruled out with the methodology employed. Twenty-four out of 73 mountains of greater than 20-kb peaks of H3K27me3 were diminished in sub-telomeric or sub-centromeric regions. Analysis of RNA expression showed 1047 genes with differential expression in WRN-/- MSCs. Of interest is that the most significantly down-regulated genes were those involved in the nuclear membrane and epigenomic organization. Co-immunoprecipitation showed that WRN formed a complex with the histone methyltransferase for H3K9me3, SUV39H1, HP1α, and LAP2β, which suggests that WRN plays a role in maintenance of heterochromatin [7].

To test the hypothesis that WRN plays a direct role in the maintenance of heterochromatin, RNA interference (RNAi) knockdown of SUV39H1 or HP1α was performed. This intervention produced a phenotype similar to the WNR-/- in MSCs, including premature senescence, as assayed by induction of p16ink4a and SA-b-galactosidase and reduction of H3K9me3 expression. Genetic inactivation of the SUV39H1 enzymatic activity by mutation of histidine 324 to lysine in ESCs resulted in MSCs that had reduced LAP2β and LBR and decreased H3K9me3 and HP1α. Mutant SUV39H1 MSCs had reduced proliferation and a similar premature aging phenotype to WRN-/- MSCs. However, no increase of DNA repair–associated proteins, H2AX, or ATM/ATR substrates were present, strongly suggesting that WRN effects on senescence are not related to DNA damage *per se*, but rather related to disorganization of the heterochromatin.

Importantly, over-expressing HP1α compensated for the absence of WRN by inhibiting induction of senescence. Interestingly, it has been reported in flies that HP1α decreases with age and that ectopic expression increases maximal life span about 12% [6]. Moreover, increased HP1α can prevent senescence in the Zempste24 model of Hutchinson–Gilford progeria syndrome (HGPS), in which a defective protease contributes to over-expression of progerin [8]. But some serious questions arise with data from earlier studies in mice: Knockout of SUV39H1 results in no apparent phenotype [9]. Similarly, knockout of CBX5, the gene that encodes for HP1α has no apparent phenotype [10, 11]. Consistent with these phenotypes, WRN-/- mice, unlike humans, have no phenotype.12 But given the results of Zhang *et al.* in human MSC's, a Werner's syndrome-like phenotype might have been expected for both SUV39H1 and CBX5 null mutants. Moreover, knockout of SUV39H1 actually extended lifespan by 60%, improved DNA repair and suppressed the premature aging phenotype in Zempste24 progeroid mice [13]. On the other hand, knockout of both genes encoding H3K9 methyltransfersase activity in mice, SUV39H1 and SUV39H2, significantly reduced viability during fetal development and in adults, [9] which may indicate that these enzymes have a different spectrum of activity in humans, that experimental errors are present in at least one of these studies or that the difference in telomere size between mice and humans plays a critical role. The longer telomeres found in mice may be the best explanation, as mouse models of Werner's syndrome (Wrn-/-) also don't exhibit any phenotype, at least without simultaneously knocking out telomerase (Terc) and only then in fourth generation Wrn-/-, Terc-/- mice that have short telomeres [12]. The shorter telomeres in human MSC's may be necessary to observe the phenotypic consequences of epigenomic mis-regulation in Wrn -/- cells. If this hypothesis is true, ectopic expression of telomerase may prevent loss of function in human WRN-/- MSCs as has been observed for human Wrn-/- fibroblasts [14] and may clarify the interaction between epigenomic dysregulation and telomere maintenance.

Is reduction of WRN or its partners in the maintenance of heterochromatin relevant to "normal" human aging? If so, we would expect a reduction of WRN, SU39H1, LAP2β, and so forth, with age and that increased expression of these proteins would slow aging or possibly reverse the effects of aging. Zhang *et al.* studied MSCs from dental pulp of children and of adults aged 58-years-old to 72-years-old. MSCs from the adults had reduced WRN, HP1α, SUV39H1, LAP2β, and H3K9me3 hetero-chromatin marks compared to the children. Future studies demonstrating restoration of expression of WRN or some of its co-factors to modulate the aging phenotype would be useful to confirm the importance of this work.

Of interest is whether the reduction of WRN is sufficient to cause reduction of stem cell function and how many other potential reversible epigenetic factors also change concurrently. What is the root cause of decreased expression of these co-factors? What other potential factors can drive change over time and what is the cause? More specifically, how important is the reduction of H3K9me3 marks? Sedivy *et al.* proposed that stochastic "damage" may be accumulate with aging, [15] although accumulation of potentially reversible regulatory errors by fallible epigenomic maintenance factors may be even more disruptive.

Maintenance of Epigenomic Marks Requires Precise Expression of Chromatin Regulators and Is Unstable with Aging

The number of heterochromatin marks and HP1a decrease with aging In *Drosophila*, similar to the nematode worm *Caenorhabditis elegans* and to mammals [6,16,17]. Levels of his- tone H3 decrease with age in *Drosophila* [9]. This is significant, because the presence of histone H3 may stabilize gene expression against fluctuation, as has been recently observed in C. *elegans* and Drosophila for the H3K36me3 mark, the absence of which negatively impacts life span in worms.18 The life span of flies carrying mutations that express HP1α at 50% of wild-type levels, is reduced by about 70%. Conversely, flies that express about 20% more HP1α than wild-type flies live longer; a 23% increase in median life span is observed, in part by suppressing ribosomal RNA (rRNA) transcription and preserving muscle structure and function. Most interestingly, flies that over-express HP1α at higher levels die during development, suggesting that HP1α levels require tight control to maintain homeostasis and optimize life span [6].

In HGPS, which results from accumulation of progerin (a misprocessed version of lamin A), heterochromatin, histone H3, and H3K9me3 decrease as in WS. Similarly, MSCs are also negatively affected, as well as vascular smooth muscle. Progerin has been hypothesized to be a possible driver of human aging, because progerin accumulates in chronologically aging human cells [19]. Is progerin connected to the H3K9 methylating complex? Indeed, lamin A and progerin physically interact with SUV39H1 to stabilize it and in- crease H3K9me3 [12]. In fact, progerin binds SUV39H1 better then lamin A. These data might suggest that progerin should help prevent the negative consequences of age-related changes to chromatin, rather than promote them, as progerin actually does. But SUV39H1 protein levels and H3K9me3 marks decrease with cell passage in HGPS cells [13]. Both lamin A and progerin also bind to H3K9me3 itself and H3K27/H3K27me3, although progerin has a reduced affinity for H3K27/H3K27me3 [20].

There are at least three possible explanations: (1) Progerin affects the HGPS phenotype independently of its effect on H3K9me3, (2) progerin's reduced binding to H3K27/ H3K27me3 is more significant functionally, or (3) progerin actually increases H3K9me3 levels transiently in a way that compromises H3K9me3 methylation similar to the effect seen in Drosophila when HP1a is over-expressed at too high levels. In all three cases, H3K9me3 methylation decreases due to decreased expression at the RNA level of complex proteins, including SUV39H1 [6]. Consistent with the third possibility, but not the first two, is that depleting Suv39h1 actually significantly extends life span in the Zempste24 null mice model of HGPS,13 perhaps by blocking the hypothesized toxicity of progerin-mediated transiently increased number of H3K9me3 marks.

It would be useful to actually track H3K9 and H3K27 marks in the Zempste24-/- Suv39h1-/- mice during development, or create a mouse where the double knockout can be induced in young mice to validate this idea. If true, two premature aging syndromes would result from altered H3K9me3 chromatin marks; in WS, the effect would be a consistent decrease of H3K9me3 marks in HPGS, a transient increase that triggers a subsequent decrease.

Together these results suggest that longevity may be directly related to the stability of the epigenome. If so, fidelity of epigenomic maintenance may predict life span in a large number of animals.

Reversal and Rejuvenation of Aged MSC Function

Macrophage migration inhibitory factor (MIF), a pro- inflammatory cytokine, has recently been reported to rejuvenate MSCs derived from bone marrow from 24-month-old rats. Treatment with MIF increased growth, restored ability of MSCs to mediate paracrine signaling, and increased resistance to hypoxia induced by apoptosis to levels near that of control 6-month-old rats. Rejuvenation was mediated by CD74-dependent activation of 5'-adenosine monophosphate (AMP)-activated protein kinase (AMPK) and FOXO3a. Small interfering RNA (siRNA) knockdown of CD74, AMPK, or FOXO3a blocked the rejuvenative effects of MIF.21 Interestingly, short 5-day periods of near fasting followed by ad libitum feeding also have been reported to rejuvenate MSCs in both mice and humans [22].

On the basis of the results of Zhang et al., we predict that H3K9me3 patterns are disrupted in old MCSs and at least partially reversed in rejuvenated MSCs. Expression of chromatin remodeling proteins, including WRN, is expected to be boosted. Whether intrinsic aging-associated changes such as chromatin remodeling at H3K9me3 sites are subject to influence by extrinsic factors is an important question that should be resolved in the near future.

Medical Implications

Numerous epigenetic changes associated with aging in animals, including mice and humans, have been identified in recent years. That at least some adult cells can be completely rejuvenated to pluripotent cells by nuclear transfer or defined factors suggests that damage or errors of metabolism or dysregulation associated with aging are potentially completely reversible. The reprogramming potential of aging adult cells points to the possibility that aging that is characterized by degradation of cell state results from degradation of the organization of chromatin and transcription and signaling networks. To the extent this is true, almost complete engineering of the aged phenotype may be possible. However, it should be remembered that full-blown cell senescence makes full reprogramming more difficult [23, 24]; only a small percentage of cells (5%–20%) in adults are actually senescent [25]. In any case, full reprogramming to a pluripotent state is not a viable path for in vivo rejuvenation, although more subtle reprogramming could be and it would be unwise to attempt reprogramming senescent cells because they may carry activated oncogenes. Rather, removal of senescent cells would probably be preferred [26, 27].

Partial rejuvenation of stem or differentiated cells by altering expression of factors such as sirtuins, nicotinamide adenine dinucleotide (NAD+) or by fasting suggests that many of the changes associated with aging are reversible. The plasticity of the epigenome and its identification as a "hallmark" of aging make it a particularly attractive ex-planation for rejuvenative effects. A key question is how many of the biochemical changes associated with aging are mediated via epigenetic mechanisms.

Histone modification is considered to be more plastic than other epigenomic makers, such as DNA methylation. H3K9me3 levels are expected to be responsive to manipulation by extrinsic factors. The recent report that MIF or periodic fasting can rejuvenate old MSCs provides the opportunity to link intrinsic and extrinsic mechanisms of aging in novel and potentially medically important ways. We predict that the H3K9me3 localization in MIF-treated or periodic-fasting- rejuvenated MSCs will reflect a youthful state.

Although, these results may have some impact on the treatment of WS, the most straightforward future treatment for this devastating condition remains virus-mediated gene therapy to introduce wild-type WRN into patients' cells and tissues. As for rejuvenation of MSCs in normal aging, it is unlikely that a pro-inflammatory cytokine like MIF will be employed as a rejuvenating agent *in vivo*. In fact, trials are underway to inhibit MIF with therapeutic antibodies as a therapy for cancer (Clinical Trial NCT01765790) and lupus (Clinical Trial NCT01541670). That a tradeoff exists between rejuvenative/regenerative and potentially inflammatory or oncogenic activities is consistent with prior work on the role of factors such as p16ink4a and p21waf in sup- pressing both regeneration and cancer. However, periodic near fasting may be a legitimate low-technology method to promote MSCs rejuvenation that bears further investigation.

Conclusion

Loss of stem cell function due to irreversible processes, such as differentiation, asymmetric cell division, senescence, or apoptosis, can only be overcome by replacing the lost stem cells. Cell reprogramming provides a possible route to regenerate lost stem cells, and MSC function has been reported to be mostly restored after conversion to iPSCs with subsequent re-differentiation [28]. However, even partial reprogramming based anti-aging therapies is unlikely in the near future.

That defined, potentially labile, epigenomic changes may help drive dysfunction associated with aging provides hope that therapeutics to slow or reverse aspects of aging may be discovered. Disorganized cell states can be reorganized. The search for extrinsic rejuvenative factors and agents is ever more likely to bear fruit.

References

1. Lopez-Ot´ın C, Blasco MA, Partridge L, Serrano M, Kroemer G. The hallmarks of aging. Cell 2013;153:1194–1217. 2. Cheng C-W, Adams GB, Perin L, Wei M, Zhou X, Lam BS, Da Sacco S, Mirisola M, Quinn DI, Dorff TB, Kop- chick JJ, Longo VD. Prolonged fasting reduces IGF-1/PKA to promote hematopoietic-stem-cell-based regeneration and reverse immunosuppression. Cell Stem Cell 2014;14: 810–823.

2. Florian MC, Nattamai KJ, Dorr K, Marka G, U¨ berle B, Vas V, Eckl C, Andra¨ I, Schiemann M, Oostendorp RA, Scharffetter-Kochanek K, Kestler HA, Zheng Y, Geiger H. A canonical to non-canonical Wnt signalling switch in haematopoietic stem-cell ageing. Nature 2013;503:392–396.

3. Carlson ME, Conboy MJ, Hsu M, Barchas L, Jeong J, Agrawal A, Schaffer DV, Conboy IM. Relative roles of TGF-b1 and Wnt in the systemic regulation and aging of satellite cell responses. Aging Cell 2009;8:676–689.

4. Marioni RE, Shah S, McRae AF, Chen BH, Colicino E, Harris SE, Gibson J, Henders AK, Redmond P, Cox SR, Pattie A, Corley J, Murphy L, Martin NG, Montgomery GW, Feinberg AP, Fallin MD, Multhaup ML, Jaffe AE, Joehanes R, Schwartz J, Just AC, Lunetta KL, Murabito JM, Starr JM, Horvath S, Baccarelli AA, Levy D, Visscher PM, Wray NR, Deary IJ. DNA methylation age of blood predicts all-cause mortality in later life. Genome Biol 2015;16:25.

5. Larson K, Yan S-J, Tsurumi A, Liu J, Zhou J, Gaur K, Gaur K, Guo D, Eickbush TH, Li WX. Heterochromatin formation promotes longevity and represses ribosomal RNA synthesis. PLoS Genet 2012;8.

6. Zhang W, Li J, Suzuki K, Qu J, Wang P, Zhou J, Liu X, Ren R, Xu X, Ocampo A, Yuan T, Yang J, Li Y, Shi L, Guan D, Pan H, Duan S, Ding Z, Li M, Yi F, Bai R, Wang Y, Chen C, Yang F, Li X, Wang Z, Aizawa E, Goebl A, Soligalla RD, Reddy P, Esteban CR, Tang F, Liu GH, Belmonte JC. Aging stem cells. A Werner syndrome stem cell model unveils heterochromatin alterations as a driver of human aging. Science 2015;348:1160–1163.

7. Liu J, Yin X, LiuB, Zheng H, Zhou G, Gong L, Li M, Li X, Wang Y, Hu J, Krishnan V, Zhou Z, Wang Z. HP1a mediates defective heterochromatin repair and accelerates senescence in Zmpste24-deficient cells. Cell Cycle 2014;13:1237–1247.

8. Peters AHFM, O'Carroll D, Scherthan H, Mechtler K, Sauer S, Schofer C, Weipoltshammer K, Pagani M, Lachner M, Kohlmaier A, Opravil S, Doyle M, Sibilia M, Jenuwein T. Loss of the Suv39h histone methyltransferases impairs mammalian heterochromatin and henome dtability. Cell 2001;107:323–337.

9. Aucott R, Bullwinkel J, Yu Y, Shi W, Billur M, Brown JP, Menzel U, Kioussis D, Wang G, Reisert I, Weimer J, Pandita RK, Sharma GG, Pandita TK, Fundele R, Singh PB. HP1-b is required for development of the cerebral neocortex and neuromuscular junctions. J Cell Biol 2008;183:597–606.

10. Brown JP, Bullwinkel J, Baron-Luhr B, Billur M, Schneider P, Winking H, Singh PB. HP1c function is required for male germ cell survival and spermatogenesis. Epigenetics Chromatin 2010;3:9.

11. Chang S, Multani AS, Cabrera NG, Naylor ML, Laud P, Lombard D, et al. Essential role of limiting telomeres in the pathogenesis of Werner syndrome. Nat Genet 2004;36: 877–882.

12. Liu B, Wang Z, Zhang L, Ghosh S, Zheng H, Zhou Z. De- pleting the methyltransferase Suv39h1 improves DNA repair and extends lifespan in a progeria mouse model. Nat Com- mun 2013;4:1868.

13. Wyllie FS, Jones CJ, Skinner JW, Haughton MF, Wallis C, Wynford-Thomas D, et al. Telomerase prevents the ac- celerated cell ageing of Werner syndrome fibroblasts. Nat Genet 2000;24:16–17.

14. Sedivy JM, Banumathy G, Adams PD. Aging by epige- netics—a consequence of chromatin damage? Exp Cell Res 2008;314:1909–1917.

15. O'Sullivan RJ, Kubicek S, Schreiber SL, Karlseder J. Re- duced histone biosynthesis and chromatin changes arising from a damage signal at telomeres. Nat Struct Mol Biol 2010;17:1218–1225.

16. Ivanov A, Pawlikowski J, Manoharan I, Tuyn J van, Nelson DM, Rai TS, Shah PP, Hewitt G, Korolchuk VI, Passos JF, Wu H, Berger SL, Adams PD. Lysosome-mediated processing of chromatin in senescence. J Cell Biol 2013;202: 129–143.

17. Blase S, Mirzaei H, Mirisola MG, Childress P, Ji L, Groshen S, Penna F, Odetti P, Perin L, Conti PS, Ikeno Y, Kennedy BK, Cohen P, Morgan TE, Dorff TB, Longo VD. A periodic diet that mimics fasting promotes multi-system regeneration, enhanced cognitive performance, and healthspan. Cell Me- tab 2015;22:88–99.

18. Li H, Collado M, Villasante A, Strati K, Ortega S, Canamero M, Blasco MA, Serrano M. The Ink4/Arf locus is a barrier for iPS reprogramming. Nature 2009;460:1136–1139.

19. Wang B, Miyagoe-Suzuki Y, Yada E, Ito N, Nishiyama T, Nakamura M, Ono Y, Motohashi N, Segawa M, Masuda S, Takeda S. Reprogramming efficiency and quality of induced pluripotent stem cells (iPSCs) generated from muscle-derived fibroblasts of mdx mice at different ages. PLoS Curr 2011;3.

20. Jeyapalan JC, Ferreira M, Sedivy JM, Herbig U. Accu- mulation of senescent cells in mitotic tissue of aging primates. Mech Ageing Dev 2007;128:36–44.

21. Baker DJ, Wijshake T, Tchkonia T, LeBrasseur NK, Childs BG, van de Sluis B, Kirkland JL, van Deursen JM. Clear- ance of p16Ink4a-positive senescent cells delays ageing- associated disorders. Nature 2011;479:232–236.

22. Zhu Y, Tchkonia T, Pirtskhalava T, Gower AC, Ding H, Giorgadze N, Palmer AK, Ikeno Y, Hubbard GB, Lenburg M, O'Hara SP, LaRusso NF, Miller JD, Roos CM, Verzosa GC, LeBrasseur NK, Wren JD, Farr JN, Khosla S, Stout MB, McGowan SJ, Fuhrmann-Stroissnigg H, Gurkar AU, Zhao J, Colangelo D, Dorronsoro A, Ling YY, Barghouthy AS, Navarro DC, Sano T, Robbins PD, Niedernhofer LJ, Kirkland JL. The Achilles' heel of senescent cells: From transcriptome to senolytic drugs. Aging Cell 2015;14:644.

23. Pu M, Ni Z, Wang M, Wang X, Wood JG, Helfand SL, Yu 658. H, Lee SS. Trimethylation of Lys36 on H3 restricts gene expression change during aging and impacts life span. Genes Dev 2015;29:718–731.

24. Scaffidi P, Misteli T. Lamin A-dependent nuclear defects in human aging. Science 2006;312:1059–1063.

25. Bruston F, Delbarre E, O¨ stlund C, Worman HJ, Buendia B, Duband-Goulet I. Loss of a DNA binding site within the tail of prelamin A contributes to altered heterochromatin anchorage by progerin. FEBS Lett 2010;584:2999–3004.

26. Xia W, Zhang F, Xie C, Jiang M, Hou M. Macrophage migration inhibitory factor confers resistance to senescence through CD74-dependent AMPK-FOXO3a signaling in mesenchymal stem cells. Stem Cell Res Ther 2015;6.

27. Brandhorst S, Choi IY, Wei M, Cheng CW, Sedrakyan S, Navarrete G, Dubeau L, Yap LP, Park R, Vinciguerra M, Di

28. Frobel J, Hemeda H, Lenz M, Abagnale G, Joussen S, De- necke B, Saric′ T, Zenke M, Wagner W. Epigenetic rejuve- nation of mesenchymal stromal cells derived from induced pluripotent stem cells. Stem Cell Rep 2014;3:414–422.

About The Authors

James W. Larrick, MD, PhD

JWLarrick@gmail.com
Founder, Managing Director,
Panorama Research Institute
1230 Bordeaux Drive
Sunnyvale, CA 94089
[Pano.com]

and

Managing Director, CMO
Velocity Pharmaceutical
Development
400 Oyster Point Boulevard
South San Francisco, CA 94080

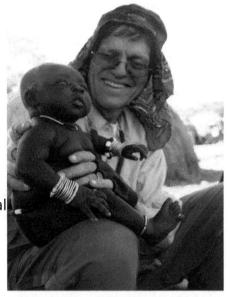

Dr. James Larrick is a biomedical entrepreneur with an international reputation in biotechnology [cytokines, therapeutic antibodies, molecular biology, pharmaceutical drug development] having written or co-authored nine books, over 250 papers/chapters and >fifty patents in his thirty year career. He has served on the editorial board of six journals. Dr. Larrick's work on therapeutic antibodies and other protein therapeutics has spanned the whole range of biopharmaceutical product development from target discovery, process science to clinical trials.

Dr. Larrick received his MD and PhD. degrees from Duke University School of Medicine, Durham, NC as a Medical Scientist Training Program scholar. After house-staff training in the Department of Medicine at Stanford University School of Medicine, he completed a post-doctoral fellowship in the Stanford Cancer Biology Research Labs working on therapeutic human monoclonal antibodies for cancer and infectious diseases. In 1982, he continued this work as a founding scientist of Cetus Immune Research Labs, Palo Alto, CA, where he became Director of Research in 1986. While at Cetus he pioneered the use of PCR for the construction of recombinant antibodies. This technology was critical to the development of antibody library cloning and the practical development of recombinant antibodies as a new class of biotherapeutics with annual revenues of >$100B. Recent work at PRI has focused on Applied Healthspan Engineering the utilization of advances in molecular medicine to preserve well-being as we age.

In 1991, Dr. Larrick founded the Panorama Institute of Molecular Medicine, a non-profit research institute situated near Stanford University and Panorama Research Inc., a biopharmaceutical incubator company. Dr. Larrick's PRI team has discovered and initiated development of a diverse, and innovative portfolio of pharmaceutical molecules addressing major unmet needs in cancer, infectious, autoimmune, cardiovascular, neurological and metabolic diseases. PRI has incubated >30 life science projects/companies. Based on this work he has co-founded more than a dozen companies. Among these are Planet Biotechnology Inc., Kalobios Inc., NuGen Technology Inc., Panolife Products Inc., PanResearch Inc., Adamas Inc., Absalus Inc. (now Teva Inc.), Humanyx Ltd., TransTarget Inc., Larix Bioscience LLC, and Galaxy Biotech LLC, etc.. Two companies have been co-founded in Europe, PanGenetics b.v. and TargetQuest b.v. To date PRI-initiated projects and/or companies have led to seven IPOs/exits. Currently Dr. Larrick serves on the Boards of several early stage companies.

Since 1998 Dr. Larrick has led the biopharma screening committees of various Bay Area angel investment groups, most recently serving on the Board of Life Science Angels. Since 2010 he has served as a managing director and Chief Medical Officer of CMEA-funded Velocity Pharmaceutical Development LLC, based in South San Francisco.

Dr. Larrick has organized and led a number of biomedical expeditions, including studies of nutrition, malaria, genetics, and high altitude adaptation among native peoples of Ecuador, Peru, Indonesia, Guatemala, Nepal, India, Tibet and China, Ethiopia and Bhutan. He has a genuine interest in fostering entrepreneurial activities and promoting healthcare among those less fortunate. Presently he helps fund and serves on the Boards of two non-profits, the Sustainable Sciences Institute (www.ssilink.org) focused on education and delivery of appropriate technology to less developed countries in Africa and Latin America and the Sankofa Center for African Dance and Culture focused on education, diagnosis and therapy of HIV/AIDS and tuberculosis in Ghana (www.thesankofacenter.org). Additional humanitarian activities (Ethiopia, Bhutan, Indonesia) are carried out via Juvare.org.

Andrew Mendelsohn, PhD

Amend@regensci.org
Head of Molecular Biology,
Panorama Research Institute
1230 Bordeaux Drive
Sunnyvale, CA 94089

and

Founder and Director of Research
Regenerative Sciences Institute

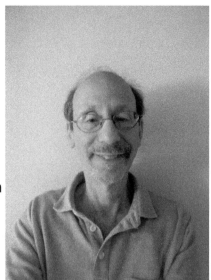

Dr. Andrew Mendelsohn has been deeply interested in the biology of aging for many years. He founded the 501(c)(3) non-profit Regenerative Sciences Institute in 1994 to pursue research at the interface of aging, regeneration, and what is now called synthetic biology. In 1997, he co-authored one of the earliest papers in synthetic biology. He has served as Director of Molecular Biology at the Panorama Research Institute, which seeks to develop state-of-the-art therapeutics and is a co-founder of Wintgen LLC which seeks to alter Wnt pathway regulation to cure macular degeneration. He serves as Director of Research at Regenerative Sciences Institute (www.regensci.org), which seeks to overcome aging by using synthetic and computational biology to engineer enhanced regeneration and rejuvenation. At the heart of our approach is the creation and insertion of new biological programs into cells to augment pre-existing incomplete regeneration mechanisms.

Index

1

2

4

5

8

A

B

C

D

E

F

G

H

M

N

nutrition 55, 135

O

obese 14-15, 178
obesity 14-15, 18-20, 55-56, 74, 81, 133, 145
Oct4 157, 159, 163
oncogene 72, 108-109, 133
oncogenes 108, 190
oncogenesis 117
oncogenic 31, 34, 108, 114, 191
orexin 55
organelle 137, 142, 170
organelles 5, 137, 166
orphan 72, 89
OSKM 157-164
osteoblasts 186
osteoporosis 186

ovarian 2, 111-113, 116
ovaries 2
over-expression 7, 108, 119-122, 173, 177, 179, 186, 188
Oxaloacetate 48
Oxidants 117
oxidation 43, 119, 130, 132-133, 162
oxidative 4, 6, 14-17, 19, 24-25, 29, 40, 42-43, 46-47, 63, 101, 105-106, 109, 112, 114-115, 118-121, 124-125, 129, 133
oxygen 6, 16, 24, 29, 45, 86, 98, 108, 118-119, 124, 137, 160
oxygenase-1 25

P

p16ink4a 159-160, 165-170, 172-173, 187, 191
p21cip 159
p21cip1 168
p21ink4a 187
p21waf 191
pain 4, 18, 138
pancreas 130, 163
pancreatic 111, 114, 116, 159, 161
parabiosis 54, 65, 75, 80-81, 91-94
paracrine 136, 138, 143, 190
paradoxes 107, 115
paraquat 60
Pard3 78
Parkinson's 28, 145
PARP 58-63, 112, 125, 130
PARP1 58-62, 64, 128
PARPs 58-59, 130
pathogenesis 19, 85
pathological 7, 32, 80, 151, 159, 178
pathology 23, 31, 35, 46, 49, 88, 130, 159, 185-186
pathway 4, 14, 19, 29, 45, 48, 58, 60, 63, 76, 80, 84, 90, 114-115, 125, 133, 141, 147, 159-160, 176, 180
pathways 3-4, 25, 27-28, 31, 42-44, 46, 60, 72, 74-77, 85, 107, 109, 114,

119, 123, 127-128, 131, 133, 144, 147, 155, 173-174, 184
Pax3 74, 81
pax7 79, 82, 160, 162, 166-168, 170-172, 177
PCG-1 23-25, 119, 124
PCNA 66-68
p-CREB 101
peptidase 15
peptide 15, 25, 187
Pericytes 81
peritoneum 87
peroxide 107, 111-112, 116
pFGFR 79
PGC1 23, 26-28, 123
PGC-1 22-30, 120-123, 131-132
PGC-1a 22-23, 26-27, 120, 132
phagosomes 167
phenylalanine 15, 17-18
pheochromocytoma 137
phosphoribosyl 125, 128-129
phosphoribosyltransferase 133
phosphoribosyl-transferase 125, 133
phosphorylation 4, 14-17, 19, 26-28, 43, 77, 79, 83, 92, 112, 118-120, 124-125, 187
placenta 136

Q

R

S

T

Lightning Source UK Ltd.
Milton Keynes UK
UKHW050038231218
334386UK00003BA/39/P

9 780991 216222